From Child Welfare to Child Well-Being

Children's Well-Being: Indicators and Research Series

Volume 1

This new series focuses on the subject of measurements and indicators of children's well being and their usage, within multiple domains and in diverse cultures. More specifically, the series seeks to present measures and data resources, analysis of data, exploration of theoretical issues, and information about the status of children, as well as the implementation of this information in policy and practice. By doing so it aims to explore how child indicators can be used to improve the development and the well being of children.

With an international perspective the series will provide a unique applied perspective, by bringing in a variety of analytical models, varied perspectives, and a variety of social policy regimes.

Children's Well-Being: Indicators and Research will be unique and exclusive in the field of measures and indicators of children's lives and will be a source of high quality, policy impact and rigorous scientific papers.

For further volumes:
http://www.springer.com/series/8162

Sheila B. Kamerman · Shelley Phipps ·
Asher Ben-Arieh

Editors

From Child Welfare to Child Well-Being

An International Perspective on Knowledge
in the Service of Policy Making

Springer

Editors
Sheila B. Kamerman
Columbia University
School of Social Work
1255 Amsterdam Avenue
New York NY 10027
USA
sbk2@columbia.edu

Asher Ben-Arieh
Hebrew University of Jerusalem
Paul Baerwald School of
Social Work & Social Welfare
Giv'at Ram
91905 Jerusalem
Mount Scopus
Israel
benarieh@cc.huji.ac.il

Shelley Phipps
Dalhousie University
Dept. Economics
Halifax NS B3H 3J5
Canada
Shelley.Phipps@dal.ca

The editors will like to thank the W.T. Grant foundation for their support of the editorial work on this book.

ISBN 978-90-481-3376-5   e-ISBN 978-90-481-3377-2
DOI 10.1007/978-90-481-3377-2
Springer Dordrecht Heidelberg London New York

Library of Congress Control Number: 2009937017

Printed on acid-free paper

Springer is part of Springer Science+Business Media (www.springer.com)

Preface

This chapter provides a brief overview of the book highlighting the modest progress from child welfare to child well-being reflected in these chapters, and the parallel movement in Kahn's career and research, as his scholarship developed over the years. It then moves to explore the relationship between two overarching themes, child and family policy stressing a universal approach to children and social protection stressing a more targeted approach to disadvantaged and vulnerable individuals including children and the complementarity of these strategies.

Introduction

To a large extent Alfred J. Kahn was at the forefront of the developments in the field of child welfare services (protective services, foster care, adoption, and family preservation and support). Over time his scholarship moved to a focus on the broader policy domain of child and family policy and the outcomes for child wellbeing. His work, as is true for this volume, progressed from a focus on poor, disadvantaged and vulnerable children to a focus on all children. He was convinced that children, by definition, are a vulnerable population group and that targeting all children, employing a universal policy as a strategy would do more for poor children than a narrowly focused policy targeted on poor children alone, As we first argued more than three decades ago (*Not for the Poor Alone*; "Universalism and Income Testing in Family Policy"), one could target the most disadvantaged within a universal framework, and this would lead to more successful results than targeting only the poor. The history of the last 50 years of child welfare is a history of this movement, from a deficit-oriented policy to a developmental model, from a targeted and selective strategy to a universal approach, from child welfare to child well being.

Kahn began his academic career in the 1950s, confronting the main issues in the child welfare field at that time. His focus in his early work, as in the early chapters in this book, was on the U.S child welfare field. Under the auspices of the Citizens' Committee for Children of New York, he prepared a report published in 1953 on the Children's Court in New York, providing an unprecedented look at the background and workings of the Court. He called the system "a dream still unrealized" that needed to focus more on rehabilitation than punishment. In 1957 he published a report entitled For *Children In Trouble* highlighting the inadequacies of the city's efforts at helping children in trouble. In the 1960s, the report entitled *A Dream Deferred*, called for a reorganization of social services to help families cope better with emergencies. He was among the early advocates of community—based social services rather than institutional or foster care and an early advocate, as well, for child allowances, urging a universal policy regime in support of the economic well-being of all children and their families.

The book begins with an essay by Kahn on how children, youth, and families have changed over time and the implications of these changes for children's life experiences and the opportunities they may have. How we are organized in the public and private sectors around children's problems, is his first overarching question. He reminds us that we should no longer focus just on the social problems of adolescents, but rather seek out positive and productive roles for them. Nonetheless, dysfunctional families will exist and still need help, and the need for substitute families remains, as we can see now in Africa, with regard to children orphaned as a consequence of HIV AIDS and the growing number of child-headed households. He concludes by raising the question: Should we work at improving the link between childhood, foster family care, and adoption by better integrating child welfare programs or should we address a broader range of social policies affecting children? Should we advance across-policy domains (income transfers, health, education, personal social services) rather than remain in one, by adopting a holistic strategy, sustaining the treatment of children within a child and family policy agenda? Families are changing and the experiences of youth are changing. Will we provide new opportunities for them? Will youth still be labeled "dysfunctional" and in need of rescue or will we stress, instead, their potential for creativity and productivity?

Ben-Arieh continues and supplements this discussion by describing the childhood social indicator movement, and the progress being made from a focus on poor and suffering children to promoting children's well being. He lays out several different theoretical frameworks, including:

- Ecological theories of child development
- The concept of children's rights
- The new sociology of childhood
- Children as the unit of analysis
- Children's quality of life
- Attention to child and family policy.

Different sources of data are now available and used, in assessing child well being. These include administrative data, census data, survey data, longitudinal data, and other large scale data bases, providing data as the target for extensive and rigorous quantitative studies as well as comparative data bases offering new insights with regard to child well—being in Europe, described subsequently by Richardson.

Ben-Arieh reminds us of the role indicators play in providing policy-relevant data and the progress that has been carried out with regard to a changed view of children and childhood, including:

– A growing emphasis on child well being rather than just on survival
– A growing emphasis on enhancing positive outcomes rather than confronting negative impacts
– A focus on children's current well being rather than their future development
– A focus on the voices of children rather than only adult perspectives.

Ben-Arieh concludes by reminding us of the explosion in the number of "state of the child" reports that have been published since the 1980s, and the emerging global interest in childhood social indicators.

The next cluster of chapters focuses specifically on the traditional child welfare system. McGowan's history of child welfare leaves us with a sense of how little has been achieved in movement towards a developmental model. She reminds us that the field is very much on the public agenda today. Yet some of the tensions that have pervaded the field in the past, still remain. Among the ongoing issues, still debated, are child saving versus family preservation, the extent to which the state should assume responsibility for problems in family life, local or state versus federal responsibility for standard setting, public versus private sector dominance in social service delivery, categorical versus integrated social service programs. She concludes by noting that the child welfare field continues to struggle with these contradictions.

Courtney's chapter highlights the need for more attention to youth transitioning out of foster care, the need for normative supports for these older adolescents, and suggests strategies for achieving a broader basis for improving the outcomes for the 18–21 year olds. Fallon et al explores three different systems for carrying out child maltreatment surveillance while Zeira reminds us of the value of practice wisdom and learning from practice in child welfare. This cluster ends with a chapter on New York City and the need for sharply honed advocacy skills to achieve political goals. Although addressing issues in New York, Nayowith provides a case history of the efforts needed to mobilize advocacy efforts, aimed at affecting child policy and doing better by children. She points out the importance of gathering the facts to provide an evidence base for mobilizing support for legislation, or opposition to proposed laws, depending on the issue.

Following this are several chapters on different theoretical perspectives, from Bruyere and Garbarino, discussing the ecological perspective coupled with a child rights perspective, both essential to an understanding of the factors shaping child well being. Staller offers us a discussion of how social problems can be deconstructed in different ways leading to various definitions of any social problem, with an intriguing review of the different ways children leaving home may be viewed: as runaway youth or missing children. The runaway youth movement was framed from the youth's perspective and took a child's rights' approach. In contrast, the missing children movement took a parents' rights approach and worried parents sought help in locating children. The policy responses take very different forms depending on which definition is favored. Staller's objective is to apply her analytic framework to how any problem has been shaped and responded to.

Coulton and Fischer focus on the development and application of child well-being indicators at the local level, referring to sub-state geographic areas or political jurisdictions, also referred to as community or neighborhood indicators. They discuss the infrastructure needed to sustain local indicators work, including both the production of child wellbeing indicators and how they are used to address policy and program. They conclude by providing several case studies that demonstrate how child wellbeing indicators have been developed and applied in selected locales.

Aber et al., focus on the range of indicators in one particular domain, namely education while Burton and Phipps turn to a different type of indicator, namely the subjective responses of children to questions about the quality of their lives. They look, in particular, at child reports of current happiness and life satisfaction for Canadian 12–17 year olds. In contrast, Gatenio-Gabel takes a very different tack. She provides a global perspective and focuses, especially, on how developing countries consider children and what kinds of policies are relevant in environments with far more limited resources. What can be expected in the way of social protection in developing countries and what does a child rights' perspective contribute?

One could certainly argue that at the heart of the book are the several chapters on economic support for child and family well-being. Kahn, in his own work and the research he carried out in the 1970s and 1980s with Kamerman, turned increasingly to a focus on the economic situation of families with children, applying a model of hypothetical families and their experiences with earnings at different levels and different national income transfer systems. Their major finding was that comparative policy studies focused on children and their families underscored the laggard status of the U.S. with regard to the economic well being of U.S. children and their families.

Here we have a series of chapters reaching similar conclusions. The Danzigers describe child poverty in the U.S., the limitations of U.S. anti-poverty policies, and the lessons learned from research and cross-national policies. Garfinkel and Nepomnaschy discuss one particular policy, namely child support. They describe the vulnerability of lone mother families and the inadequacies of U.S., policies; and they end with some international comparisons from Europe, underscoring the better situation for the children in these families in several European countries. They point to the financial support provided in many European countries that guarantee a minimum level of financial support to children in lone parent families, when the non-custodial parent fails to pay support, pays it irregularly or not at all. And they note the relevant discussion of these policies by Kamerman and Kahn (1988).

Phipps concentrates here on policies affecting very young children in Canada, those under age 3. She stresses the role of maternity and parental leave policies cross nationally, and compares the Canadian policies with those available in eight other rich countries. She concludes that although Canadian income transfers play a vital role in reducing the depth of poverty experienced by very young children, the full package of cash transfers in other countries leaves more very young children in poverty in Canada than in most of the other countries in this study.

While using the LIS data base, Gornick and Jantii discuss the role of employment and earnings on childrens' economic well being and the importance of labor market behavior and government tax and cash transfers. They suggest that demographic differences across countries are less vital for child poverty outcomes than earnings and transfers.

Bradshaw, Richardson, and Saunders each write about international developments in child and family well being, drawing on several large scale data sets for their analyses and focusing in particular on economic well-being. Bradshaw provides an introduction to the study of child benefit packages and illustrates their value using the model family methodology employed earlier by Kahn and Kamerman (1983). In his chapter, Bradshaw describes the methods involved in using this approach to compare child benefit packages. Hypothetical (model) families of different types are assigned a specified level of earnings and the specified package of cash and tax transfers they would qualify for in different countries. The outcomes for children and their families are compared cross-nationally.

Richardson focuses on the changes in child well being in Europe, between 2003 and 2006. He reminds us that child well being is an increasingly important topic in research and policy circles at the European level and points out that European policy makers are looking beyond income poverty measures to assess childrens' well being. Other issues addressed include the work/family balance and human capital investment in future generations. He discusses the outcomes for children across multiple dimensions of well being, beyond income or material well being, including health, education, subjective well being, risk and safety, and housing.

The final chapters advance the agenda moving toward discussion of child well being: in France, in Europe, and internationally with regard to ECEC and family policies. In this context, earlier, Kamerman and Kahn (1991) highlighted the special problem of providing care and support for very young children and their families, reminding us of the need to link maternity and parental leave policies with ECEC policies and programs, to understand the importance of policies affecting the very young, an issue addressed by both Fagnani and Moss.

Fagnani reminds us that along with the Nordic countries, France leads the European Union—indeed the world—in public childcare provision and benefits aimed at reducing child care costs for families. OECD has also shown that family spending has the greatest focus on childcare services in France and the Nordic countries. As a matter of fact, the progressive arrival of mothers in the labor market since the 1970s influenced French family policy decision makers to introduce a whole range of services for parents in paid employment, which has in turn enabled a growing number of mothers to gain access to jobs. This has helped to place the question of the work/family life balance firmly onto the policy agenda. She concludes that, while couched in terms of the "best interest" of the child, French child and family policy is in fact the result of the combined forces of labor market pressures and demands for a mother's right to paid work.

In these years Kahn and Kamerman also explored the role of services in a child and family policy package (ECEC), along with time for parenting (leaves) and money (cash and tax benefits). Obviously, there are gaps here. An almost 60 year history of scholarship (40 of which was joint) covering a range of policies affecting children and their families, cannot be covered in one book. The themes mentioned above are pervasive. In addition, there are others, including: the importance of a strong role for government despite the significance of the voluntary sector and the market, especially in the social service field; the role of federalism; the impact of gender role changes and the impact of demography, both aging and fertility; the importance of political will; and, finally, the need for a holistic approach to social policy (services integration? family policy? social protection policy?) rather than a cluster of disparate categorical silos.

The book covers a remarkable range of issues and scholarship, and so did Alfred Kahn's scholarship and career.

Sheila B. Kamerman
New York, USA

References

Kahn, A. J., & Kamerman, S. B. (1983). *Income transfers for families with children:* An *eight-country study.* Philadelphia, PA: Temple University Press.

Kahn, A. J., & Kamerman, S. B. (1988). *Child support: From debt collection to social policy.* Newbury Park, CA: Sage.

Kamerman, S. B., & Kahn, A. J. (1988). Social policy and children in the U.S. and Europe. In J. L. Palmer, T. Smeeding, & B. B. Torrey (Eds.), *The vulnerable* (pp. 351–380). Washington, DC: Urban Institute Press.

Kamerman, S. B., & Kahn, A. J. (1991). *Child care, parental leave, and the Under 3s. Policy innovation in Europe.* New York: Auburn House.

Alfred J. Kahn (1919–2009)

Alfred J. Kahn, Professor Emeritus at the Columbia University School of Social Work and world-renowned social policy scholar and educator.

Kahn received his B.S.S. in 1939 from the City College of New York, his Masters of Social Work in 1946 from Columbia University School of Social Work. Dr. Kahn was the recipient of the first social work doctorate awarded by the School in 1952, and the first in New York State, as well. He taught at the Columbia University School of Social Work for 57 years, from 1947 to 2004. Those who studied, social services, child welfare, family policy, poverty and its causes and impacts, and social policy generally will remember the monumental comparative work of Dr. Kahn, who along with Professor Sheila Brody Kamerman, shaped the discourse in many fields for decades. Program and policy recommendations advanced by Dr. Kahn and Dr. Kamerman were embraced by many international NGOs and were brought to life in social welfare programs around the world. His ideas also contributed to the development of graduate social work education.

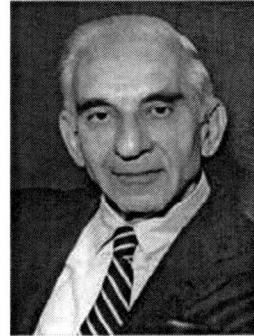

Dr. Kahn was a passionate advocate for children and their families. As an advocate, he favored universal social benefits and services, rather than means-tested, saying that they ought to be "good enough for every American, not for the poor alone." He was a consultant to federal, state, and local agencies, international organizations, and foreign governments. In this role, he shared his expertise on family policy, cash benefits and social service programs, local community social service planning and coordination, and issues of equality and equity.

Dr. Kahn was also an author and co-author, editor and co-editor, producing more than 25 books and 300 articles and chapters that have continuing relevance and a palpable impact worldwide.

Early in his research career, "the one-man watchdog organization who monitored the social services offered by the city and state of New York", as he was called in *The New York Times* (February 21, 2009), Dr. Kahn served as a consultant to New York's Citizens Committee for Children (CCC). In this capacity, he provided leadership to research staff and community lay leaders, and authored some 15 studies of city and state programs concerned with truancy, youth, police, children's courts, protective services, and child guidance programs for at-risk youth. The widely-publicized and discussed results offered blueprints for reform at the local and national levels. They were also the foundation for a 1963 volume, *Planning Community Services for Children in Trouble,* with a foreword by Eleanor Roosevelt, board member. Among his special roles, Dr. Kahn, was the United States participant and rapporteur in a 1967 U.N. "Expert Group on Social Policy and Level of Living in the Nation" and a 1969 U.N. "Expert Group on Training Social Welfare Personnel for Development Planning."

In the early 1980s, Dr. Kahn chaired the influential Committee on Child Development Research and Public Policy of The National Academy of Science. He was the recipient of awards and honors from various universities and professional associations in recognition of his pioneering work in cross-national child and family policy research.

Dr. Kahn's remarkable work in the academic and policy making fields' through out the years will continue to influence and guide professionals, researchers and social-policy advocates for many years to come.

Contents

Contributors

Lawrence J. Aber Institute for Human Development and Social change, New York University, New York, NY, USA

Asher Ben-Arieh Paul Baerwald School of Social Work and Social Welfare, Hebrew University of Jerusalem, Jerusalem, Israel

Juliette Berg Department of Applied Psychology, New York University, New York, USA

Jonathan Bradshaw Department of Social Policy and Social Work, University of York, York, UK

Edmund Bruyere Center for the Human Rights of Children, Developmental Psychology Loyola University, Chicago, USA

Peter Burton Department of Economics, Dalhousie University, Halifax, Nova Scotia, Canada

Claudia J. Coulton Center on Urban Poverty and Community Development, Mandel School of Applied Social Sciences, Case Western Reserve University, Cleveland, OH, USA

Mark E. Courtney School of Social Work, University of Washington, Seattle, WA, USA

Sandra K. Danziger School of Social Work and Gerald R. Ford School of Public Policy, University of Michigan, Ann Arbor, MI, USA

Sheldon Danziger National Poverty Center, Gerald R. Ford School of Public Policy, University of Michigan, Ann Arbor, MI, USA

Jeanne Fagnani Centre d'Economie de la Sorbonne-Team Matisse, University of Paris, France

Barbara Fallon Centre for Research on Child and Families, McGill University, Canada

Robert L. Fischer Center on Urban Poverty and Community Development, Mandel School of Applied Social Sciences, Case Western Reserve University, Cleveland, OH, USA

John Fluke American Humane Association, Englewood, CO, USA

Shirley Gatenio Gabel Graduate School of Social Services, Fordham University, New York, USA

James Garbarino Center for the Human Rights of Children, Developmental Psychology Loyola University, Chicago, USA

Irwin Garfinkel School of Social Work, Columbia University, New York, USA

Erin Godfrey Department of Applied Psychology, New York University, New York, USA

Janet C. Gornick Luxembourg Income Study; Political Science and Sociology, The Graduate center, City University of New York, USA

Markus Jäntti Luxembourg Income Study, Swedish Institute for Social Research, Stockholm University, Stockholm, Sweden

Alfred J. Kahn School of Social Work, Columbia University, New York, USA

Sheila B. Kamerman School of Social Work, Columbia University, New York, USA

Bruce MacLaurin Social Work, University of Calgary, Calgary, Canada

Brenda G. McGowan School of Social Work, Columbia University, New York, USA

Peter Moss Thomas Coram Research Unit, Institute of Education University of London, London, UK

Gail B. Nayowith Laurie M. Tisch Illumination Fund, New York, NY, Gnayowithe Lmt, illumination, Fund.org. USA

Lenna Nepomnyaschy School of Social Work, Rutgers University, New Brunswick, NJ, USA

Shelley Phipps Canadian Institute for Advanced Research and Department of Economics, Dalhousie University, Halifax, Nova Scotia, Canada

Dominic Richardson OECD Social Policy Division, Paris, France

Peter Saunders Social Policy Research Centre, University of New South Wales, Sydney, Australia

Karen M. Staller School of Social Work, University of Michigan, Ann Arbor, MI, USA

Lil Tonmyr Injury & Child Maltreatment Section, Public Health Agency of Canada, Ottawa, ON, Canada

Catalina Torrente Department of Applied Psychology, New York University, New York, USA

Nico Trocmé Centre for Research on Children and Families, School of Social Work, McGill University, Canada

Ying-Ying Yuan Walter R. McDonald & Associates, Inc., Sacramento, CA, USA

Anat Zeira Paul Baerwald School of Social Work and Social Welfare, The Hebrew University of Jerusalem, Jerusalem, Israel

Part I
Opening Chapters

From "Child Saving" to "Child Development"?

Alfred J. Kahn

What next for the field we now know as "child welfare"? Federal pressure, federal funding, court actions, periodic citizen advocacy and occasional citizen or agency recourse to the courts have created a system of sorts, a system constantly undergoing change or viewed as poorly implemented. Now, the leadership of our public social services, supportive citizens and foundations, policy researchers, and, ultimately, federal, state and local governments need to think ahead strategically. Their potentially field-altering question becomes: how are we to be organized as private and public sectors around youth concerns? What kind of evolution of child welfare are we to advocate and implement? How are we to organize, finance, conduct and empower what is indisputably an important branch of social work? Pursued far enough, the question becomes: does it make optimum sense that the child welfare systems of London, Washington, Minneapolis, and San Francisco serve as the models for cities such as Harare, Kabul, New Delhi, and Johannesburg?

The question is complicated by the fact that our traditional service system now competes with a new series of systems. What grew out of child welfare, as it evolved from child saving, now must joust with other modes of planning for children and youth, and there are some interesting choices to be made. Take virtually any state cross-section of agencies assigned management and planning tasks for children and youth and the need for some decisions becomes clear.

Historically, and today, the primary child welfare task is to manufacture or mandate alternate parenting for children with an atypical life course. But today, this may be a task assigned elsewhere in state government, outside the purview of child welfare agencies.

I came into social work via a public assistance social investigator job, but had my real training (field work integrated with theory) in a child mental health unit early in the evolution of child guidance in this country. Then, by chance, I was able to add a cultural-dimension (Jewish child guidance). Next, most fortuitously, came a long and intensive immersion in local public child welfare and child policy, which soon had an advocacy component. It was a modest step from public child welfare

A.J. Kahn (✉)
School of Social Work, Columbia University, New York, USA

S.B. Kamerman et al. (eds.), *From Child Welfare to Child Well-Being*, Children's
Well-Being: Indicators and Research 1, DOI 10.1007/978-90-481-3377-2_1,
© Springer Science+Business Media B.V. 2010

advocacy to broader social policy training in a social work doctoral program. I thus located my career, teaching throughout, consulting nationally and internationally, engaging in research worldwide, writing extensively books, articles, and papers. In similar vein, I am most honored and pleased to join my esteemed colleagues in the explorations within this volume. I am deeply interested in how disparate societies organize themselves to deliver social welfare benefits and services. And, for many decades, I have closely monitored and assessed child welfare and children's services.

Children have almost always been the objects of a considerable degree of societal attention. They in fact have reliably constituted one of the few domains in which a laissez faire world does not generally enforce a "hands off" policy, since children are so vulnerable. But which children generate attention, what kinds of attention, with how much diversity in response at a given moment, and with what consequences—if such consequences have been noted? These pages will sketch the process preliminarily. What follows is in roughly chronological order. No attempt has been made to engage in adequate research, documentation, illustration or geographic coverage. A full accounting would be lengthy. A brief scholarly overview must forgo considerable complexity. Nonetheless, a preliminary effort would appear justifiable as an introduction to current discussion and perhaps as an initial instigator for future action. Change is underway—"hands off" is not an optimal response. The fundamental question is: what does the future hold for the field of child welfare?

Today, in what is considered primary care, we identify modern constructions or evolutions, and even family sub-structures, out of earlier child-related activity. There are tribal groups (God's Army, for example) which in primary relationships retain an earlier child-parent pattern: without a family in its modern sense, the children and youth are organized for shared tasks (hunting, food production, caring for the wounded, and burials, etc.). Recall Oliver Twist and his rag-tag family organized around begging and petty thievery. Youth are characteristically recruited to augment the work force. Recruits are acquired out of battles, by kidnapping, by purchase, and even, occasionally, by volunteering. The desire someday or in some way to reassemble one's own tribe provides the skeleton for larger enterprises, areas or infrastructures. And tribal leadership requires some relationship bounds. A dynamic process is continuously in play and can be recognized currently in the parallel of the united foster care youth with the returning soldier-warrior.

It is not possible to talk of child policy without mention of infanticide. No one was measuring need or matching numbers of childbirths to what society tasks required. Thus, if there were too many children and youth, the surplus was liquidated. The social rationales and mechanisms were often ingenious. Or more benign options were adopted. Children deemed not usable were left to die soon after birth. Later, in a brilliant after-thought, a child disposal system (basket at the church compound gates) was set up to recruit priests, nuns, and monks. Indeed, there was child saving, but we should recall that, from the most primitive times until the Renaissance or later, the number of infanticides far outpaced deployment as a member of the useful (farming), dangerous (soldering), or meritorious (priesthood).

From about the time of the Renaissance until modern times, most periods could be characterized as "child saving" in the modern sense of the term. Either the solution was assigned merit (join the priesthood) or the children were assigned places in residential schools or in adjuncts of religious facilities where they would have regular religious instruction and practice and were defined as "saved". Infanticide did not disappear, but became less visible or more acceptable, and the society was encouraged to earn religious merit by creating these child rescue opportunities.

We thus introduce a period, several hundred years in duration, perhaps as long as from 1700 to 1900, which subsumes a diversity of institutions, facilities, programs and actions which develop or come to be in favor. Most current child welfare is created out of this collaboration. It is possible to blame or praise depending on the choice of illustration. Most of our chapter illustrations reflect a stage in these developments.

There was no precise beginning moment when children joined other hunters and gatherers, laborers, or soldiers who could (or can) be taken in by a family in a semi-permanent relationship and be "adopted". The boundary between this status and other family members was, or could be, narrow. Family continuity and solidarity were valued and sought. Loyalties mattered. People wanted heirs. They created family lines and trees, even when they knew they could not, or likely would not, survive. But the adoption concept was differentiated and given its own identity. At various paces, the process might entail a financial transaction, a religious ritual, or a public ceremony. Then why not recruitment? Soon there were also agents and agencies "in the business". There were set procedures and legal documents. Within adoption (also at one time carefully separated) there was foster care, a kind of lesser adoption. Programs were allowed to develop in which all kinds of workable roles might be structured. Where widespread, a foster agency could identify an extended family and dominate a residential charter of public housing. (It took building demolition to "liberate" the members!)

Central goals were, and are, the critical component- to affirm, or reaffirm, crisis architecture for what had over several thousand years emerged as a family. Within family, relationships were defined as having religious and mystical significance, with spiritual support from God. Child welfare built on family sociology, tribal economy, and military structures. For illustration, see the Old Testament or Shakespeare.

But now something else is occurring. Child and youth policy become child, youth and mastering basic math. In short, something has been added into the previous standard: becoming a viable middle-school youth who can behave appropriately and learn becomes a young person's modern role. It may be specialization in math, computers, language, second language, engineering—or much else. It is as though family coherence has been overtaken by individual success, and one must now master some new individualized skill set as a prerequisite to a role in contemporary society. Witness the thousands of industrious youth now at work in China and India. Do they not illustrate a new pattern?

New dimensions enter child and youth policy because children, family, and society are changing. To monitor the quality of education ("No Child Left Behind"),

American classes are evaluated as producers of educational excellence. Now, to assess our relative success with regard to family stability, we monitor a school's unmarried parent rates. To gauge successful citizenship, we look for evidence of civic involvement (such as election volunteering and HIV-prevention counseling).

Note the shift. Our indicators have become math and English achievement and civic participation, alongside unmarried parenthood- with a shift of emphasis to learning and proactive societal behavior. These newer indicators are offered as an alternative to foster care. The goal is no longer family and its substitutes, no longer foster care to save a family, but rather, an institutional path to advance family well-being. It is not merely child saving, but enhancing child well-being by substantively addressing goals within the very context of the schoolroom. Are these inclusions in the basic classroom the equivalent of what affluent parents provide their Ivy League-bound middle school youth, rather than a preventive to child welfare?

Is this the case? Do middle class parents and children in sufficient numbers still fight the old battles: avoid unwed parenthood; strive for functional families; keep up with school work; live at home through high school; carry on in college; identify and pursue one's life's work?

Because the issue is no longer family viability alone, our society is adapting. Child welfare arises from the Social Security Act and family welfare structures and programs within the states. Many states are attempting to create integrated child welfare structures and programs. At the present time, we are grappling with economic problems by reverting to a middle class work ethic, but that is simply not enough. The new model becomes laissez-faire capitalism, gradually being exemplified by China and India, whose economic leadership begins to take on considerable skill and expertise. It is a transitional phase, where "no child is left behind" and everybody learns the requisite skills to become a participating member of the labor force. Soon, the "underdeveloped" countries will be competing with the labor force of the "developed" world. Social relationships at the middle school level are the heirs to the middle class family neighborhood of the Golden Age. We are creating a new and empowered youth generation of distinctive individuals, not a device to enhance, protect, or substitute for the family. Broken families are not the focus for curative intervention. Stated differently: Developing countries following a late-capitalism welfare state model want all of their citizens appropriately trained and skilled. Everyone is to work. Individualism is nurtured.

It is as if a generation has skipped the hunter-gatherer-soldier phase to leap into a family structure with enriched content and expanded boundaries. Child welfare planners are no longer merely helping to solve a structural problem facing families, but also entering into the next societal task. Welfare state laissez faire is focusing on productive youth roles, as advanced industrial societies experiment with finding a suitable place in society for middle school youth. One need not be a social problem to be part of this process, but the hundreds of thousands of dysfunctional, unrelated (un-family-related) youth—dysfunctional youth who would formerly acquire a family tie via foster care—have a new opportunity. It could be a crucial development, a society with millions of youth growing into individualized, functional roles (mathematician, linguist, engineer, entertainer, athlete, etc.), the possibilities keep expanding.

To put our question differently: are we about to improve the arc of childhood, foster care, and adoption by better integrating child welfare programs with the Social Security Act? Or will we look upon our newest middle school generation as having roles very similar to previous generations? Will our newest generation take on new roles and create its own distinctive place in a society in which young people create a different world, where competence and success are gauged on the basis of work skills and achievements? Society will be re-shaping families. Youth of all classes will engage in varied and significant tasks. State government will be responsible to families. We are referring to the equivalent of what, at present, only affluent middle class parents are able to provide their Ivy League-bound children. Now, every young person will have the opportunity to experience and be positively shaped by the process. At-risk young people will no longer be negatively labeled dysfunctional and in need of rescue. The emphasis will no longer be on the problems, rather the limitless potential, of each wondrously individual child.

From Child Welfare to Children Well-Being: The Child Indicators Perspective

Asher Ben-Arieh

Al Khan was among the first to study children's welfare in a comparative way and to monitor the status of children over time. As early as the 1940th Kahn was involved in one of the pioneering efforts to study the "state of children" in New York through his collaboration with the Citizen Committee for Children (Ben-Arieh, 2006). Similarly, some 40 years ago, Al and Sheila Kamerman were the first to examine child welfare across developed countries (Kamerman & Kahn, 1978).

But it is not only his path breaking efforts that single out Kahn as one of the leading scholars in our field. In my eyes, it was also his ability to foresee where the field was heading, to identify the changes underway, and to lead the way forward that singles him out for special recognition. Indeed, the field of child welfare has dramatically changed in the last decades. As my colleagues who contributed to this volume so brilliantly show, we have indeed moved from saving poor and suffering children to promoting children's well-being.

As history so often conspires, about the same time as Kahn and Kamerman began their venture into comparative child welfare studies, the social indicators movement sprung to life in a vibrant and clear voice. Its first signs of life began in the 1960s amid a climate of rapid social change. At the time, there was a sense among social scientists and public officials that well measured and consistently collected social indicators could offer a way to monitor the condition of groups in society in the present and over time, including the conditions of children and families (Aborn, 1985; Land, 2000).

Today, after more than 50 years, not only have we witnessed a shift from child welfare to child well-being, but, as I will attempt to show in this chapter, we have seen child indicators undergo a dramatic change. Truly, most of these changes have occurred only in the last 25 years, but they are no less dramatic because of it, and they are in line with changes in the broader field of child welfare. These changes have not occurred in isolation. They are the consequence of the work and efforts of many around the globe. I have been lucky to be in the center of the child indicators

A. Ben-Arieh (✉)
Paul Baerwald School of Social Work and Social Welfare, Hebrew University of Jerusalem, Jerusalem, Israel
e-mail: benarieh@cc.huji.ac.il

S.B. Kamerman et al. (eds.), *From Child Welfare to Child Well-Being*, Children's Well-Being: Indicators and Research 1, DOI 10.1007/978-90-481-3377-2_2,
© Springer Science+Business Media B.V. 2010

movement during the last 20 years. I am even luckier to have had Al along with me, curious and enthusiastic as ever and always looking into the future trying to understand and foresee not only where we are, but where we should be going.

1 Child Social Indicators

The rapidly growing use of and interest in childhood social indicators is in many ways a reaction to the rapid changes in family life and the growing demand from child development professionals, social scientists and the public for a better picture of children's well-being. It is also the consequence of both the demands for more accurate measures of the conditions children face and the quest for outcome measures designed to address those conditions (Ben-Arieh & Wintersberger, 1997; Casas, 2000; Forssén & Ritakallio, 2006; Lee, 1997).

Beyond these general explanations, I would argue that the emergence of the child indicators movement be attributed to "new" normative and conceptual theories as well as methodological advancements. Since the early 1970s, three major normative or theoretical developments have contributed to the emergence and rapid development of the child indicators movement: (1) the ecological theories of child development; (2) the normative concept of children's rights; and (3) the new sociology of childhood as a stage in and of itself.

Similarly, three methodological issues supported the development of the child indicators movement: (1) the emerging importance of subjective perspectives; (2) the call for using the child as the unit of observation; and (3) the expanded use of administrative data and the growing variety of data sources.

Finally, and particularly in recent years, the call for more policy-oriented research contributed to the child indicators movement. These theoretical, methodological, and policy impetuses are discussed in more depth below.

2 "New" Normative and Theoretical Approaches

Theories and normative approaches to children welfare abound. Many have contributed to this effort and many more continue to work in this field. Yet, I single out three such approaches that not only influenced the child welfare field at large but had a particular impact on the child indicators movement.

2.1 The Ecology of Child Development

Today, children's capabilities are understood in the context of their development and well-being. These are dynamic processes, influenced by a multitude of factors. Children interact with their environment and thus play an active role in creating their well-being by balancing the different factors, developing and making use of resources, and responding to stress. Bronfenbrenner's bio-ecological model of human development (Bronfenbrenner & Morris, 1998) conceptualizes child development on the basis of four concentric circles of environmental influence, with time as an underlying factor, recognizing both individual changes over time and historic time.

The child, with all his or her personal characteristics, interacts first and foremost with the family, but also a range of other people and systems: friends, neighbors, health care, child care, school, and so forth. These direct interactions compose the child's *micro-system*, and this is the level with the strongest direct influence on children. Connections between the different structures within the micro-system, for example between parents and school, occur in the *meso-system*. One level up, the *exo-system* represents the societal context in which families live, including parents' social networks, the conditions in the local community, access to and quality of services, parents' workplace, and the media. The exo-system affects the child mainly indirectly by influencing the different structures within the micro-system. The *macro-system*, finally, points to the wider societal context of cultural norms and values, policies, economic conditions, and global developments. The different systems are dynamic and interdependent, influencing one another and changing over time (Lippman, 2004; Olk, 2004; Stevens, Dickson, Poland, & Prasad, 2005).

In interacting with the different systems and subsystems, children and their families encounter both barriers and facilitators. These barriers and facilitators can, in many respects, be considered indicators of child well-being. Together with the various outcomes at the different levels, this ecological perspective had immense impact on the child indicators movement and its development (Bradshaw, Hoscher, & Richardson, 2007).

2.2 Children's Rights as Human Rights

The United Nation's Convention on the Rights of the Child (CRC) offers a normative framework for understanding children's well-being. Its four general principles fit closely with conceptualizations of child well-being. The first of these is nondiscrimination. Article 2 of the CRC argues for recognizing the life situations and well-being of excluded groups of children, such as those with disabilities, children in institutions, or refugee children, and to disaggregate available data by age, gender, ethnicity, geography, and economic background. The second principle, the best interest of the child (article 3), itself implies a child focus and strengthens children's role as citizens in their own right. From this principle comes the imperative to use the child as a unit of analysis.

The complexity of children's lives is reflected in the third principle, that of survival and development (article 6). The CRC promotes a holistic view of child development and well-being, giving equal weight to children's civic, political, social, economic, and cultural rights, and stressing that these rights are interrelated, universal, and indivisible. Concepts of child well-being accordingly must be

multidimensional and ecological. The fourth principle calls for respecting the view
of the child (article 12), acknowledging children's rights to be heard and to have
their view taken into account in matters that affect them (Santos Pais, 1999).

These views of children's rights contributed to the child indicators movement in
several important ways. First, they have placed children on the agenda, thus calling
for more data on their life and well-being. Second, they call for indicators to monitor
the implementation of the CRC and the fulfillment of children's rights. Third, by the
breadth of topics and issues covered, these views demand indicators in sub domains
and areas of interest that were not measured or monitored before.

2.3 The "New" Sociology of Childhood

One of the most important concepts that had shaped the child indicators movement
is that of childhood as a stage in and of itself. The discourse on child well-being is
thus also one of well-being and well-becoming (Frones, 2007). The more traditional
perspective was one that looked on child well-being in terms of children's future,
focusing on their education and future employability. The "new" perspective on
child well-being focuses on children's current (during childhood) life situation.

Although one can argue that it is reasonable to develop indicators of child well-
being that focus on children as "future adults" or members of the next generation,
such approaches often fail to consider the life stage of childhood, a stage that has
its own sociological characteristics (Alanen, 2001; Olk, 2006; Qvortrup, 1999). The
CRC, for example, makes clear that children's immediate well-being is important in
its own right. Children's present life and development and future life chances thus
must be reconciled in conceptualizations of well-being by looking both into the
conditions under which children are doing well and child outcomes across a range
of domains (Ben-Arieh et al., 2001).

3 The New Methodological Perspectives and the Child Indicators Movement

Just as the new theories and normative methods created the context in which
the child indicators movement flourished, three methodological perspectives contributed to its rapid evolution during the last 30 years. These methodological
changes are naturally linked to the theories and concepts presented above, but they
also have individual merits and warrant a separate discussion.

3.1 The Emergence of the Subjective Perspective

Prout (1997) argued that "large-scale social phenomena and small-scale inter subjective action implicate each other such that the complexity of the social world

cannot be expressed through a simple asymmetry of objective social structure and subjective actors". Yet, much research on children's lives has until recently focused on objective descriptions, treating children as passive objects who are acted on by the adult world. As the child indicators movement accepted and built on the theoretical foundations outlined above, it became clear that a new role for children had emerged, one that coupled the search for objective measures with a subjective view of childhood (Casas, González, Figuer, & Coenders, 2004; Mareš, 2006).

This has proved particularly important given that studies have shown, especially during adolescence, that parents do not always accurately convey their child's feelings (Shek, 1998; Sweeting, 2001). Further, studies have shown that including the perspectives of children is important not only because they differ from those of the adults, but because doing so respects children as persons, better informs policymakers, provides a foundation for child advocacy and enhances legal and political socialization of children (Melton & Limber, 1992).

The child indicators movement, which traditionally was based on aggregate statistics, bloomed as new indicators sought to capture children's own account of their lives and living conditions. The field quickly realized that although there are areas in which indirect information may be superior—such as on the household economy as reported by parents, or grades from school records—in most instances, and particularly for crucial indicators such as mental well-being and social relations, children's own reports are necessary (Lohan & Murphy, 2001; Ohannessian, Lerner, Lerner, & Voneye, 1995; Shek, 1998).

3.2 Children as the Unit of Observation

If children have basic rights and their childhood is worthy of study by itself, then making the child the unit of observation becomes apparent (Jensen & Saporiti, 1992). The child indicators movement thus began incorporating child-centered indicators, ones that begin from the child and move outward, separating, at least for measurement purposes, the child from his or her family. Sen (1997) has argued for measures that reflect the life a person is actually living rather than the resources or means a person may have available. Sen's approach takes into account personal choices, constraints, circumstances, and abilities to achieve a preferred living standard. Applying Sen's approach to the assessment of a child's living conditions highlights the need to focus on the child, rather than the household or community, as the unit of analysis (Ben-Arieh et al., 2001).

An informative example can be drawn from Sauli's (1997) work on families in Finland. If researchers use the family as the unit of analysis, one-half of the families with children are one-child families. However, using the child as the unit of analysis reveals that only one-fourth of them live without siblings. If the field is to gain an accurate picture of children and their experience, it must develop indicators that focus on the child as the unit of observation. This also means disaggregating information in traditional databases to more reliably assess their well-being.

3.3 The Emergence of Administrative Data and the Variability of Data Sources

The richness of children's lives and their domains of well-being mean that any single source of information will be incomplete. Therefore, the field sought three different sources of information: administrative data, census and surveys, and social research (longitudinal and ad hoc). Although researchers had used the latter two systematically and regularly in the past, administrative data emerged in the "era of information" during the second half of the twentieth century and contributed to the evolution of the child indicators movement.

Administrative data, even though collected primarily for purposes other than research, are a powerful resource for research (Goerge, 1997). The data, maintained by organizations that serve children and families daily, are an important source of information on the conditions of children. Until recently, administrative data were confined to paper files. However, as information systems were computerized and became more accessible, administrative data emerged as a rich source of information for developing indicators of children's well-being. For example, administrative data, by definition, cover the population of individuals or families with a particular status or receiving a particular service. In addition to service receipt, the files often contain information on their address or neighborhood, thus contributing to the development of indicators at the regional or local level and the consequent "small region monitoring" (Banister, 1994).

Further, administrative data may be the best option for quickly developing more timely or new community and local indicators of children's well-being. Given the expense of new or continuing social surveys, and given that much administrative data already exist, this source is ideal for the short-term development of indicators that can be used to inform the public and policymakers.

4 The Policy Context

Finally, the growing demand that indicators be devised and used in ways that (hopefully) enhance their impact beyond academic pursuits has contributed to the emergence of the field. In that regard, some indicators and measurements have clearly led to new policies and programs for children and some have not (Ben-Arieh & Goerge, 2006). It is also evident that the same indicator, when used in certain contexts, has led to desired outcomes while in others, it did not. The effort to develop better policy-oriented indicators led to a thorough examination of existing indicators and to better data collection, including across new domains of life (Titeler & Ben-Arieh, 2006).

5 The Development of the Child Indicators Movement

The child indicators movement went through six major changes during the past 25 years: (1) Early indicators tended to focus on child survival, whereas recent indicators look beyond survival to child well-being; (2) Early indicators primarily focused on negative outcomes in life, while recent indicators look at positive outcomes in a child's life; (3) Early indicators emphasized children's "well-becoming", that is, their subsequent achievement or well-being; recent indicators focus on children's current well-being; (4) Early indicators were derived from "traditional" domains of child well-being, primarily those of professions, while recent indicators are emerging from new domains that cut across professions; (5) Early indicators focused on the adult's perspective, whereas new indicators consider the child's perspective as well; (6) Recent years have seen efforts to develop various composite indices of children's well-being (Bradshaw et al., 2007; Lippman, 2007). This evolution of child well-being indicators has occurred virtually everywhere, although at varying paces (Ben-Arieh, 2002, 2006). I detail these changes below.

5.1 From Survival to Well-Being

Much attention has been paid to children's physical survival and basic needs, focusing often on threats to children's survival, and the use of such indicators has spurred programs to save children's lives (Ben-Arieh, 2000; Bradshaw et al., 2007). Infant and child mortality, school enrollment and dropout, immunizations, and childhood disease are all examples of indicators of basic needs. However, a fundamental shift occurred when the focus moved from survival to well-being. Researchers argued in the late 1990s for indicators that moved beyond basic needs of development and beyond the phenomenon of deviance to those that promote child development (Aber, 1997; Pittman & Irby, 1997). Indeed, the field moved from efforts to determine minimums, as in saving a life, to those that focus on quality of life. This move was supported by efforts to understand what constitutes "quality of life" and its implications for children (Casas, 2000; Hubner, 1997, 2004).

5.2 From Negative to Positive

Measures of risk factors or negative behaviors are not the same as measures that gauge protective factors or positive behaviors (Aber & Jones, 1997). The absence of problems or failures does not necessarily indicate proper growth and success (Ben-Arieh, 2005; Moore, Lippman, & Brown, 2004). Thus, the challenge became developing indicators that hold societies accountable for more than the safe warehousing of children and youth (Pittman & Irby, 1997). As Resnick (1995, p. 3) states: "children's well-being indicators are on the move from concentrating only on trends of dying, distress, disability, and discomfort to tackling the issue of indicators of sparkle, satisfaction, and well-being."

However, children's positive outcomes are not static. They result from interplay of resources and risk factors of the child, his or her family, friends, school, and in the wider society. These factors are constantly changing, and children, with their evolving capacities, actively create their well-being by mediating these different factors.

5.3 From Well-Becoming to Well-Being

In contrast to the immediacy of well-*being*, well-*becoming* describes a future focus (i.e., preparing children to be productive and happy adults). Qvortrup (1999) laid the foundation for considering children's well-being, rather than only well-becoming, claiming that the conventional preoccupation with the next generation is a preoccupation of adults. Although not a necessarily harmful view, anyone interested in children and childhood should also be interested in the present as well as future childhood. In other words, children are instrumentalized by the forward-looking perspectives in the sense that their "good life" is postponed until adulthood. As such, perspectives of well-becoming focus on opportunities rather than provisions (De Lone, 1979).

Accepting the arguments of Qvortrup and others to concentrate on the well-being of children does not deny the relevance of a child's development toward adulthood. However, focusing on preparing children to become citizens suggests that they are not citizens during childhood, a concept that is hard to reconcile with a belief in children's rights. It is not uncommon to find in the literature reference to the importance of rearing children who will be creative, ethical, and moral adult members of community. It is harder to find reference to children's well-being in their childhood, even indicators of poverty or health, which on the surface are indicators of current well-being, are discussed in a context that is forward-looking: the outcomes of child poverty are diminished future prospects. Indeed, both perspectives are legitimate and necessary, both for social science and public policy. However, the emergence of the child-centered perspective, and its focus on children's well-being, introduced new ideas and energy to the child indicators movement.

5.4 From Traditional to New Domains

Studies have shown that the above three shifts are interrelated and are both the reason and the outcome of each other (Ben-Arieh, 2006). Until recently when measuring the state of children, researchers concerned themselves with traditional domains, those which were defined either by profession or by a social service (i.e., education, health, foster care). Looking at children's well-being rather than only well-becoming naturally brings into focus new domains of child-well being, such as children's life skills, children's civic involvement and participation, and children's culture (Ben-Arieh, 2000).

5.5 From an Adult to a Child Perspective

When we take into account the four changes outlines above, efforts to study children's well-being must ask at least some of the following questions: What are children doing? What do children need? What do children have? What do children think and feel? To whom or what are children connected and related? What do children contribute? Answering such questions will create a better picture of children as human beings in their present life, the positive aspects of their life, and it will do so in a way that values them as legitimate members of their community and the broader society (Ben-Arieh et al., 2001).

It is, however, evident that most of the data that already exist or data we collect using traditional methods do not help us very much in seeking answers to this set of questions. A good example would be the remarkable work by Land and colleagues, who studied children's well-being in the United States during the last quarter of the twentieth century (Land, Lamb, & Mustillo, 2001). Their reliance on existing databases led them to use traditional indicators of children's well-being, and thus their work has limited potential in answering such questions as outlined above.

To better answer such questions, we must focus on children's daily lives, which is something that children know the most about. Studies have found, for example, that parents do not really know how children spend their time (Funk et al., 1989) or what they are worried about (Gottlieb & Bronstein, 1996). Hence, to answer such questions, we must involve children in such studies, at least as our primary source of information.

5.6 Toward a Composite Index of Child Well-Being

Although expanding data on children provides policymakers and the media important information (Brown & Moore, 2003), this increasing supply of information has also led to calls for a single summary number to capture the circumstances of children. Such a composite would, it is argued, facilitate easier assessment of progress or decline. Moreover, it might be easier to hold policymakers accountable if a single number were used. In addition, it would be simpler to compare trends across demographic groups and different localities and regions (UNICEF, 2007). As noted above, the latter half of the twentieth century witnessed enormous growth in the data available to track and compare trends in children's development over time. As a result, researchers have attempted to develop summary indices (Ben-Arieh, in press; Moore, Vandivere, Lippman, McPhee, & Bloch, 2007).

6 The Current Status of the Child Indicators Movement

It is time now to turn to where the field stands today. I would argue that the current field of child indicators can be generally characterized by ten features:

(1) Indicators, their measurement, and use are driven by the universal acceptance of the CRC;
(2) Indicators have broadened beyond children's immediate survival to their well-being (without necessarily neglecting the survival indicators). Yet, in this regard, developing countries (appropriately) tend to focus more on survival

indicators, while more developed countries tend to focus on other aspects of children's lives;

(3) Efforts are combining a focus on negative and positive aspects of children's lives;

(4) The well-becoming perspective—a focus on the future success of the generation—while still dominant, is no longer the only perspective. Well-being—children's current status—is now considered legitimate as well;

(5) New domains of child well-being have emerged. Thus, a focus on children's life or civic skills, for example, is more common, fewer efforts are profession- or service-oriented, and many more are child-centered;

(6) The child as the unit of observation is now common. Efforts to measure and monitor children's well-being today start from the child and move outward;

(7) Efforts to include subjective perceptions, including the child's, are growing. Recent efforts acknowledge the usefulness of both quantitative and qualitative studies, as well as mixed methods;

(8) Local and regional reports are multiplying, and this trend seems here to stay. Although especially notable in North America and other Western countries, this geographic focus will eventually (and probably already) penetrate to non-Western regions and countries;

(9) Numerous efforts to develop composite indices are underway at all geographic levels, (local, national, and international);

(10) There is an evident shift toward an emphasis on policy-oriented efforts. A major criterion for selecting indicators is their usefulness to community workers and policymakers. Policymakers are often included in the process of developing the indicators and discussing the usefulness of various choices.

The child indicators field has evolved. The various reviews of the field support this claim. The volume of activity is clearly rising, and new indicators, composite indices, and State of the Child reports are emerging.

7 Future Perspectives

The field is clearly growing. The doubling in the number of "State of the Child" reports alone since the 1980s is an indicator of this growth (Ben-Arieh, 2006). Although the growth of these reports may be nearing its peak in the West, it is safe to say that its growth will likely continue in non-Western and non-English-speaking countries, where the emergence of State of the Child reports is still relatively new. Studies have also found that most of these reports are a one-time affair. Although there are several long-standing and well-known periodicals (such as *The State of the World's Children*, *Kids Count*), they are still the minority. It is possible that, eventually, the growing number of reports will lead to established periodicals, rather than a series of one-time reports (Ben-Arieh, 2006). Similarly, perhaps more local and regional reports will emerge in these countries, as they have in the West (O'Hare & Bramstedt, 2003).

Although the field has indeed changed dramatically during the last 30 years, we are still in the midst of the process. None of the above shifts has reached its final destination. However, all have definitely left the station. Therefore, the first reasonable conclusion is that the field will continue to move in these directions. Some have claimed that the continuation of the trends described here will eventually lead to the creation of a new role for children in measuring and monitoring their own well-being. In a field that looks beyond survival and to the full range of child well-being, including children and their own perspectives would be a natural evolution. Indeed incorporating children's subjective perceptions is both a prerequisite and a consequence of the changing field of measuring and monitoring child well-being. This in turn will lead to making children active actors in the effort to measure and monitor their own well-being rather than being an object to study (Ben-Arieh, 2005).

Finally, the field is maturing and getting more organized. What started in the last decades of the twentieth century with several international and national projects (see for example http://multinational-indicators.chapinhall.org; Hauser, Brown, & Prosser, 1997; Ben-Arieh et al., 2001) had developed by 2006 into the International Society for Child Indicators (ISCI) (www.childindicators.org) and the launch of the *Child Indicators Research* journal. These accomplishments and advances will no doubt continue apace.

References

Aber, J. L. (1997). Measuring child poverty for use in comparative policy analysis. In A. Ben-Arieh & H. Wintersberger (Eds.), *Monitoring and measuring the state of children: Beyond survival. Eurosocial Report No. 62* (pp. 193–207). Vienna: European Centre for Social Welfare Policy and Research.

Aber, L. J., & Jones, S. (1997). Indicators of positive development in early childhood: Improving concepts and measures. In R. M. Hauser, B. V. Brown, & W. R. Prosser (Eds.), *Indicators of children's well-being* (pp. 395–408). New York: Russell Sage Foundation.

Aborn, M. (1985, August). *Statistical legacies of the social indicators movement.* Paper presented at the annual meeting of the American Statistical Association, Las Vegas, NV.

Alanen, L. (2001). Childhood as a generational condition. In L. Alanen & B. Mayall (Eds.), *Conceptualizing child-adult relations* (pp. 26–49). London: Falmer.

Banister, J. (1994). *FDCH congressional testimony.* Washington, DC: US Congress.

Ben-Arieh, A. (2000). Beyond welfare: Measuring and monitoring the state of children-new trends and domains. *Social Indicators Research, 52*(3), 235–257.

Ben-Arieh, A. (2002). Evaluating the outcomes of programs versus monitoring well-being: A child-centered perspective. In T. Vecchiato, A. N. Maluccio, & C. Canali (Eds.), *Evaluation in child and family services: Comparative client and program perspective.* New York: Aldine de Gruyter.

Ben-Arieh, A. (2005). Where are the children? Children's role in measuring and monitoring their well-being. *Social Indicators, 74*(3), 573–596.

Ben-Arieh, A. (2006). Is the study of the "State of Our Children" changing? Revisiting after five years. *Children and Youth Services Review, 28*(7), 799–811.

Ben-Arieh, A. (2008). "Indicators and indices of Children's well being: toward a more policy oriented perspective" *European Journal of Education 43*, (pp. 37–50).

Ben-Arieh, A., & Goerge, R. (Eds.) (2006). *Indicators of children's well-being: Understanding their role, usage, and policy influence.* Dordrecht, Netherlands: Springer.

Ben-Arieh, A., Kaufman, H. N., Andrews, B. A., Goerge, R., Lee, B. J., & Aber, J. L. (2001). *Measuring and monitoring children's well-being*. The Netherlands: Kluwer.

Ben-Arieh, A., & Wintersberger, H. (Eds.) (1997). *Monitoring and measuring the state of children: Beyond survival. Eurosocial Report No. 62*. Vienna: European Centre for Social Welfare Policy and Research.

Bradshaw, J., Hoscher, P., & Richardson, D. (2007). An index of child well-being in the European Union. *Social Indicators Research, 80*(1), 133–177.

Bronfenbrenner, U., & Morris, P. (1998). The ecology of developmental processes. In W. Damon & R. Lerner (Eds.), *Handbook of child psychology: Theoretical models of human development* (Vol. 1, 5th ed.). New York: John Wiley.

Brown, B., & Moore, K. (2003). Child and youth well-being: The social indicators field. In R. Lerner, F. Jacobs, & J. Wertlieb (Eds.), *Handbook of applied developmental science: Promoting positive child, adolescent, and family development through research, policies, and programs*. Thousand Oaks, CA: Sage.

Casas, F. (2000). Quality of life and the life experience of children. In E. Verhellen (Ed.), *Fifth international interdisciplinary course on children's rights*. Belgium: University of Ghent.

Casas, F., González, M., Figuer, C., & Coenders, G. (2004). Subjective well-being, values, and goal achievement: The case of planned versus by chance searches on the Internet. *Social Indicators Research, 66*, 123–141.

De Lone, R. H. (1979). *Small futures: Children, inequality, and the limits of liberal reform*. New York: Harcourt Brace Jovanovich.

Forssén, K., & Ritakallio, V. (2006). First births. A comparative study of the patterns of transition to parenthood in Europe. In J. Bradshaw & A. Hatland (Eds.), *Social policy, employment and family change in comparative perspective* (pp. 161–177). New York: Edward Elgar.

Frones, I. (2007). Theorizing indicators. *Social Indicators Research, 83*(1), 5–23.

Funk, J., Hagan, J. & Schimming, J (1999) "Children and electronic games: A comparison of parents' and children's perceptions of children's habits and preferences in a United States sample" *Psychological Reports, 85*(3), 883–888.

Goerge, R. M. (1997). The use of administrative data in measuring the state of children. In A. Ben-Arieh & H. Wintersberger (Eds.), *Monitoring and measuring the state of children: Beyond survival. Eurosocial Report No. 62* (pp. 277–286). Vienna: European Centre for Social Welfare Policy and Research.

Gottlieb, D. & Bronstein, P. (1996). Parent's perceptions of children's worries in a changing world. *Journal of Genetic Psychology, 157*(1), 104–118.

Hauser, R. M., Brown, B. V., & Prosser, W. R. (Eds.) (1997). *Indicators of children's well-being*. New York: Russell Sage Foundation.

Hubner, E. S. (1997). Life satisfaction and happiness. In G. G. Bear, K. M. Minke, & A. Thomas (Eds.), *Children's needs II: Development, problems, and alternatives* (pp. 271–278). Bethesda, MD: National Association of School Psychologists.

Hubner, E. S. (2004). Research on assessment of life satisfaction of children and adolescents. *Social Indicators Research, 66*, 3–33.

Jensen, A. M., & Saporiti, A. (1992). *Do children count?* Vienna: European Centre for Social Welfare Policy and Research.

Kamerman, S. B., & Kahn, A. (Eds.) (1978). *Family policy: Government and families in fourteen countries*. New York: Columbia University Press.

Land, K. (2000). Social indicators. In E. F. Borgatta & R. V. Montgomery (Eds.), *Encyclopedia of sociology, revised edition* (pp. 2682–2690). New York: Macmillan.

Land, K., Lamb, V. L., & Mustillo, S. K. (2001). Child and youth well-being in the United States, 1975–1998: Some findings from a new index. *Social Indicators Research, 56*, 241–320.

Lee, B. J. (1997). The use of census and surveys: Implications for developing childhood social indicator models. In A. Ben-Arieh & H. Wintersberger (Eds.), *Monitoring and measuring the state of children: Beyond survival. Eurosocial Report No. 62* (pp. 301–308). Vienna: European Centre for Social Welfare Policy and Research.

Lippman, L. (2004). *Indicators of child, family and community connections.* Washington, DC: Office of the Assistant Secretary for Planning and Evaluation, US Department of Health and Human Services.

Lippman, L. (2007). Indicators and indices of child well-being: A brief American history. *Social Indicators Research, 83*(1), 39–53.

Lohan, J. A., & Murphy, S. A. (2001). Parents' perceptions of adolescent sibling grief responses after an adolescent or young adult child's sudden, violent death. *Omega-Journal of Death and Dying, 44*(3), 195–213.

Mareš, J. (2006). *Kvalita života u dětí a dospívajících I.* Brno: MSD.

Melton, G., & Limber, S. (1992). What children's rights mean to children: Children's own views. In M. Freeman & P. Veerman (Eds.), *The ideologies of children's rights* (pp. 167–187). Dordrecht: Martinus Nijhoff.

Moore, K. A., Lippman, L., & Brown, B. (2004). Indicators of child well-being: The promise for positive youth development. *ANNALS, AAPSS, 591*, 125–145.

Moore, K. A., Vandivere, S., Lippman, L., McPhee, C., & Bloch, M. (2007). An index of the condition of children: The ideal and a less-than-ideal U.S. example. *Social Indicators Research, 84*, 291–331.

Ohannessian, C. M., Lerner, R. M., Lerner, J. V., & Voneye, A. (1995). Discrepancies in adolescents and parents perceptions of family functioning and adolescent emotional adjustment. *Journal of Early Adolescence, 15*(4), 490–516.

O'Hare, W. P., & Bramstedt, N. L. (2003). *Assessing the KIDS COUNT composite index: A Kids Count working paper.* Baltimore, MD: Annie E. Casey Foundation.

Olk, T. (2004). German children's welfare between economy and ideology. In A. M. Jensen, A. Ben-Arieh, C. Conti, D. Kutsar, M. N. G. Phádraig, & H. W. Nielsen (Eds.), *Children's welfare in an ageing Europe* (Vol. 2). Oslo: Norwegian Centre for Child Research.

Olk, T. (2006). Welfare states and generational order. In H. Wintersberger, L. Alanen, T. Olk, & J. Ovortrup (Eds.), *Childhood, generational order and the welfare state. Exploring children's social and economic welfare* (pp. 59–90). Odense: University of Southern Denmark Press.

Pittman, K., & Irby, M. (1997). Promoting investment in life skills for youth: Beyond indicators for survival and problem prevention. In A. Ben-Arieh & H. Wintersberger (Eds.), *Monitoring and measuring the state of children: Beyond survival. Eurosocial Report No. 62* (pp. 239–246). Vienna: European Centre for Social Welfare Policy and Research.

Prout, A. (1997). Objective vs. subjective indicators or both? Whose perspective counts? In A. Ben-Arieh & H. Wintersberger (Eds.), *Monitoring and measuring the state of children: Beyond survival. Eurosocial Report No. 62* (pp. 89–100). Vienna: European Centre for Social Welfare Policy and Research.

Qvortrup, J. (1999). The meaning of child's standard of living. In A. B. Andrews & N. H. Kaufman (Eds.), *Implementing the U.N. convention on the rights of the child: A standard of living adequate for development.* Westport, CT: Praeger.

Resnick, M. (1995). *Discussant's comments: Indicators of children's well-being. Conference papers* (Vol. 2). Madison: University of Wisconsin-Madison, Institute for Research on Poverty, Special Report Series.

Santos Pais, M. (1999). *A human rights conceptual framework for UNICEF. UNICEF Innocenti Essay 9.* Florence, Italy: UNICEF Innocenti Research Centre.

Sauli, H. (1997). Using databases for monitoring the socioeconomic state of children. In A. Ben-Arieh & H. Wintersberger (Eds.), *Monitoring and measuring the state of children: Beyond survival. Eurosocial Report No. 62* (pp. 287–299). Vienna: European Centre for Social Welfare Policy and Research.

Sen, A. (1997). *On economic inequality.* Oxford: Oxford University Press.

Shek, D. T. L. (1998). A longitudinal study of Hong Kong adolescents' and parents' perceptions of family functioning and well-being. *Journal of Genetic Psychology, 159*(4), 389–403.

Stevens, K., Dickson, M., Poland, M., & Prasad, R. (2005). *Focus on families: Reinforcing the importance of family. Families with dependent children – Successful outcomes project. Report on literature review and focus groups.* Wellington, New Zealand: Families Commission. Available at http://www.familiescommission.govt.nz/download/focus-on-families.pdf

Sweeting, H. (2001). Our family, whose perspective? An investigation of children's family life and health. *Journal of Adolescence, 24*(2), 229–250.

Titler, J., & Ben-Arieh, A. (2006). So where should the research go? Some possible directions and their research implications. In A. Ben-Arieh & R. Goerge (Eds.), *Indicators of children's well-being: Understanding their role, usage and policy influence.* Dordrecht, Netherlands: Springer.

UNICEF. (2007). *Child poverty in perspective: An overview of child well-being in rich countries. Innocenti Report Card 7.* Florence, Italy: UNICEF Innocenti Research Center.

Part II
Child Welfare

An Historical Perspective on Child Welfare

Brenda G. McGowan

The field of child welfare has changed dramatically in the United States over the years. There are multiple reasons for this transformation. Some directly reflect changing concepts of childhood, historic debates regarding the importance of child saving versus family preservation, and differing views about public responsibility for children. Other reasons derive from changes in the larger society including the size and composition of the child population, growth in the economy, and alternating views of the powers and responsibilities of different levels of government.

This chapter will present an overview of the development of child welfare services in the United States over time. It will examine the ways that concepts of children's rights and needs have evolved, the impact of increased understanding of child development on service provision, the administrative and legislative provisions introduced to meet changing family and children's needs, and many of the factors that have blocked attainment of these policy objectives.

1 The Early Years

There were no organized services for children during the 17th and 18th centuries. The family was the basic economic unit in the Colonial era, and children who lived beyond 4–5 years were expected to contribute to the work of the family. Most of the types of problems we would later come to view as child welfare problems, if they arose at all, were assumed to be the responsibility of extended family or voluntary associations and local towns and communities.

B.G. McGowan (✉)
School of Social Work, Columbia University, New York, USA

Portions of this chapter were published previously in "Historical Evolution of Child Welfare Services" by B.G. McGowan published in *Child Welfare: Current Dilemmas, Future Directions.* B.G. McGowan and W. Meezan, eds., Peacock Publishers, 1983; and *Child Welfare for the Twenty-First Century.* G.P. Mallon and P.M. Hess, eds., Columbia University Press, 2005.

Social provisions for the two groups of children that were expected to require attention from public authorities, orphans and children of paupers, derived from the English Poor Law tradition. These children were generally handled in one of four ways: outdoor relief, farming-out, almshouses, or indenture. Some dependent children were cared for through informal arrangements organized by relatives, neighbors, and church groups. Also, a few orphanages for children were established during this early period, the first founded by the Ursuline Convent in New Orleans in 1727. However, dependent young children were most commonly placed in public almshouses until they reached the age of eight or nine and then they were indentured until they reached majority.

In sum, during the first two centuries the provisions for dependent children were meager local arrangements made to insure that children received a minimum level of subsistence and a religious upbringing and that they were taught the values of industriousness and hard work. As Hillary Rodham [Clinton] commented:

> In the eighteenth century, ... the term children's rights would have been a *non sequiter*. Children were regarded as chattels of the family and wards of the state, with no recognized political character or power and few legal rights. (Rodham, 1973).

2 Increasing State Responsibility for Children: The Nineteenth Century

During the 19th century large-scale social changes led to significant improvements in the country's social provisions for different groups of children. The importation of large numbers of slaves reduced the number of requests for indentured white children, and the eventual abolition of slavery created opposition to the very concept of indenture. The Industrial Revolution and the emergence of a bourgeois class in which the labor of children and women was not required at home led to a focus on the developmental and educational needs of young children. Major economic growth freed funds for the development of private philanthropies. Massive waves of immigrants created large pools of needy Catholic and Jewish children. And new industries led to more dangerous labor from parents and youth and new environmental hazards for low income families.

The 19th century witnessed increased assumption of state responsibility for dependent children. Two early reports, the Yates Report issued by the New York secretary of state and one issued by the Massachusetts Committee on Pauper Laws, documented the evils of outdoor relief and indenture for children and concluded that dependent children were best cared for in almshouses. A major expansion of almshouse care followed the publication of these reports, but the potential harms to children posed by confining them with all classes of dependent adults were not foreseen. By mid-century investigating committees in many states had concluded that the conditions in these almshouses were wretched for children and were calling for special facilities under public or private auspices for young children. As a New York State Senate Select Committee noted in its report on the state almshouses, these are "the worst possible nurseries, contributing to an annual accession to our population of three hundred infants, whose present destiny is to pass their most impressible years in the midst of such vicious associations as will stamp them for a life of future infamy and crime" (New York State Senate, 1857. Cited in Bremner, 1970 , pp. 648–649).

There was a dramatic increase in the number of institutions for orphans and dependent children established, some following, and some even prior to, the issuance of these reports. Although commonly called orphanages, these facilities were designed not only for orphans, but also for all children whose parents were unable to provide adequate care. Black children not sold as slaves were excluded from most of the private orphanages, but several separate facilities were established for these children, the first of which was the Philadelphia Association for the Care of Colored Children established by the Society of Friends in 1922 (Billingsley & Giovanni, 1972).

2.1 Free Foster Home Movement

Public recognition of the poor conditions for children in almshouses also led to another, very significant reform effort, the free foster home movement. In 1853 Charles Loring Brace organized the Children's Aid Society, and by the end of the century Children's Aid Societies were established in most of the major cities in the Eastern part of the country. Brace was convinced that the best way to save poor children from the evils of the City was to place them in Christian homes in the country. He assumed that these homes could provide the children solid moral training and teach good work habits. Hence he recruited large numbers of free foster homes in the Midwest and upper New York State and sent trainloads of children to these locations. By 1879 Children's Aid Society had sent approximately 40,000 destitute and homeless children to homes in the country (Bremner, 1970–74).

A parallel development was the Children's Home Society movement. These statewide child-placing agencies, organized under Protestant auspices, were also designed to provide free foster homes for children. First founded by Martin Van Buren Van Ardsale in Illinois in 1883, this program spread rapidly. By 1916 there were 36 Children's Home Societies in Midwestern and Southern states (Thurston, 1930).

The free foster home movement was a major reform and led to the foster care model of care so prevalent for dependent children today. However, it was not without its critics for two reasons. First, although foster care was conceptually different from indenture, in practice foster children were often expected to pay for their bread and board through free labor. Investigations of the foster families were minimal so many reports were made about children receiving poor treatment. Second, no provision was or could be made to insure children received instruction in their own religion. This caused some Roman Catholic and Jewish leaders to oppose the movement because they thought the children placed in Protestant homes were likely to lose their religious foundation. This concern led to the establishment of separate child care institutions for Roman Catholic and Jewish children and later debates about the relative advantages of foster home versus institutional care (Wolins & Piliavin, 1964).

Paralleling the reforms in service provision for dependent children were changes in the administration of services. The states gradually began to assume responsibility for administering and funding the service provisions for children originally adminis-tered by voluntary organizations and local towns and communities. Different states adopted distinct models of administration with different balance between foster home and institutional care, different allocation of responsibility between state, county, and local government, and different degrees of reliance on voluntary versus public programs.

2.2 Early Child Protective Services

The earliest child protective services were started in the 19th century. The legal prin-ciple of *parens patriae*, derived from its use in England to justify state intervention in the family, was used to authorize government intervention to protect children. In the Colonial era the responsibility of local government to protect dependent and neglected children was recognized, and various laws were passed acknowledging this responsibility in principle, but no laws authorizing the right of the state to remove children for protective reasons were passed until the early 19th century (Pecora, Whittaker, Maluccio, & Barth, 2000).

Widespread attention to the problem of child abuse was first drawn in 1874 with publicity surrounding the case of a child named Mary Ellen Wilson and the subse-quent founding of the New York Society for the Prevention of Cruelty to Children. A mission worker visiting in the child's neighborhood was horrified when she saw the conditions in which this child was living. After seeking help to no avail from the police department and a children's organization, she contacted Henry Bergh, founder of the Society for the Prevention of Cruelty to Animals. He sought written testimony from the mission worker and contacted an attorney, Elbridge Gerry, who brought the case to court under an obscure doctrine of habeas corpus. After Mary Ellen was removed from the home and her caretaker was sentenced, Bergh and Gerry worked to establish the New York Society for the Prevention of Cruelty to Children in 1875 (Jalongo, 2008). In its first year of operation the Society estab-lished a telephone link with the police department, received authorization to act on behalf of the state attorney general and the county district attorney, and investigated several hundred complaints, prosecuted 68 criminal cases, and rescued 72 abused and neglected children (http://www.nyspcc.org/beta_history/nyspcc_story.html "The NYSPPCC Story." retrieved 10/25/08).

Similar societies were quickly established in other parts of the country. By 1900 there were more than 250 such societies (Bremner, 1970–74). Newspaper accounts of the early meetings of these agencies indicate that the founders saw their primary mission as prosecuting parents, not providing direct services to children or parents. Yet, in recognition of the many harmful conditions in which children were living, the NYSPCC and other societies began to sponsor a number of laws designed to protect children from all forms of neglect and exploitation, not merely the prevention of abuse in children's own homes.

2.3 Provisions for Delinquent Youth

There are interesting parallels and differences in the way American society cared historically for delinquent youth and dependent and neglected children. Under English common law tradition, children over the age of seven who committed criminal offenses were treated the same way as adults and subject to harsh cruel punishments such as whipping, banishment, and even death. The early colonies adopted similar procedures and continued to use various types of severe corporal for children until the 18th century when the concept of confinement was introduced. By the beginning of the 19th century, many juvenile offenders were confined in almshouses with adults and dependent children. This practice ultimately led to public pressure to create special public facilities for delinquent youth, and many of these were established, all of which emphasized strict discipline and hard work. Some of these facilities, often termed reform schools, were experimental in nature, designed to aid in the reformation of troubled youth. Yet they all had to derive much of their income from the contracted labor of the youths, which frequently resulted in corruption, exploitation and brutal treatment of the inmates. As a leading juvenile authority of the time commented:

> While flogging had long been abolished in the Navy and the use of the "cat" in the state prisons, it is still thought necessary in order to realize a fair pecuniary return from the children's labor, for the contractor to inflict severe corporal punishment for deficiency in imposed tasks. (Letchworth, 1882. Cited in Bremner, 1970–74, p. 291).

There were many investigations and exposes of the conditions in these reform schools, and gradually voluntary community-based methods such as probation were developed for delinquent youth. Then the first juvenile court was established in Illinois in 1899. The concept of the juvenile court spread quickly throughout the country and had a major impact on the development of children's services in the 20th century. These are non-criminal courts derived from the English chancery courts that exercise the privilege of the state as *parens patriae* and do not require rigid rules of evidence to permit state intervention in children's lives (Bremner, 1970–74, pp. 440–441; See also Abbott, 1938, pp. 331–332). Although originally designed to rule on youth offenders, they gradually assumed a significant role in the processing of dependent, neglected and abused children.

3 Late Nineteenth Century: Progressive Era Influences

Until the latter part of the 19th century state intervention in a child's life usually occurred only when it was perceived that the child threatened the social order because she or he lacked proper family and religious upbringing and/or had committed delinquent acts. Two developments of the last quarter of the century, the Charity Organization Society and the settlement house movement, greatly expanded services for children and families. Though their friendly visitors, the Charity Organization Societies sought out poor families to certify them as worthy of help and to provide role modeling, advice, and moral instruction. Although they ministered to families on a case by case basis, they gradually came to the recognition that poverty was often the result of social forces outside the individual's control and began to focus on these social forces as well.

This recognition merged with the philosophy underlying the settlement house movement, a middle class movement designed to humanize the cities. The early settlers placed a strong emphasis on investigating and addressing poor social conditions. For example, some of the leaders of this movement were the prime movers behind the establishment of the juvenile court and laws against child labor. They also provided a range of developmental services for children and parents such as day care, language classes, playgrounds, and family life education. Thus by the end of the century, services had been expanded to protect children and to provide for some of their needs within their own homes and communities.

At the same time states had begun to introduce policies and procedures for licensing and regulating residential child care facilities. Participants at the National Conference of Charities and Corrections in the 1890s highlighted the importance of state supervision of child care institutions.

As Grace Abbott wrote:

> It was pointed out that the state should know where its dependent children are, its agents should visit and inspect institutions and agencies at regular intervals—including local public as well as all private agencies—and both should be required to make full reports to the State. (Abbott, 1938, pp. 17–18).

The developments at the end of the 19th century set the stage for what would become the hallmarks of the child welfare field during the 20th century: Bureaucratization, professionalization and expanded state intervention in the lives of children. Bremner commented:

> As the state intervened more frequently and effectively in the relations between parent and child in order to protect children against parental mismanagement, the state also forced children to conform to public norms of behavior and obligation. Thus the child did not escape control; rather he experienced a partial exchange of masters in which the ignorance, neglect, and exploitation of some parents were replaced by presumably fair and uniform treatment at the hands of public authorities and agencies. The transfer of responsibilities required an elaboration of administration and judicial techniques of investigation, decision, and supervision. (Bremner, 1970–74, p. 117).

3.1 White House Conference on Children

The first major event of the 20th century influencing child welfare services was the White House Conference on Children in 1909. The delegates, reflecting the sentiments of the Progressive Era, went on record as supporting the following principle:

> Home life is the highest and finest product of civilization . . . Children should not be deprived of it except for urgent and compelling reasons. Children of parents of working character, suffering from temporary misfortune, and children of reasonably efficient and deserving mothers who are without the support of the normal breadwinners should as a rule be kept with their parents, such aid being given as may be necessary to maintain suitable homes for the rearing of the children.

Mother's Pensions and other types of programs providing public aid to children were established, first in 1911 in Illinois as Funds for Parents and in 20 other states within the next two years (Abbott, 1938, pp. 164–166). Unfortunately, the acts authorizing these funds faced some opposition as potentially harmful to the welfare of children, and the funds were very limited and provided on a restricted, somewhat arbitrary basis. Therefore, they did little to fully implement the aspirations enunciated at the White House Conference, but the principle set forth set a framework for future directions in the field.

3.2 U.S. Children's Bureau

The U.S. Children's Bureau was established in 1912 as a consequence of intense lobbying by leaders of the settlement house movement, child labor and women's groups, voluntary service agencies, and the state boards of charities and corrections. It was given little initial funding, but a very broad mandate to "investigate and report . . . upon all matters pertaining to the welfare of children and child life among all classes of our people . . . ." (U.S. Statutes at Large, 37, 1912. Cited in Parker & Carpenter, 1981). The establishment of the Bureau demonstrated for the first time Congressional recognition that the federal government has a responsibility for the welfare of children. The first leader of the Children's Bureau, Julia Lathrop, provided skilled leadership, gained widespread public support and greatly expanded its budget and range of activities.

The initial bill establishing the Bureau was opposed by some who feared federal intrusion into states' rights. And the Sheppard-Towner Act of 1921, which gave the Bureau responsibility for administering grants-in-aid to the states for maternal and child health programs, was vehemently opposed by some who again feared violation of states' rights and intrusion on family privacy. Despite periodic attacks, the Children's Bureau served as the primary federal agency representing interests of children for many years. Program emphasis evolved over time as the leaders changed from those concerned with broad social issues to ones more focused on issues and problems in child health and child welfare. However, it continued to carry out its primary functions of investigation, advocacy, public education, research, and standard-setting until it was reorganized as a subdivision of the U.S. Department of health, Education, and Welfare in 1969 and lost its leadership role.

4 Developments of the Early Twentieth Century

During the first three decades of the 20th century, there were a number of administrative changes that built on the actions of the late 19th century. More state departments were established for the delivery of child welfare services, some shifted to county-based systems of care away from the earlier local town or city based systems, and the states began to assume more responsibility for standard-setting, licensing, and regulation of public and voluntary child care facilities. Significant progress was made in establishing civil service standards for the hiring and promotion of personnel in public child welfare positions. Two major national voluntary organizations devoted to research, standard-setting, agency accreditation, and knowledge dissemination were established during this period: American Association for Organizing Family Social Work (later the Family Service Association of America and now Family Service America) in 1919; and the Child Welfare League of America in 1920. And the long notable history of child welfare research was initiated with the publication in 1924 of Sophie Van Theis' outcome study of 910 children placed in foster care in New York.

Juvenile court activities expanded during this period. By 1919 all but three states had passed juvenile court legislation, and the jurisdiction of the court had been expanded in many locations (Abbott, 1938, pp. 614–620). The first court clinic was established in Chicago in 1909, and the child guidance movement was initiated a few years later with the founding of the Judge Baker Clinic in Boston. Protective services for children also expanded during this period, moving away from the earlier focus on prosecution of parents to emphasis on services to children and parents in their own homes.

The debate over the relative merits of foster homes versus institutions continued into the 1920s (Bremner, 1970–74, p. 247), but both continued to expand. The one very new service initiated during this period was adoption as a child welfare service. Informal adoptions had occurred since the colonial era. Laws providing for the transfer of parental rights from biological parents to adoptive parents were passed in the mid-19th century, but recognition of the importance of protecting the interests of children in these transactions did not develop until the early 20th century. Minnesota passed the first law in 1917 requiring that judges refer all non-relative adoption cases to a voluntary or public welfare agency for investigation prior to approval of the adoption petition (Abbott, 1938, pp. 34–36).

4.1 Provisions for Black Children

Because black children were often excluded from the child welfare services developed for white children in the late 19th and early 20th century, the black community had to develop a whole separate system of care for dependent children. This was done through a variety of informal arrangements, as well as orphanages, old folks and children's homes, and day nurseries (Billingsley & Giovanni, 1972, p. 51). The National Urban League established in 1910 took a very active advocacy role in pushing for equitable distribution of child welfare services; and the massive migration of blacks to urban areas after World War I forced increased recognition of the needs of black children. Also greater openness to black children developed in the traditional child welfare system as the number of public facilities increased (Billingsley & Giovanni, 1972, pp. 74–75). Thus, by 1930 the participants at the White House Conference were able argue that black children should be entitled to the same standards of care as white children and should be served through the existing child welfare system (Billingsley & Giovanni, 1972, pp. 74–76).

4.2 Social Security Law

The early 20th century trends in child welfare had a definite impact on the scope and nature of programs developed to help American families cope with the problems they experienced in the aftermath of the Depression of 1929. It has often been suggested that the first days of the Roosevelt administration in 1933 changed the entire social fabric of the country by redefining the role of the federal government in addressing social welfare problems. Certainly, the Social Security Act of 1935 had a major impact on the structure and financing of child welfare services. Two components of this law, both of which stemmed from recommendations of the Children's Bureau, had a major impact on the subsequent development of child welfare services.

Title IV, Grants to States for Aid to Dependent Children, of the Social Security Law sought to extend the concept of mothers' pensions by providing federal matching funds for grants to fatherless families; requiring a single state agency to administer the program; and mandating coverage of all political subdivisions in each state. It was designed as a federal grant-in-aid program and permitted state autonomy in setting eligibility standards, determining payment levels, and developing administrative and operational procedures. (The program, later named Aid to Families of Dependent Children (AFDC), was eventually extended to families with a permanently and totally disabled parent, and, at state option, to families with an unemployed parent).

The other major component of the Social Security Act affecting the provision of child welfare services was Title V, Part 3, Child Welfare Services. This program was designed not only to help children in their own families, but also to benefit those in substitute care by ". . . enabling the United States, through the Children's Bureau, to cooperate with State public welfare agencies in establishing, extending, and strengthening, especially in predominantly rural areas, public welfare services . . . for the protection and care of homeless, dependent, and neglected children, and children in danger of becoming delinquent . . ." (Title V, Part 3, Social Security Act. Cited in Bremner, 1970–74, p. 615). Although the funding for this program was quite modest, states quickly took advantage of this relatively permissive legislation to obtain federal funding for child welfare services.

5 Post World War II Era: Expansion of Services

The time from the late 30s to the late 50s was a period of relative consolidation and growth for the field. The Children's Bureau and the Child Welfare League of America both made major progress in setting and monitoring standards for service provision. Many states expanded professional educational opportunities for child welfare staff. The total number and rate of children placed in foster home and institutional care declined (Low, 1966, Cited in Bremner, 1970–74) while the proportion of children receiving services in their own homes, the total public expenditures for child welfare, and the total number of professional staff in public child welfare increased significantly during this period (Richan, 1978).

One change in the nature of service provision during this period was that many voluntary agencies established special programs for unmarried mothers and for adoption of infants. The other important change was a marked shift in the types of institutional care provided to dependent youth, as many of the traditional child care facilities began to be converted into various types of residential treatment centers. To illustrate, in 1950, 45% of the white children in residential care were in institutions for dependent children, and 25% were in institutions for the mentally disabled. By 1960 only 29% were in child care institutions, and 36% were in facilities for the mentally disabled. Although the distribution of nonwhite children showed a similar trend, in 1960 over half of the nonwhite children (54%) were confined in correctional facilities compared to only 25% of the white children (Low, 1965. Cited in Billingsley & Giovanni, 1972). This suggests that the trend toward individualized treatment planning was not strong enough to counter patterns of racially discriminatory treatment.

Several important studies published in the 1950s regarding the needs of "multiproblem," "disorganized," and "hard-to-reach" families served primarily to stimulate experimentation with different types of clinical services, not any examination of the structure of services (See, for example, Buell, 1952; Geisman & Ayers, 1958; New York City Youth Board, 1958). The field at that time was relatively small, and quality and coverage, uneven. Tight system boundaries made it difficult for many children and families to gain access to service, while it was difficult for others to be discharged from care. Some of the voluntary agencies provided intensive high quality, specialized services while many public agencies struggled to provide minimum care and protection. Services were geared almost entirely toward placement, and individual casework was the primary service modality. But the publication of a study by Maas & Engler (1959), *Children in Need of Parents*, ultimately forced an examination of the structure and focus of child welfare services. This study of children in foster care in nine communities posed many of the questions raised repeatedly since that time about children in "limbo," children who had drifted into foster care, had no permanent family ties, and were not being prepared for adoptive placement.

6 The 1960s and 1970s

The inauguration of the Kennedy administration in 1961 ushered in an era of tremendous social ferment and change. To recap briefly, the 1960s witnessed the rediscovery of poverty as a public issue; the War on Poverty under the Johnson administration; the expansion of the civil rights movement, leading to the passage of the 1964 Civil Rights Act; the emergence of the concept of black power and the racial conflicts of the late 1960s; the development of the welfare rights movement and the establishment of other related types of clients' rights groups; the burgeoning of a youth culture that symbolized many challenges to traditional American values and mores; and the perpetuation of an unpopular war in Vietnam that contributed to the growing distrust and alienation of large segments of the population from governmental institutions.

In this context of social reform several advisory committees and task forces composed of leading social welfare experts and policymakers in the Kennedy administration were formed to study public welfare policy and consider needed changes in public assistance and social service programs. The 1961, 1962 and 1967 amendments to the Social Security Act reflected the recommendations of these advisory bodies, particularly in relation to the expansion of provisions for public social services.

6.1 AFDC-Foster Care

The 1961 Amendment, called AFDC-Foster Care, was initiated to address a problem that had arisen in Louisiana after the state passed a "suitable home law" saying that children in homes where there was an illegitimate birth would no longer be entitled to AFDC (then called ADC). The burden of this state law fell very disproportionately on black children so a wide range of advocacy groups mobilized to fight the way Louisiana was implementing this law. Eventually, the Secretary of the Department of Health, Education and Welfare issued a new ruling stating that if a child were judged to be living in an "unsuitable home", the state had an obligation to improve the conditions at home and maintain AFDC payments or to remove the child from the home. This ruling and the Congressional amendment that quickly followed gave increased support to the view that children are entitled to protective services from the state and that families receiving welfare should receive social services (Lindhorst & Leighniger, 2003). Moreover, the law authorized use of AFDC funds for the costs of foster care for AFDC-eligible children removed from their homes because of a judicial determination of need. Although this amendment received little public notice at the time of its original passage, it may have done more than any subsequent legislation to increase the number of children entering foster care because it is the only open-ended federal funding for child welfare services.

6.2 1962 and 1967 Amendments to the Social Security Law

The 1962 Amendment to the Social Security Law provided 75–25% federal matching funds for state/local expenditures for social services for current, former, and potential welfare recipients. The 1967 Amendments replaced the original Title V with Title IVB, Child Welfare Services Program, and authorized the use of Title IVA funds for purchase of service from voluntary agencies. These Amendments set a policy framework for subsequent developments in this field.

The clear intention of the social welfare leaders involved in the deliberations around the 1962 and 1967 amendments was to develop a comprehensive public service system that would meet the service needs of low-income families, diminish the dysfunctional separation between child welfare and family service programs, and insure children in families on AFDC the services and benefits available to children in foster care. It was hoped that the development of comprehensive public social services for families and children would help to alleviate many service delivery problems and inequities.

Unfortunately, this goal was doomed because of the unrealistic expectations, conflicting objectives, hopes, and fears that quickly developed among advocates and skeptics alike around the concept of expanded public social services. Social welfare leaders failed to anticipate the degree to which legislative intent and rational social planning could be undermined by restrictive federal and state administrative regulations; political and bureaucratic constraints; and the intransigence of established interest groups in the family and children's service field. Political and civic leaders supported the concept of expanded social services on the assumption that they would help to reduce welfare rolls. They were then sorely disillusioned when welfare costs continued to multiply as a consequence of changing demographic patterns, relaxed eligibility requirements, and increased "take-up" among potential AFDC recipients.

Direct service providers and consumers were led to believe that the expansion of public funding would enhance the quality and quantity of service provision, and they were frequently frustrated, often enraged, when these expectations were not fulfilled. Civil rights and consumer groups, concerned about the potential for social control and invasion of privacy inherent in any effort to tie public assistance to service provision, became increasingly wary of efforts to expand state intervention in family life. And welfare rights activists and leaders of the War on Poverty, committed to the concept of maximum feasible participation of the poor, disparaged the so-called service strategy as a naïve attempt to solve the problems of poverty via the provision of casework services (Wickenden, 1976).

Despite the ambivalence about the potential costs and benefits inherent in an expanded public social service delivery system, federal and state funding for social services expanded rapidly, especially after passage of the 1967 Amendment permitting purchase of service from voluntary agencies, and expectations rose. Many child welfare agencies attempted to respond to the opportunities posed by this changing perception of public family service by expanding their range of service provision, initiating demonstration projects, developing more specialized child care facilities, and expanding staff training.

6.3 New Expectations and Demands

At this same time the child welfare field was confronted with new demands and expectations from various client groups. Foster parent and adoptive parent groups began to organize, demanding more equitable treatment and expanded programs for adoptive and foster care children with "special needs." The movement toward deinstitutionalization for youngsters in correctional facilities, psychiatric hospitals and school for retarded children created whole new pools of children that child welfare agencies were expected to serve. The emergence of the child advocacy movement in the late 60s created pressure for child welfare workers to engage in social action aimed at improving the quality of services and resources provided by all types of child-serving organizations. And legal rights groups concerned about parents' and children's rights began to challenge policies and procedures regarding movement of children in and out of placement and the quality and accessibility of substitute care arrangements. As these pressures on the field were increasing, the Children's Bureau, the only federal agency with an established record of commitment to improving child welfare services, was decimated by the reorganization of the Department of Health, Education and Welfare in 1969.

The social context shifted again somewhat in the 1970s. Self-help and advocacy groups representing a wide range of interest groups began to organize to demand their rights. Calls for affirmative action and equal treatment for women and minorities replaced the push for civil rights and equal opportunity. Concern was growing about the national economy due to rampant inflation and unemployment. "Middle America" began to react. The Nixon Administration ushered in the era of new federalism. And in 1972 Congress imposed a $2.5 billion ceiling on funding for social services.

Title XX of the Social Security Act was passed in 1975, redefining historical concepts regarding the appropriate objectives, decision-making responsibility, organizational and funding patterns of social services in this country. It also significantly expanded eligibility for publicly funded social services by providing for more families above the poverty line. The components of this act that impacted most directly on the child welfare field were the assignment to the states of greater responsibility for service planning and program development; a reduction in the range of federal regulations governing service provision; a mandate for increased public participation in assessment of service needs; and diminished provisions for categorical programs for special populations at risk. Perhaps more significant, as Austin commented on the implications of Title XX: "The financing, regulation, and management of human services has become a major domestic policy issue in the United States" (Austin, 1980, p. 19). This development had enormous implications for child welfare because it placed on the public agenda the question of appropriate responsibility for the care of dependent and neglected children.

In the l970s child welfare agencies started to be attacked for their failure to keep children out of placement, minimize costs while maintaining appropriate resources for children who must be placed in temporary substitute care, and move children back into their own families or into permanent adoptive homes as quickly as possible (See, for example, Fanshel & Shinn, 1978; Bernstein, Snider & Meezan, 1975; Strauss, 1977; Knitzer, Allen, & McGowan, 1978; Persico, 1979). The tenor of these critiques built on the research Maas and Engler published in 1959 regarding the problems of children in limbo.

Efforts to reform the delivery of child welfare services during this period were directed primarily toward revising the statutory base governing state intervention in family life and increasing the requirements for public accountability of service providers. For example, by 1977 twenty states plus the District of Columbia had instituted some type of formal judicial, court-administered, or citizen review (Chappell & Hevener, 1977). Many others followed, and the trend toward developing increasingly complex systems for internal case monitoring and program review became virtually universal.

6.4 Introduction of Permanency Planning

Three other developments of the late 1970s also contributed to the major shift in child welfare policy that occurred in 1980. One was a new focus on the concept of permanency planning. This was precipitated not only by the theoretical writings of J. Goldstein, Solnit, Goldstein, & Freud, (1973, 1979) on the concept of psychological parenting, but also by the reports of successful demonstration projects designed to prevent placement and/or promote permanence for children in foster care through reunification or adoption (Jones et al., 1976; Burt & Balyeat, 1974; Maybanks & Bryce, 1979; Pike, 1976; Emlen, L'Ahti, & Downs, 1978). A second important development was passage of the Indian Child Welfare Act of 1978. Congress enacted this law in response to concerns raised about the high proportion of Indian American children removed from their families and placed in foster homes, institutions and adoptive homes outside the Native American communities. The law specified that all court hearings involving Native American children must be held in tribal courts and that tribes have a right to participate in state court hearings. The Indian Child Welfare Grant program was established with specific guidelines for placement and family reunification. Another significant development was a series of Senate subcommittee hearings focused first on issues of adoption, and later, on broader foster care issues (Allen & Knitzer, 1983, p. 119).

6.5 Child Abuse Prevention and Treatment Act of 1974

Two of the major laws that continue to direct child welfare services today were passed in this era. The first, the Child Abuse Prevention and Treatment Act of 1974 (P.L. 93-247), grew out of extensive publicity about the "the battered child syndrome" aroused by an article in the *Journal of the American Medical Association* in 1962. Although the country had long had protective services for children, this was the first time widespread public and professional attention was drawn to the problem. In the mid-60s a number of states passed mandatory reporting laws, but P.L. 93-247 represented the first federal recognition of this problem. The law itself provided a small amount of funding to states for research and demonstration projects, but it stipulated that in order to qualify for funding, the states had to pass laws requiring mandatory reporting of suspected and known cases of maltreatment, and confidentiality and immunity for reporters. All of the states quickly passed such legislation. However, the law did not clearly define child abuse or neglect. This lack of a clear operational definition has created numerous problems over time for clients, social workers, and judges as interpretations of the law have varied across time, geographic areas, and personnel. Although the law has consistently been funded at low levels and has focused almost entirely on child abuse reporting, not prevention, it has served to focus enormous public attention on the problems of child abuse and neglect.

6.6 Adoption Assistance and Child Welfare Act of 1980

The other important child welfare legislation growing out of the issues raised in the 1970s was the Adoption Assistance and Child Welfare Reform Act of 1980, P.L. 96-272. This act essentially reversed the trend toward a diminished role for the federal government in the funding and structuring of social services and addressed directly many of the problems research had documented in the child welfare system. The act introduced the concept of permanency planning as the primary objective of child welfare policy, mandating a series of mechanisms designed to redirect funds from foster care to prevention and adoption services. It adopted what Allen & Knitzer (1983) termed a carrot and stick approach by creating new Title IVB funds for preventive services, setting a cap on funding for foster care that was to become effective once the funding for IVB reached specified levels, and providing open-ended funding for adoption subsidies for children defined as "hard to place." In addition, PL 96-272 mandated that states make "reasonable efforts" to prevent foster placements, provide due process for all parties involved in such placements, and require placement for children in "the least detrimental alternative." Other components of the law were directed at increasing state planning and accountability by requiring state inventories of all children in placement longer than 6 months; the development of state plans for foster care and adoption services; routine collection of aggregate and case data to monitor implementation of these plans; and individual case reviews of all children in placement longer than 6 months and judicial review after 18 months. No effort was made to address the inherent conflicts between the provisions of this law and those of the Child Abuse Prevention and Treatment Act of 1974.

7 1980s–1990s: Reducing Expectations

After President Reagan was inaugurated in 1981, there were a number of efforts to fold the funding for this law into a block grant and eliminate funding for the Child Abuse Prevention and Treatment Act of 1974. Although these efforts failed, the actions of the Reagan administration had other effects on child welfare services. A block grant for social services was folded into the Omnibus Budget Reconciliation Act Congress passed in 1981. This law compounded many of the drawbacks of Title XX by decreasing federal monitoring and regulation and reducing service standards. Although funding for P.L. 96-272 was kept out of the block grant, the child welfare field experienced indirect effects during this period because many families in which children were at risk of placement were unable to receive some of the services they needed. They also suffered increased poverty due to cutbacks in entitlement programs such as AFDC and Medicaid. Consequently, families tended to put off routine, early intervention services and to arrive at child welfare agencies in greater need than they might have had they received help earlier.

Although the number of children in foster care leveled off briefly after passage of P.L. 92-272, reports of child abuse and neglect increased markedly, as did foster placements, during the later 1980s. There is no consensus as to the reasons for these trends. The reduction in available family social services could have contributed, as could the cutbacks in entitlement programs. Some argued that these increases were the result of increased reporting, suggesting that there was no real increase in the problem of child maltreatment, simply an increase in the degree to which suspected cases were reported. Others attributed these trends to increased maternal substance abuse, increased family homelessness, or increased poverty. Still others blamed the dramatic increase in kinship foster care that occurred following the U.S. Supreme Court decision in *Miller vs. Youakim* (1979), stating that children living in relatives' homes are entitled to the same level of foster care payments as children living with non-kin.

7.1 Family Preservation Programs

A number of programs were initiated in the 80s and early 90s to demonstrate "reasonable effort" to prevent placement. There were many variations in the type and duration of these services, but they were all generally described as family preservation services. The program that ultimately received the most attention, Homebuilders, was started in Tacoma, Washington, under the auspice of the

Behavioral Sciences Institute. The Edna McConnell Clark Foundation invested heavily in this program model, called intensive family preservation services, and helped to organize a loose coalition of national organizations to work on policy implementation of this model at the state level. It also provided funding in the late 80s for a group of states to engage in strategic implementation of this type of services. By the early 90s this group had made progress in implementing intensive family preservation services at the state level and had generated support for this service as a significant component of child welfare services (Farrow, 2001). In 1993 Congress passed legislation for the Family Preservation and Support Services Program, P.L. 103-66. This law provides some funding for both family preservation and family support services. (Family preservation services are designed to prevent, through intensive brief services, the imminent placement of children in foster care, whereas family support services are expected to provide a range of open-ended primary prevention services to families that request such assistance).

Although family preservation programs continued to expand during the 1990s, several forces converged to raise concern about the value of these services (McGowan & Walsh, 2000). These included, first, the continued rise in child abuse and neglect complaints, leading to increased numbers of foster placements. Second, in contrast to earlier reports of the success of intensive family preservation services, carefully designed studies began to document some of the limitations of this model of service. (Schuerman et al., 1994; Nelson, 1997). Third, conservative lay commentators began to stir public anger about the dramatic rise in kinship foster care and the possibility of relatives of "bad" parents receiving money from the state to care for the children of their relatives (MacDonald, 1994, 1999). Fourth, the resurgence of conservative political forces began to legitimize public attacks on families in poverty dependent on AFDC who may have difficulty providing proper care for their children (MacDonald, 1994). Finally, public exposes about a few isolated cases in which children in families that received family preservation services were later abused by their parents precipitated widespread debate about the relative value of family preservation versus child protection and the need to give priority to children's safety (Ferro, 2001). Although intensive family preservation and family support services continue to this day and have helped innumerable numbers of families and children, they have lost some of their initial excitement and funding support as a result of these charges.

7.2 Personal Responsibility and Work Opportunities Act of 1996

The Personal Responsibility and Work Opportunities Act of 1996. P.L. 104-193, eliminated the concept of financial entitlement under AFDC and replaced this with the Temporary Assistance for Needy Families (TANF). The program passed with no real consideration of its potential impact on families in need of child welfare services. The law has a number of provisions that make it more difficult for high risk families in poverty to maintain their children safely at home. As Courtney (1997) commented: "The passage of P.L. 104-193 marks the first time in U.S. history when federal law mandates efforts to protect children from maltreatment, but makes no guarantee of basic economic supports for children." To illustrate, the law imposes a 5-year lifetime limit on receipt of TANF funds, imposes strict work requirements on parents receiving TANF, prohibits individuals convicted of drug-related offenses after passage of the law from receiving TANF or Food Stamp benefits for life, and permits states to establish a family cap that denies cash benefits to children born into families already receiving TANF.

7.3 Adoption and Safe Families Act of 1997 (ASFA)

The most significant change in child welfare policy after the Adoption Assistance and Child Welfare Reform Act of 1980 was the passage of the Adoption and Safe Families Act of 1997, which amends Title IVE of the Social Security Law. Reflecting some of the same conservative sentiments that led to the passage of the welfare reform act the preceding year, the enactment of this law, frequently referred to as ASFA, makes the safety of children the priority in all decision-making. It diminishes the emphasis on family preservation, and promotes speedy termination of parental rights and adoptive placement when parents cannot quickly resolve the problems that led to placement. Although the law reaffirms the concept of permanency planning and re-authorized the Family Preservation and Support Services program, renaming it promoting Safe and Stable Families program, it specifies a number of circumstances under which states are not required to make "reasonable effort" to preserve or reunify families. It mandates a permanency hearing after a child has been in care for 12 months and every 12 months thereafter and requires states, with certain exceptions, to file a termination of parental rights petition in cases in which a child has been in care 15 of the past 22 months. This means that parents who cannot resolve the problems that led to placement and may require longer treatment, e.g., substance abusers, are at risk of having their rights terminated; no matter what the age of the child or the degree of parent-child attachment.

In some ways this law seemed designed primarily to promote adoptions, providing additional funding for states that increase their number of completed adoption and authorizing the Department of Health and Human Services to provide technical assistance to states and localities to help them reach their adoption targets. As Halpern (1998) commented, this law indicates that "Congress believes adoption is the new panacea for the problems of foster care." States that do not comply with its provisions risk losing a portion of their Title IVE and Title IVB funds. The law reaffirms the importance of making reasonable efforts to maintain children at home, but specifies that agencies are not required to do so when keeping a child a home might place him/her in jeopardy.

On a positive note, the law signals a willingness to increase the federal role in child welfare services and to demand state accountability by mandating the Department of Health and Human Services (HHS) to develop outcome measures to monitor state performance. The Department, in response, developed national standards with benchmark indicators of success to measure performance on six statewide data indicators. These are identified as recurrence of maltreatment; incidence of child abuse and/or neglect in foster care; foster care re-entries; stability of foster care placements; length of time to achieve reunification; and length of time to achieve adoption.

8 The Twenty-First Century

During the past decade there have been relatively few policy shifts in child welfare. One important bill, enacted in response to increasing concerns raised about the serious social problems of many of the children aging out of foster care, e.g., homelessness, substance abuse, unemployment, is the John H. Chafee Foster Care Independence Program, Title 1 of the Foster Care Independence Act of 1999, P.L. 106-169. This program was established to provide funds to states to aid youth up to age 21 make the transition to adulthood more successfully. It allows states to provide a wide range of services including room and board, educational and training programs, Medicaid, employment services, and financial support to these youngsters.

The only other policy innovation of recent years in child welfare was the enactment of the Intercountry Adoption Act of 2000, P.L. 106-279. This legislation signaled the United States' support and ratification of the provisions of the Hague Convention on Protection of Children and Cooperation in Respect to Intercountry Adoption. It places responsibility for intercountry adoptions and implementation of the standards set by the Hague Convention within the U.S. Department of State.

The several other laws passed in this period have essentially responded to various critiques raised about the child welfare system and attempted to strengthen the policy provisions surrounding child protective services, foster care and adoption services. To illustrate, the President signed the most recent law, Fostering Connections to Success and Increasing Adoptions Act, in October 2008. This act was the culmination of work by a bipartisan group of advocates and elected officials. Among other provisions, the law extends assistance to youth aging out of foster care, continues federal assistance for subsidized guardianship by caregivers in states that opt to authorize such care; provides funds to aid with family group decision-making models; expands training funds for child welfare workers; and extends and expands adoption incentives.

8.1 Child and Family Services Reviews

The most significant administrative change of the past decade has been the implementation in 2000 of a new federal process of monitoring state child welfare programs on the basis of on site reviews of cases known as Child and Family Services Reviews. Administered by the Administration for Children and Families within the U.S. Department of Health and Human Services, these reviews are designed to examine child welfare practices at the ground level and determine the effects of these practices on the children and families involved. The reviews are based on the conviction that although policies and procedures are essential to an agency's capacity to support positive outcomes, day-to-day practices actually determine the outcomes. As implemented, the reviews have become the federal government's prime mechanism for promoting improvements in child welfare services nationally.

Published reports regarding the results of these reviews have identified a number of problems in different states' capacity to achieve the outcomes identified by the Department of Health and Human Services. Many of the foundations, research and advocacy groups working to improve child welfare services have reached similar conclusions regarding the various factors that hinder quality service provision. Some of the recommendations of these groups have been addressed, others not. For example, the Pew Commission on Children in Foster Care (2004) called for a number of improvements in the juvenile and family courts, and several of these have been addressed, in part by the Deficit Reduction Act of 2005. On the other hand, the Pew Commission and a group titled Fostering Results (McDonald, 2004) both called for changes in federal financing mechanisms, saying current rules stifle innovation and change. A small number of states have been granted permission to seek waivers to use Title IVE funds for non foster care purposes, but there have been no real changes in the rules.

Problems that have been identified repeatedly in the past decade as contributing to deficiencies in service delivery include the disproportionate treatment of African American children and families; low salaries, poor training, and high rates of turnover among child welfare workers; lack of permanency planning for many children who remain overlong in foster care; and continued inadequate preparation and resources for youths aging out of foster care. A number of programmatic initiatives have been introduced to address these problems and others. These include the Family-to-Family and Making Connections programs introduced by the Annie E. Casey Foundation, various types of community partnerships, family group decision-making, new training models for child welfare staff, and parent and youth organizing. In addition, there have been vast improvements in systems of data collection and analysis on the state and federal levels. These are all promising initiatives. Child welfare services seem better today than they were a generation ago, but cautiousness must be indicated because so many reforms are being implemented so quickly. It is difficult to assess their potential collective impact.

9 Conclusion

The field is very much on the public agenda today, as evidenced by the extensive media attention that surrounds every incident of egregious child maltreatment and the recent passage of the Fostering Connections to Success and Increasing Adoptions Act. This bodes well for future attention to the continuing problems in child welfare. Yet, some of the tensions that have pervaded the field such as child saving versus family preservation, the degree to which the state should assume responsibility for problems in family life, and local versus federal responsibility for standard-setting are likely to persist. As Sealander commented in her book, *The Failed Century of the Child*, "The 'century of the child' failed in part because ideas central to attempts to improve childhood also enshrined contradictions in American culture." (2003, p. 356). The child welfare field continues to struggle with these contradictions.

More troubling, as this brief review of the history of child welfare services demonstrates, the field has been caught in a repetitive pattern of one step backward for every two steps forward. We have definitely moved beyond the early belief that the best way to save children from maltreatment was to place them in foster care indefinitely. We now have clear knowledge about the importance to children of maintaining family ties and giving them a secure, relatively permanent home. Yet, every effort to expand services designed to maintain children in their own homes has faltered to some degree. And in recent years we see an increased push toward the use of adoption as a means of rescuing children from poor parenting rather than the provision of needed supports to parents unable to provide adequate care.

Similarly, we have learned that children's developmental opportunities are dependent on the provision of adequate family and community resources. Yet, there is minimal public funding for the income and other supplementary supports required by many families who enter the child welfare system, and many child welfare agencies continue to operate in relative isolation from other community facilities.

Alfred Kahn was a major contributor to the literature and debates on child welfare services during the second half of the twentieth century. From his early days as a consultant for Citizens' Committee for Children of New York, he was always trying to push the field forward. One of his earliest books, *Planning Community Services for Children in Trouble*, published in 1963, reflected some of the insights he had gained through this work regarding the many deficiencies in child welfare and other related service systems. Based on his research and observations about services in New York City, he began to argue for greater service integration and coordination across the country. From that point forward Kahn remained consistently ahead of the field, arguing for more services to families above the poverty line, a more developmental perspective in the provision of child welfare services, and the value of learning from the experiences of service providers in other countries. Had the field followed his lead, we might not still be struggling with the many problems created by the deficit model that continues to characterize child welfare services today.

References

Abbott, G. (1938). *The child and the state* (Vols. 1–2). Chicago: University of Chicago Press.
Adoption and Safe Families Act. (1997). P.L. 105–89.
Adoption Assistance and Child Welfare Act. (1980). P.L. 96-272.
Allen, M. L., & Knitzer, J. (1983). Child welfare: Examining the policy framework. In B. G. McGowan, & W. Meezan (Eds.), *Child welfare: Current dilemmas, future directions* (pp. 93–141). Itasca, IL: Peacock Publishers.

Austin, D. M. (1980). Title XX and the future of social services. *The Urban and Social Change Review, 13*(Summer), 19.

Bernstein, B., Snider, D., & Meezan, W. (1975). *Foster care needs and alternatives to placement.* Albany, NY: New York State Board of Social Welfare.

Billingsley, A., & Giovanni, J. (1972). *Children of the storm: Black children and American child welfare.* New York: Harcourt Brace Jovanovich.

Bremner, R. (Ed.) (1970–1974a). *Children and youth in America: A documentary history* (Vols. 1–3). Cambridge, MA: Harvard University Press.

Buell, B. (1952). *Community planning for human services.* Westport, CT: Greenwood Press.

Burt, M., & Balyeat, R. (1974). A new system for improving care of neglected and abused children. *Child Welfare, 53*, 167–179.

Chappell, B., & Hevener, B. (1977). *Periodic review of children in foster care: Mechanisms for reviews.* Newark, NJ: Child Service Association.

Child Abuse Prevention and Treatment Act. (1974). P.L.93-247.

Courtney, M. E. (1997). Welfare reform and child welfare services. In S. B. Kamerman & A. J. Kahn (Eds.), *Child welfare in the context of " welfare reform"* (pp. 1–35). New York: Cross National Studies Program, Columbia Universit School of Social Work.

Emlen, A. C., L'Ahti, J., & Downs, S. W. (1978). *Overcoming barriers to planning for children in foster care.* Washington, DC: U.S. Government Printing Office.

Family Preservation and Support Services Program. (1993). P.L. 103-66.

Fanshel, D., & Shinn, E. (1978). *Children in foster care: A longitudinal investigation.* New York: Columbia University Press.

Farrow, F. (2001). *The shifting policy impact of intensive family preservation services.* Chicago: Chapin Hall Center for Children at the University of Chicago.

Foster Care Independence Act. (1999). P.L. 106-169.

Geisman, L. L., & Ayers, B. (1958). *Families in trouble.* St. Paul, MN: Greater St. Paul Community Chests and Councils.

Goldstein, J., Solnit, A. J., Goldstein, S., & Freud, A. (1973). *Beyond the best interests of the child.* New York: Free Press.

Goldstein, J., Solnit, A.J., Goldstein, S., & Freud, A. (1979). *Beyond the best interests of the child*, 2nd ed., N.Y.: Free Press.

Halpern, R. (1998). Abandoning family preservation in a rush to adoption. *Interdisciplinary report on at risk children & families, 1*(1), 10–11.

Indian Child Welfare Act. (1978). P.L. 95–608.

Jalongo, M. L. (2008). The story of Mary Ellen Wilson: Tracing the origins of child protection in America. *Early Childhood Education Journal, 34*(1), 1–4.

Jones, M.A., Newman, R., & Shyne, A.W. (1976). *A Second chance for Families: Evaluation of a program to reduce foster care.* N.Y.: Child Welfare League of America.

Kahn, A. J. (1963). Planning community services for children in trouble. New York: Columbia University Press.

Knitzer, J., Allen, M. L., & McGowan, B. (1978). *Children without homes.* Washington, DC: Children's Defense Fund.

Lindhorst, T., & Leighniger, L. (2003). " Ending welfare as we know it" in 1960: Louisiana's suitable home law. *Social Service Review, 77*, 564–584.

MacDonald, H. (1994). *The ideology of family preservation. The Public Interest*, 115, 45–60.

Maas, H., & Engler, R. (1959). *Children in need of parents.* New York: Columbia University Press.

MacDonald, H. (1999). Foster care's underworld. *City Journal, 9*(Winter), 44–53.

Maybanks, S., & Bryce, M., eds. (1979). *Home-based services for children and families.* Springfield, Il: Charles C. Thomas, publisher.

McGowan, B. G., & Walsh, E. M. (2000). Policy challenges for child welfare in the new century. *Child Welfare, 79*, 11–27.

Miller vs. Youakim. (1979). 440 U.S. 125.

Nelson, K. E. (1997). Family preservation – What is it? *Children and Youth Services Review, 19*, 101–118.

New York City Youth Board. (1958). *Reaching the unreached family* (Youth Board Monograph No. 5). New York: New York City Youth Board.

Parker, J. K., & Carpenter, E. M. (1981, March). Julia Lathrop and the children's bureau: The emergence of an institution. *Social Service Review, 55*, 62–79.

Pecora, P., Whittaker, J. K., Maluccio, A. N., & Barth, R. H. (2000). *The child welfare challenge.* New York: Aldine de Gruyter.

Persico, J. (1979). *Who knows? Who cares?: Forgotten children in foster care.* New York: National Commission on Children in Need of Parents.

Personal Responsibility and Work Opportunities Act. (1996). P.L. 104–193.

Pew Commission on Children in Foster Care. (2004). *Recommendations to overhaul children's foster care system.* Washington, DC: Pew Commission.

Pike, V. (1976). Permanent planning for foster children: The Oregon project. *Children Today, 6,* 22–41.

Promoting Safe and Stable Families Amendment. (2001). P.L. 107–133.

Richan, W. C. (1978). *Personnel issues in child welfare services.* Washington, DC: U.S. Department of Health, Education and Welfare.

Rodham, H. (1973). Children under the law. *Harvard Educational Review, 43*(4), 483–514.

Schuerman, J.K., Rzepnicki, T.L., & Littell, J.H. (1994). *Putting Families First: An experiment in family preservation.* N.Y.: Aldine de Gruyter.

Strauss, G. (1977). *The children are waiting: The failure to achieve permanent homes for foster children in New York City.* New York: New York City Comptroller's Office.

The NYSPPCC Story. (http://www.nyspcc.org/beta_history/nyspcc_story.html retrieved 10/25/08).

Thurston, H. W. (1930). *The dependent child.* New York: Columbia University Press.

Van Theis, S. (1924). *How foster children turn out.* New York: Charities Aid Association.

Wickenden, E. (1976, December). A perspective on social services: An essay review. *Social Service Review, 50*, 574–588.

Wolins, M., & Piliavin, I. (1964). *Institution or foster Care*: A century of debate. N.Y.: Child Welfare League of America.

Testing Practice Wisdom in Child Welfare

Anat Zeira

Many practice decisions are based on what is known as practice wisdom. While in our everyday lives, we use such knowledge to make both simple and complex decisions, professionals, such as Child Protection Officers have to decide for example, whether or not to remove a child from home. Thus, they often base their decisions on their "individual theory of practice that represents the worker's attempt to conceptualize what he is doing" (Bloom, 1975, p. 66). This knowledge however, is implicit and is not available for utilization in practice or research. It is therefore important to conceptualize this source of knowledge, and to explore its potential for utilization in practice and policy (Collins, Amodeo, & Clay, 2008).

1 What is Practice Wisdom?

Lynn and Kevin need to decide which of the two neighborhood schools is more suitable for their five-year old son, Daniel. To make this decision, they ask neighbors and visit the schools on open house days. They also gather practical information (e.g., cost, distance from home), and discuss their values and beliefs about education. Finally, they reach a decision. Their decision-making process is based on their knowledge as parents and could be called practice wisdom. Professionals reach their practice decisions using a similar process (Schon, 1983). For both layman and professionals, however, the information included in this process is not always available in an explicit manner. If we asked Lynn and Kevin how they chose the school for Daniel, we probably would not get a detailed description of how they reached their decision. Yet, people know much more about their decision making process than they usually express but the limited ability of human beings to hold all information needed, results in applying short cuts in decision making processes. Instead of a well explicated process of reaching a decision, people make use of heuristics, which are short cuts that create a body of knowledge of its own and is stored in the minds of people (DeRoose, 1990).

A. Zeira (✉)
Paul Baerwald School of Social Work and Social Welfare, The Hebrew University of Jerusalem, Jerusalem, Israel

S.B. Kamerman et al. (eds.), *From Child Welfare to Child Well-Being*, Children's Well-Being: Indicators and Research 1, DOI 10.1007/978-90-481-3377-2_4,
© Springer Science+Business Media B.V. 2010

The term practice wisdom appears in the literature of social work as a type of knowledge that practitioners possess (Chu & Tsui, 2008). Literature on social work practice reveals other expressions for practice wisdom, like "tacit knowledge" (Imre, 1984), "felt knowledge" (Duehn, 1981), "intuition" (Carew, 1987) or "common sense" (DeRoose, 1990). This term is often diminished and misused to describe a second best source of knowledge that has no empirical validity (Nelsen, 1993). Yet, it is the result of a trial-and-error process that social workers experience with their clients (Nelsen, 1993). Workers collect and store information in their minds, use it in their practice and share it with others in different ways (e.g., field instruction, case conferences). Practice knowledge is not necessarily systematically accumulated, although there are attempts to do so. For example, Ivanoff, Blythe, & Tripodi (1994) describe a model of research-based practice that is employed within the problem-solving framework. Their model consists of four sequential phases (assessment, planning interventions, implementing interventions and follow up) and "is a heuristic device to specify decisions and activities of social work practitioners" (p. 10). Practice wisdom develops through a similar process (DeRoose, 1990), but the problem-solving process inherent in practice wisdom is not fully explicated.

Nonetheless, practice wisdom is valid to a certain degree. Its validity is gained through success, as the worker keeps in mind what worked and what did not work and replicates it as needed (Nelsen, 1993). Instead of repeating the complete process that led them to the specific conclusion, workers use heuristics or practice wisdom the next time they need to reach a similar decision.

2 Applications of Practice Wisdom

The term practice wisdom is sometimes used for research purposes (Nelsen, 1993; Scott, 1990; Carew, 1987), while others use it to clarify issues of knowledge building and philosophy of science, as well as to bridge the gap between research and practice (Klein & Bloom, 1995; Goldstein, 1990; Krill, 1990). Practice wisdom may also be seen as a micro knowledge base of interventions that solely serves practitioners (Mullen, 1988). The term has also been used to describe knowledge that clearly is not based on theory or research findings.

Within the domain of practice research, it has been suggested that practice wisdom can serve a source for generating hypotheses for empirical studies (Nelsen, 1993). Practice wisdom contains relevant information about what practitioners need to know to accomplish treatment goals and help their clients. For example, practice wisdom suggests that engaging an alcoholic client in a self-help group has a positive effect on the client's relationship with his or her family members.

Practitioners report that they often use practice wisdom in their daily case decision making (Mullen, 1983). "Personal intervention models" developed by

Mullen (1988) refer to intervention strategies that social workers accumulate and apply for attaining outcomes to specific client problems. When creating a "personal intervention model", social workers integrate this sporadic knowledge, acquired through their continued professional experience and learning from various sources of information, into a body of knowledge that is available to them. Mullen (1983) found that practitioners include practice wisdom in "personal intervention models" more often than other sources of knowledge (such as theory or knowledge derived from research findings on effective interventions).

Unfortunately, practice wisdom is caught in the debate over qualitative vs. quantitative approaches to generate knowledge in social work. I suggest that an approach will be adopted according to its merit for the specific research goal. Research of an exploratory nature that aims for example at learning characteristics of a new population (e.g., children of HIV positive parents), can benefit form employing qualitative methods; an explanatory research, aimed at explaining a phenomenon, would better use rigor quantitative methods. Klein & Bloom (1995) attempted to use practice wisdom to resolve the dispute between the qualitative and quantitative approaches. They argue: "practice wisdom is a significant component of both quantitative and qualitative knowledge and thus links empirical knowledge and practice" (p. 803). Thus, point out that practice wisdom represents the bridge between positivistic and phenomenological philosophies.

The growing attention to practice wisdom as a worthy source of information has led to some suggestions on how to benefit from it, mainly for research purposes. Nelsen (1993), for instance, suggests using practice wisdom to generate hypotheses that will be more relevant to practitioners. The potential of practice wisdom for research is largely due to the fact that it is rooted in problem solving models. It basically represents the private problem-solving model of each practitioner (i.e., what to do with a specific client problem). Such cognitive models contain the expected order of events in treatment (Bloom, Fischer, & Orme, 1995), that eventually result in hypotheses that reflect the practitioner's solutions to client problems.

Using practice wisdom in research raises the question of validity. To a certain extent, this knowledge is valid, although the validity is not necessarily empirical. Based on their experience, practitioners usually know when to terminate an intervention and/or replace it with another one. Because the accumulation of practice wisdom is grounded on a problem-solving process, Reid (1994) argues that it is valid, scientific practice.

Learning from the experience of social workers in innovative ways expands our practice knowledge (Schon, 1983). It is possible to uncover practice wisdom and turn it into an explicit source of information. Furthermore, it is worthwhile to look at how practitioners arrive at their practice decisions and reveal their reasoning. Practice knowledge should be derived from all available sources of information and approaches. As long as the integrity of the methods is maintained, and knowledge is related to the complexity of the human being and interactions within the human society, the path for new directions of arriving at practice knowledge widens.

3 Why Test Practice Wisdom?

Over the years there has been a call for systematic formulation of practice wisdom in social work but little has been done about it (Davis, 2007). To date, theories or empirical evidence have received greater attention as the focus of research activities. Debates over the concept and meaning of evidence-based practice in social work with children and families even amplify the important role practice wisdom plays in developing guidelines accountable practice (Zeira et al., 2008). Here, several arguments for evaluating practice wisdom are explicated.

3.1 Practice Wisdom is a Good Source of Knowledge

What makes a source of knowledge good for practice research? For one thing, it has the quality one looks for when trying to understand the complexity of the helping process in that it covers a wide variety of cases. Practice knowledge represents a wide range of problems and clients with which social workers deal daily. Moreover, practice knowledge reflects the content of the real world, as it relates to actual clients and situations, as opposed to using "artificial" case vignettes that presumably represent clinical situations. For example, workers are given a standard situation (that may be based on real events), and are asked to relate to them as if they were their real cases. Naturally, these vignettes lack the complexity and richness of information embraced in real practice events.

Practice wisdom opens a window into successful practice. Practitioners generally know, although some may say intuitively, what works for their clients. They continually make decisions about intervention plans, altering an intervention, adding another intervention or terminating an intervention. Unfortunately, practitioners neither articulate their deeds nor their rationale. The apparent overall success of their work, though not always empirically evident, is the proof that there is something in what they do. This body of knowledge needs to be tested in order to make what is already there explicit and empirically evident. This claim finds support in the history of social work where, as early as the days of Mary Richmond, practice wisdom had gained respect as a source of developing knowledge for the profession (DeRoose, 1990). This direction is also in accord with Nelsen's (1993) claim that much of what social workers do is not researchable, (e.g., practice wisdom) yet it can't be meaningless.

Practice wisdom also is a good source of knowledge because it can be phrased in operational terms. If we can help practitioners identify and describe what they do that works, we can get a hold of information with a great potential for transition into operational definitions. For example, let's look at a successful intervention process with alcoholic single mothers. If this intervention is explained in the form of a detailed description, a list of activities that has achieved success in treatment can be developed. In turn, these activities can be measured (e.g., in terms of duration and extent). As Klein & Bloom (1995) suggest, "practice wisdom exhibits a qualitative dimension in the form of operational definitions." There is little doubt that this is the form of knowledge that is most desired in order to give the profession the solid base it needs.

3.2 Practice Wisdom Helps Bridge the Gap Between Research and Practice

Traditionally, evaluating treatment effectiveness is conducted by using what is called the "positivistic" approach, in which hypotheses are based on theories or previous research findings. A classic example of such an investigation is the study conducted by Wills, Faitler, & Snyder (1987) that compared the effectiveness of two alternative treatment models for dealing with marital problems (insight-oriented vs. behavioral therapy). The hypotheses were deductively formulated (i.e., based on theories), and an inherent assumption was that the two treatment models were distinct. Therefore, they were expected to yield somewhat different outcomes. The findings of this research, however, were inconclusive. Neither treatment model was significantly superior. These findings are typical of many treatment outcome studies and raise two separate issues. The first issue is methodological concerns related to integrity in implementing a treatment model. Was each therapy or intervention implemented as intended? Due to the complexity of the treatment variables under investigation, accurate measurement is not possible. The other issue has to do with the low utilization of findings of outcome studies by practitioners. These findings were simply irrelevant for practitioners because they were conducted "in vitro" (Mullen, 1985; Ruckdeschel, 1985). Despite efforts to utilize randomized controls trials in social work research, the setting of real practice poses issues about the situations of the client that are sometimes ignored when they are presented in theoretical terms (Mahrer, 1988; Zeira et al., 2008). Also, hypotheses based on theory tend to include abstract terms and hence be phrased in more general, conceptual terms (Gendlin, 1986).

As mentioned in the previous section, practice wisdom contains assumptions (or hypotheses) about things that work. This knowledge is stored in the practitioners' minds and reflected in their professional activities and has the potential to be explicated and then phrased in operational terms. Once phrased operationally, it can serve as a solid basis for formulating specific hypotheses. This source of knowledge increases the relevancy of hypotheses under investigation because their origin is in actual social work practice (Mahrer, 1988).

One of the most widely discussed issues related to social work practice research concerns the gap between research and practice. It is often claimed that research endeavors do not meet practice needs (Gambrill, 1994). Practitioners do not use research findings partly because they can't apply them in their practice (Rosen, 1994). There is no definite conclusion in this debate and several directions of research (e.g., single-case methodologies) have been developed to address this gap.

I would like to suggest that the gap between practice and research could be bridged by taking information that implicitly exists in practice and making it useful via research. Let me explain how it can be done. If we agree that practitioners hold knowledge regarding effective interventions, this will provide the "what" component for research on the intervention process. Researchers have knowledge on the "how to" component of the same endeavor. If we can find a way to combine the potential contribution of each party, we can increase the usefulness of research findings due to the fact that they originate in the field of practice. So, why not let practitioners dictate the content, and researchers contribute the methods and rules? This will enhance the relevance of the research to both practice and research as well as make a contribution to theory (Argyris, 1985).

3.3 Practice Wisdom Helps Practitioners Describe What They Do

The core of the social work profession lies in field settings, not in the halls of the academia. One important role of practice research is to provide front line workers with tools and knowledge to better serve their clients (Blythe & Tripodi, 1989). An important part of this endeavor should be to help practitioners better document their practice.

This is especially necessary for the work of professionals in child welfare, where officers of the law are responsible for the well-being of children and must keep records of there various activities. Systematic documentation of professional activities, especially the components of the intervention process, is crucial also to accumulating practice knowledge (Benbenishty, 1992). To date, there is not enough evidence from direct practice (Fook, 1996; Gambrill, 1994). The reason for this situation is partly because practitioners normally do not volunteer to provide a systematic description of their reflections and activities that are of a demanding nature. As a result, their experiences are lost and others cannot benefit from them. Recognition of this source of knowledge may encourage people in the field, whose daily efforts are meaningful, to describe what they do and keep track of their actions (Dybicz, 2004). When workers are able to say explicitly what they did and provide a rationale for their actions, it creates a knowledge base for the profession. Such documentation is also crucial for policy makers in child welfare that will be able to select best practices. The contribution of researchers must be in creating tools to facilitate systematic description of practice activities. When cooperation is achieved between field people and academics, both sides will benefit. I believe that by exposing practice wisdom to systematic investigation, we can develop a better understanding of the nature of practice.

4 Explicating Practice Wisdom

In this part, I would like to suggest a method for explicating practice wisdom. First, I review the challenge of collecting data on direct practice by practitioners for practice decisions. Second, I suggest a conceptual framework that allows generating specific hypotheses based on social workers' practice wisdom. Last I illustrate a training program in which workers used this method and discuss promoting and preventive factors for its dissemination.

4.1 Collecting Data on Direct Practice

Direct practice data contains evidence from actual practitioners' treatments. In order to investigate practice wisdom, we first need to have data on activities, thoughts, motives, and rationales that are part of the daily routine of practitioners. There are several different ways of collecting direct practice information (Reid & Smith, 1989). These can generally be categorized into three groups: observations, interviews, and self-administered tools (Neuman, 1995; Rubin & Babbie, 1989 and Grinnell, 1988, to name a few).

Self-administered tools (also known as "paper and pencil" measures) are most useful to collect data on outcomes. For example in parent education projects may monitor parenting skills using simple self-report scales (e.g., Corcoran & Fischer, 2000). However, such tools must be relevant to both the practitioner and to the client (Edwards & Reid, 1989). The benefits of self-administered tools will be increased if two steps are taken. The first is to adopt a structured form that provides practitioners with a physical framework. The second is to follow a conceptual framework of the treatment process that allows different practitioners to document their practice yet sharing the same concepts. For example, suppose that workers in a welfare agency wish to explore their tacit knowledge. Instead of their usual "free form" case documentation, they select a set of structured forms that is based on an agreeable conception of practice (a specific conception of practice will be suggested later in this chapter). This group of workers now shares the same form and concepts in describing their interventions (i.e., the different phases of the process, their sequence and interrelations). In a way, they speak the same language and now have a better ability to share their knowledge on the agency level.

4.2 Combining Qualitative and Quantitative Methods

As noted earlier in this chapter, practice wisdom is stored in practitioners' minds and hidden in their decision making process and is not available like other types of knowledge that serve the profession. Since each worker has a unique way of arriving at case decisions, a common denominator needs to be found, in order to operationalize and measure this knowledge. Practice wisdom is shared by practitioners in some form, such as case conferences, supervision or client's case records within an agency setting. For example, by reflecting what they know from their past experiences and predicting how a case can be resolved. In other words, they think back to what has worked for them in the past with similar client problems or goals. Unfortunately, as Gingerich (1995) has noted, most of this practice wisdom is lost because practitioners lack the means to elicit and describe that knowledge.

In the process of implementing specific interventions, practitioners have certain considerations related to specific client situations and characteristics that usually exist in an implicit manner. It is difficult for practitioners to articulate and trace the formal steps with which they have derived at a decision. This recognition has two implications: first, it makes it difficult to articulate practice activities; and second, since these considerations are unique, they will not be included in hypotheses derived from theories (Fook, 1996).

Describing practice wisdom requires information that reflects the richness and complexity of practice activities (Parton, 2000). To preserve all that is encompassed in practice, we need to combine qualitative and quantitative approaches to data collection and analysis (Allen-Meares & Lane, 1990). Practitioners, for example, could construct a structured "paper-and-pencil" form to record practice events in their own words. This allows some flexibility in data collection and analysis while maintaining systematic criteria of the procedure.

4.3 Conceptualizing the Intervention Process

Rosen (1992) introduced Systematic Planned Practice (SPP) which has been applied in a number of research projects and is described in details elsewhere (Rosen, 1992, 1994) and later was the basis for the development of practice guidelines (Rosen & Proctor, 2003). SPP is also a framework for planning the entire intervention process. It is based on the notion that professional intervention involves conscious and rational decisions (Rosen, Proctor, & Livne, 1985). SPP refers to future activities that reflect the intentions of the workers without the compromises made due to daily concerns, such as caseload or lack of time. This conception is especially useful with regard to developing goals in treatment and has been used in past research to explicate social workers' practice wisdom (Zeira, 2000; Zeira & Rosen, 2000). A treatment plan is comprised of three basic components: the client problems, the expected outcomes, and the intervention strategies (Rosen & Proctor, 1978) and is undertaken in phases. Figure 1 delineates the different phases according to SPP guidelines.

As illustrated in Fig. 1, the first phase represents the identified problem. The assertion of the outcomes is the second phase and is based on the formulation of the identified problem. Outcomes are differentiated according to their role in the process: Ultimate outcomes are those objectives whose attainment represents a successful termination when treating a problem. To attain an ultimate outcome, the worker might take several intermediate outcomes which are steps on the way to the ultimate outcome. The last phase of the treatment plan pertains to selecting appropriate intervention strategies for each one of the outcomes.

By asking practitioners to document their treatment plans with SPP, major decision points in treatment can be traced. In that sense, a treatment plan resembles a cognitive map (Bitonti, 1993) or other models of cognitive schemata. Formulation of each phase of SPP is based on providing a rationale. Hence, the treatment plan

Problems	Ultimate Outcomes	Intermediate Outcomes	Interventions
1. parent-child relationships	1. improve parent-child relationships	1. talk not shout	a. communication skills
			b. legitimization
		2. plan the next day	a. discussing tasks
			b. assigning tasks
		3. establish timetable	a. discussing alternatives
			b. report in log
			c. discussing the log

Fig. 1 Treatment plan for the first presented problem of the Bar-On family

creates an opportunity for the practitioner to explicate the sequence of events that leads him or her to a decision about the specific intervention for a specific outcome with a specific client. It unfolds the different phases of the treatment process, as each phase leads the practitioner to the next one. This is a self-administered tool to be implemented by practitioners as part of their daily activities. It is also a source of reliable data on actual practice decisions of social workers that later can lead to generation of specific hypotheses about their practice.

4.4 Generating Specific Hypotheses

Ivanoff et al. (1994) stress that "An intervention hypothesis states the predicted relationship between an intervention and an expected consequence of that intervention" (p. 67). By indicating what is the best solution for a client's problem practitioners are implicitly formulating several hypotheses. Every practitioner, however, uses different language and style to describe her or his activities. In order to generate specific hypotheses across practitioners, we need to overcome their personal differences. Hence, the next step in explicating practice wisdom is to find a common denominator among practitioners by analyzing the contents of the treatment plans that were prepared according to SPP guidelines.

Content analysis procedure refers to the identification of category systems in a given text (Reid & Bailey-Dempsey, 1994). Content analysis of a treatment plan requires developing categories for the problems, outcomes and interventions included in the treatment process. For example, categories for client problems may include interpersonal (i.e., relationships), emotional (i.e., depression), behavioral (i.e., delinquency) and environmental (i.e., poverty). The three components of the treatment plan (i.e., the identified client problem, the desired outcomes and the intervention strategies that are thought to best achieve the desired outcomes) are conceptually related to one another. Categories are the common denominator we are looking for to overcome personal differences in language and style among practitioners (Zeira & Rosen, 1999).

Describing the treatment process with categories yields a map for a specific client. This map represents the case decision-making process for one client by one practitioner. Because all maps share the same framework, it provides the opportunity to look across practitioners and to search for similarities and differences. Above all, these maps can generate several specific hypotheses on treatment interventions. When looking at the maps across all the practitioners in an agency, we can learn, for example, what are the most common (or frequent) problems or outcomes they deal with, and what are the interventions they would most likely use to achieve successful outcomes. The advantage of this procedure is its ability to retain the clinical meaning of the practitioners' intentions and thoughts, as well as the richness and complexity that actual data can offer. Moreover, this approach may provide insights to developing innovative intervention programs.

5 Implications for Practice Research and Policy

Child welfare practice comprises a wide variety of activities including critical life decisions such as a child removal from his/her birth parents. Typically these activities require more advanced skills on behalf of the workers. It may also sometimes require implementing new policy guidelines or practice initiatives (Zeira, 2004). Tacit knowledge, or practice wisdom, of the practitioners is thus a valuable source of information to make informed decisions.

Explicating and aggregating tacit knowledge, whether on the agency level or in a group of agencies, also increases the validity of practice decisions and the probability that the selected intervention will solve the identified problem. Child Welfare Officers are in a better position to interpret and implement policy favorably for a given client. Because practice wisdom includes a variety of personal and organizational factors (e.g., the worker's own views of the policy, the explicit or implicit pressure to close case, etc.) its explication may serve as guiding principles for both stakeholders and practitioners who wish to design intervention protocols, that are less influenced for example by the workers' personal biases.

Such an approach, as will be illustrated below, does not require funding. Instead, it requires an organizational decision to use a common language that is based on the practice wisdom of the organization's workers. This act is in accord with the notion of accountable practice (Rosen, 1992) where workers are expected to first, show the linkage between their professional acts and the desired outcomes, and second to be able to articulate the ineterventive path. Therefore, explicating practice wisdom, especially in child welfare, implies better management of practice decisions and proper implementation of policies.

The mechanism to explicate practice wisdom involves both researchers that can provide the conceptual and methodological grounds and stakeholders that can enforce the requirements for eliciting practice knowledge. It requires training the workers to use the set of forms (e.g., Fig. 1) and creating a forum that will discuss their contents. This is not different from other training or supervision activities. In fact, Collins, Amodeo, & Clay (2007) argue that training improves intervention, especially in child welfare services. When practice wisdom is used a basis for that training, it gives the context with which the activities are anchored. Supervision of Child Welfare Workers becomes much more effective because it includes the supportive conditions required to facilitate effective training (Collins et al., 2007).

Despite the limited external validity of practice wisdom, it has merit to shaping and implementing new policies. Explication of practice wisdom according to SPP guidelines can serve as the model that tells a story of multiple cases. For example, what are the possible alternative to increase a child's well being and which contextual factors are similar and which are unique? A response to these issues that is based on the practice wisdom of workers and that uses valid instruments to measure its activities allows a scholarly analysis of the way workers implement policies.

6 Case Illustration

The following illustration demonstrates how knowledge from one's own practice can generate specific hypotheses by applying the method and guidelines suggested above. Extracting and aggregating of several such applications portrays the practice wisdom.

6.1 The Client Unit

The client unit is a multi-problem family that voluntarily approached a social welfare agency that serves a lower-middle class neighborhood. In the assessment interview, Mrs. and Mr. Bar-On revealed that they couldn't handle their four children (ages 13, 10, 7 and 3) any longer. Mr. and Mrs. Bar-On fight all the time, their children do not listen to them, they can't pay the rent and the oldest child is spending time with "bad kids". They feel their life is in a mess and they want help. When asked, Mrs. and Mr. Bar-On said their most urgent problem is the children's behavior. They felt that if the family atmosphere was more pleasant, they would be able to handle the other issues. The worker, impressed by their motivation for change, set the following priorities for treatment: (1) parent-children relationships; (2) marital relationship; (3) the behavior of the oldest child; and (4) financial issues. For the purpose of this illustration we will focus only on the first presented problem.

6.2 The Treatment Plan

Devoted to SPP guidelines, the worker prepared a treatment plan using the form presented above. Figure 1 describes the treatment plan for the first presented problem of the Bar-On family. The plan illustrates the conceptual link between the actions of the worker (the interventions) and the purposes of this act (the desired outcomes). In order to help the family resolve the presented problem in parent-child relationship, the practitioner formulated an ultimate outcome indicating that Mrs. and Mr. Bar-On will improve their relationship with their children. Obviously, this outcome is stated in broad terms and needs to be more specific for the worker to articulate an intervention plan. Therefore, the worker formulated three intermediate outcomes (shown on the third column of Fig. 1) that would lead to the desired improvement of the relationships of the Bar-On's with their children: (a) family members will talk to each other rather than shout; (b) family members will plan the course of the following day in order to avoid chaotic behaviors; and (c) family members will establish a timetable and routine that will allow for direct interaction between them.

In order to achieve those outcomes, the worker needs to select intervention strategies (shown on the last column of Fig. 1). This is the core of social work practice—what the worker chooses to do in order to improve the client's situation. The worker decides to base her intervention on a family system model (e.g., Reid & Epstein, 1977). This choice is anchored in the belief that all family members are part of the treatment process and that relationships within a family can improve only if family members will learn to share their feelings and thoughts with each other. Working with the family as a system may also take a form of dyadic meetings, or the worker may work separately with the children for a while.

The worker applies task-centered oriented techniques to establish a routine for the family meetings and to create an atmosphere of trust. She might achieve that goal by supporting and encouraging the family members, in order to reach an agreement on number of sessions, and their location and duration. Then, the major intervention strategies may follow. For the first intermediate outcome: "Family members will talk to each other rather than shout;" the worker thought that helping *improve their communication skills* (e.g., looking at each other while talking to each other, paying attention to the tone of speech, telling about positive events) along with *legitimization* (i.e., of thoughts, feelings or behaviors) would be effective. The second intermediate outcome "Family members will plan the course of the following day;" would be best achieved, according, to our worker by *tasks* that family members will accomplish between sessions. Such tasks could be for each family member to list his or her schedule for the next week. Preceding the task assignments are *discussions* aimed at deciding on the content of the task assignment. To address the third outcome "Family members will establish timetable and habits to allow for direct interaction;" the worker believes that *discussing the alternatives* separately with each family member is an effective technique, along with helping family members *reach a series of decisions* on what, when and how they wish to do together and then have them *report in a log* what they actually did. In the log each family member will write his or her wishes and thoughts. The content of the log can later serve as a basis for *further discussions* in future sessions. The intermediate outcomes put together with consequent interventions create a sequence that explicates the worker's treatment plan. If a written and explicit rationale is added, it may reveal the worker's decision making process when working with a family.

7 Summary

Treatment plans created by workers are a good source of knowledge that can yield "mini-hypotheses" on effective interventions. An example of such a mini-hypothesis is "improving communication skills between family members enhance quiet speaking among them" presented above. The knowledge base for such hypotheses rests on the expertise and practice knowledge of the worker. Granted, the hypotheses need to be refined, and perhaps more specific to allow for other workers access to this information.

We may take our worker a step further and suggest the assumption, that the Bar-On family parent-child relationship problems will improve as a result of her intervention be tested. Testing hypotheses generated by workers will provide empirical evidence to their practice, which can be later part of the agency's practice model (Zeira, 2000). Single-subject designs (SSD) are most useful for that matter, and benefit both the practitioner and the client (Ivanoff et al., 1994). These designs can be represented by visual means, and graphs can actually help the client see the changes (Bloom et al., 1995). All in all, workers who work in this manner do not have to radically alter their practice. In the illustration above, the worker gave the Bar-On family the best help she could provide based on her knowledge, belief and experience, her own practice wisdom. The researcher has only helped her explicate what she already knows and does as part of her daily routine with clients. What does it take? It asks for cooperation between the worker, who holds the practice knowledge, and the researcher, who provides the tools and framework to allow the explication.

Despite continuous efforts to integrate between practice and research in social work, further attempts for increased collaboration are still needed. Recognition of practice wisdom as a suitable source of knowledge and empirical efforts to confirm its validity are welcome. This type of cooperation between field workers and academia can enrich and promote social work practice knowledge. In child welfare where every practice decision has short and long-term impacts on the life of children and adolescents, such efforts are especially challenging.

References

Allen-Meares, P., & Lane, B. A. (1990). Social work practice: Integrating qualitative and quantitative data collection techniques. *Social Work, 35,* 452–458.

Argyris, C. (1985). Making knowledge more relevant to practice: Maps for action. In E. E., Lawler, S. A., Mohrman, G. E. Ledford, & T. G. Cummings (Eds.), *Doing research that is useful for theory and practice* (pp. 79–125). San Francisco: Jossey-Bass.

Benbenishty, R. (1992). An overview of methods to elicit and model expert clinical judgment and decision making. *Social Service Review, 65,* 598–616.

Bitonti, C. (1993). Cognitive mapping: A qualitative research method for social work. *Social Work Research & Abstracts, 29,* 9–16.

Bloom, M. (1975). *The paradox of helping.* New York: John Willey & Sons.

Bloom, M., Fischer, J., & Orme, J. (1995). *Evaluating practice: Guidelines for the accountable professional.* Boston: Allyn & Bacon.

Blythe, B. J., & Tripodi, T. (1989). *Measurement in direct social work practice*. Newberry Park, CA: Sage.

Carew, R. (1987). The place of intuition in social work. *Australian Social Work, 40*, 5–9.

Chu, W. C., & Tsui, M. (2008). The nature of practice wisdom in social work revisited. *International Social Work, 51*, 47–54.

Collins, M. E., Amodeo, M., & Clay, C. (2007). Training as a factor in policy implementation: Lessons from a national evaluation of child welfare training. *Children and Youth Services Review, 29*, 1487–1502.

Collins, M. E., Amodeo, M., & Clay, C. (2008). Planning and evaluating child welfare training projects. *Child Welfare, 87*, 69–86.

Corcoran, K., & Fischer, J. (2000). *Measures for clinical practice: A sourcebook*. New York: The Free Press.

Davis, D. (2007). Why do MSW students evaluate practice the way they do? An evidence-based theory for clinical supervisors. *The Clinical Supervisor, 26*, 159–175.

DeRoose, Y. (1990). The development of practice wisdom through human problem-solving processes. *Social Service Review, 64*, 276–287.

Duehn, W. D. (1981). The process of social work practice and research. In R. M. Grinnell (Ed.), *Social work research and evaluation* (pp. 11–34). Itasca, IL: Peacock.

Dybicz, P. (2004). An inquiry into practice wisdom. *Families in Society, 85*, 197–203.

Edwards, R. L., & Reid, W. J. (1989). Structured case recording in child welfare: An assessment of social workers' reactions. *Social Work, 34*, 49–52.

Fook, J. (1996). The reflective researcher: Developing a reflective approach to practice. In J. Fook (Ed.), *The reflective researcher* (pp. 1–10). Sydney: Allen & Unwin.

Gambrill, E. (1994). Social work research: Priorities and obstacles. *Research on Social Work Practice, 4*, 359–388.

Gendlin, E. T. (1986). What comes after traditional psychotherapy? *American Psychologist, 41*, 131–136.

Gingerich, W. J. (1995). Expert systems. In R. L. Edwards (Ed.), *Encyclopedia of Social Work* (pp. 917–925). Washington, DC: NASW.

Goldstein, H. (1990). The knowledge base of social work practice: Theory, wisdom, analogue, or art? *Families in Society: The Journal of Contemporary Human Services, 71*, 32–43.

Grinnell, R. M. (1988). *Social work research and evaluation*. Itasca, IL: Peacock.

Imre, R. W. (1984). The nature of knowledge in social work. *Social Work, 29*, 41–45.

Ivanoff, A., Blythe, B. J., & Tripodi, T. (1994). *Involuntary clients in social work practice*. New York: Aldine de Gruyter.

Klein, W. C., & Bloom, M. (1995). Practice wisdom. *Social Work, 40*, 799–807.

Krill, D. (1990). *Practice wisdom: A guide for helping professionals*. Newberry Park, CA: Sage.

Mahrer, A. R. (1988). Discovery-oriented psychotherapy research. *American Psychologist, 43*, 694–702.

Mullen, E. J. (1983). Personal practice models. In A. Rosenblatt & D. Waldfogel (Eds.), *Handbook of clinical social work* (pp. 623–649). San Francisco: Jossey-Bass.

Mullen, E. J. (1985). Methodological dilemmas in social work research. *Social Work Research & Abstracts, 21*, 12–20.

Mullen, E. J. (1988). Constructing personal practice models. In R. M. Grinnell (Ed.), *Social work research and evaluation* (pp. 503–533). Itasca, IL: Peacock.

Nelsen, J. (1993). Testing practice wisdom: Another use for single-system research. *Journal of Social Service Research, 18*, 65–82.

Neuman, L. H. (1995). *Social research methods*. Boston: Allyn & Bacon.

Parton, N. (2000). Some thoughts on the relationship between theory and practice in and for social work. *British Journal of Social Work, 30*, 449–463.

Reid, W. J. (1994). The empirical practice movement. *Social Service Review, 68*, 165–184.

Reid, W. J., & Bailey-Dempsey, C. (1994). Content analysis in design and development. *Research on Social Work Practice, 4*, 101–114.

Reid, W. J., & Epstein, L. (1977). *Task centered practice*. New York: Columbia University Press.

Reid, W. J., & Smith, A. D. (1989). *Research in social work*. New York: Columbia University Press.

Rosen, A. (1992). Facilitating clinical decision making and evaluation. *Families in Society: The Journal of Contemporary Human Services, 73*, 522–530.

Rosen, A. (1994). Knowledge use in direct practice. *Social Service Review, 68*, 561–577.

Rosen, A., & Proctor, E. (1978). Specifying the treatment process: The basis for effectiveness research. *Journal of Social Service Research, 2*, 25–43.

Rosen, A., & Proctor, E. (2003). *Developing practice guidelines for social work intervention: Issues, methods and research agenda*. New York: Columbia University Press.

Rosen, A., Proctor, E., & Livne, S. (1985). Planning and direct practice. *Social Service Review, 59*, 161–167.

Rubin, A., & Babbie, E. (1989). *Research methods for social work*. Belmont, CA: Wadsworth.

Ruckdeschel, R. A. (1985). Qualitative research as perspective. *Social Work Research & Abstracts, 21*(2), 17–21.

Schon, D. (1983). *The reflective practitioner*. New York: Basic Books Inc.

Scott, D. (1990). Practice wisdom: The neglected source of practice research. *Social Work, 35*, 564–568.

Wills, R. S., Faitler, S., & Snyder, D. K. (1987). Distinctiveness of behavioral vs. insight-oriented marital therapy: An empirical analysis. *Journal of Consulting and Clinical Psychology, 55*, 685–690.

Zeira, A. (2000). Generating empirical knowledge on the basis of practice wisdom. *Society and Welfare, 20*, 265–290 (Hebrew).

Zeira, A. (2004). New initiatives in out-of-home placements in Israel. *Child and Family Social Work, 9*, 305–307.

Zeira, A., & Rosen, A. (1999). Intermediate outcomes pursued by practitioners: A qualitative analysis. *Social Work Research, 23*, 79–87.

Zeira, A., & Rosen, A. (2000). Unraveling "tacit knowledge": What social workers do and why they do it. *Social Service Review, 74*, 103–123.

Zeira, A., Canali, C., Vecchiato, T., Jergeby, U., Thoburn, J., & Neve, E. (2008). Evidence-based social work practice with children and families: A cross national perspective. *European Journal of Social Work, 11*, 1–18.

Understanding Child Maltreatment Systems: A Foundation for Child Welfare Policy

Barbara Fallon, Nico Trocmé, John Fluke, Bruce MacLaurin, Lil Tonmyr, and Ying-Ying Yuan

1 Introduction

How many children are maltreated in the population is a subject of debate in the literature. There is agreement only that the true extent of child maltreatment is unknown. The scope of this problem is estimated from self-report surveys or reports to child welfare services and/or police, but many incidents of abuse or neglect are never admitted or reported (Cicchetti & Carlson, 1989; MacMillan, Jamieson, & Walsh, 2003). Estimates indicate that between half to four fifths of all victims of maltreatment are not known to child protection services (Bolen & Scannapieco, 1999; Sedlak & Broadhurst, 1996). The tip-of-the-iceberg analogy easily comes to mind when one thinks of the scope of child maltreatment (Sedlak & Broadhurst, 1996; Trocmé et al., 2005).

The question of how to measure identified child maltreatment is one with which more and more jurisdictions are grappling. Although there are continued efforts in North America to create uniform approaches to the measurement of child maltreatment, there are enormous inconsistencies and variations in definitions used in child welfare legislation and by agency officials and researchers (Runyan et al., 2005). The purpose of this chapter is to focus on the different approaches used to determine the extent of reported child maltreatment in the United States and Canada. These jurisdictions have comprehensive population surveys and administrative maltreatment data available through a number of sources including administrative data and

B. Fallon (✉)
Centre for Research on Child and Families, McGill University, Canada

The CIS is completed by a national team of researchers from University sites, and funded by the Public Health Agency of Canada, with support from the Provinces and Territories. NCANDS is federally sponsored by the Children's Bureau in the Administration of Children, Youth and Families (ACYF) in the Administration for Children and Families (ACF) in the U.S. Department of Health and Human Services, and receives technical support from Walter R. McDonald & Associates, Inc., with assistance from the American Humane Association. The various NIS studies have been conducted by Westat under contract to the US Department of Health and Human Services. The opinions expressed here concerning CIS, NIS, and NCANDS are those of the authors and not of the funders or other groups conducting such studies.

Slightly revised version from *Child Abuse & Neglect: The International Journal,* forthcoming (2009), Elsevier sample surveys. This chapter compares the three major child maltreatment surveillance methods being used in North America to assist researchers and policy analysts with interpreting these datasets as well as help officials from other countries in developing surveillance systems that are appropriately adapted to their needs. Al Kahn was a pioneer in the field of cross-national child and family policy research. His commitment to the rights of children and in particular, the rights of children involved in the child welfare system began with a commitment to collecting and understanding data. This legacy has served as a foundation for this chapter.

Before discussing the three North American child maltreatment surveillance systems, an overview of the key measurement issues associated with the measurement of reported child maltreatment is provided. Self-report surveys are not the subject of this chapter as the focus will be on administrative data and sample surveys in order to assist with the interpretation of the various models. However, self-report survey data are the primary source for estimates of the prevalence of childhood maltreatment and have also been used to estimate the incidence of maltreatment (Finkelhor, Ormrod, Turner, & Hamby, 2005).

2 Key Measurement Issues

Understanding the definitional issues associated with measuring the phenomenon of child maltreatment is essential to understanding the difference in surveillance approaches. One of the difficulties in comparing child abuse and neglect reports is that statistics are rarely presented with enough detail to allow one to consider all the data collection issues and their potential impact on measurement. Maltreatment statistics can vary considerably in the forms of maltreatment being reported. The failure to document multiple forms of maltreatment can lead to underestimating some forms of maltreatment (MacMillan et al., 1997; English et al., 2005) even among reported children. Some measures include only cases where the child has been harmed, while others also consider children maltreated if they are at substantial risk of harm.

Research on rates of child maltreatment can focus on the annual incidence, which is the number of cases in a single year; or on childhood prevalence, which is the number of children maltreated during childhood. At what point a child is identified as maltreated is fundamental to understanding the limitations of data estimating the epidemiology of child maltreatment. Further, many children who are maltreated are not reported or not investigated, and many cases investigated by child welfare authorities are not substantiated (Trocmé et al., 2005; Sedlak & Broadhurst, 1996; USDHS, 2008).

How a child maltreatment event is measured is an important construct when comparing international rates of maltreatment. If provided in the aggregate, child welfare investigations can use either a child-based or family-based method of tracking cases. For child-based methods, each investigated child is counted as a separate investigation, while for family-based investigations the unit of analysis is the investigated family regardless of the number of children investigated. At the child welfare agency/office level, the number of children investigated for maltreatment may be hard to discern depending on the data collection and aggregation methods as children investigated several times in a year are often counted several times, each time as a separate investigation depending on the agency and jurisdiction. Finally, the characteristics of children and their circumstances that are investigated by child welfare authorities varies depending on the jurisdiction. Therefore, at minimum, comparisons across jurisdictions requires that the data be disaggregated.

There are several methods by which child maltreatment surveillance data can be obtained, of which we will highlight two types: professional survey methodology, and administrative data extraction.

2.1 Surveys of Professionals

Surveys of professionals are surveys that are conducted with child protection workers regarding their investigations of alleged child maltreatment. Serial surveys are those that repeat the same questions at different points in time. In North America, two serial studies collect data regarding the extent and nature of child maltreatment using surveys of child protection workers. In Canada, two cycles of the Canadian Incidence Study of Reported Child Abuse and Neglect (CIS-1998, 2003) have been completed, and the results of the third CIS cycle will be released in the fall of 2010. The Public Health Agency of Canada is committed to funding the CIS in 5-year cycles. In the United States, three National Incidence Study of Child Abuse and Neglect (NIS-1979, 1984, 1993) studies have been completed and the results of the fourth study will be released in 2009. Both the CIS and the NIS are examples of serial, cross-sectional surveys. A new sample of children reported to child welfare services is selected for each study. Conclusions about changes in rates and reported maltreatment are made based on a comparison of samples drawn from each study.

2.2 Administrative Data Extraction Methodology

The National Child Abuse and Neglect Data System (NCANDS) is a continuous data collection activity with an annual acquisition cycle (U.S. Department of Health and Human Services, 2008). NCANDS is supported by the US Federal government to collect annual statistics on child maltreatment known to the State public child welfare agency. States submit data on investigations and assessments of allegations of child maltreatment based upon extracts from their adminstrative data systems. Almost all States provide data at the child level. The next section of the chapter describes the specific methods employed for each of these data collection efforts.

2.2.1 Canadian Incidence Study of Reported Child Abuse and Neglect (CIS)

In Canada, most child abuse and neglect statistics are kept on a provincial or territorial basis. However, because of differences among provincial and territorial definitions of maltreatment, and in methods for counting cases, it is not possible to aggregate provincial and territorial statistics. The lack of comparability of provincial and territorial data has hindered the ability of governments and social service providers to improve policies and programs that address the needs of maltreated children. The 1998 Canadian Incidence Study of Reported Child Abuse and Neglect (CIS-1998) was the first study in Canada to estimate the incidence of child abuse and neglect reported to and investigated by the Canadian child welfare system. The Public Health Agency of Canada is committed to continuing a five-year cycle of data collection.

A stratified cluster sampling design is used first to select a representative sample of child welfare offices and then to sample cases within these offices. In 2003, from a total of 400 child welfare offices in Canada, 63 were randomly selected: 55 sites provided detailed information about the investigations and an additional 8 child welfare offices in Québec provided information about the form and substantiation level of the investigated maltreatments. Québec child welfare offices were included on the basis of availability of data from a common information system that was implemented in the province just prior to data collection for the CIS-2003. The fields contained in this system were mapped onto the CIS-2003 questions. While this approach provided a basis for deriving selected national estimates that include Québec, there was not sufficient correspondence between the fields and the CIS-2003 questions to include the Québec sample in all tables.

Cases opened for investigation at the randomly selected sites between October 1 and December 31, 2003, were eligible for inclusion. In several Aboriginal jurisdictions and in Québec, data collection included cases opened in January 2004. This adjustment was made to accommodate late enrolment of some Aboriginal sites and to allow for a data adjustment period in Québec's new information system. Three months was considered to be the optimum period to maintain participation and compliance with study procedures. Consultation with service providers indicated that activity during the study period is typical of the whole year, although potential seasonal effects in the types of cases investigated were not examined. However, an examination of reported maltreatment in a 12-month time frame at a large Canadian child welfare agency revealed that the volume of cases fluctuated but the type of reported maltreatment reported monthly remained consistent throughout the year (Fallon, 2005).

The CIS collects information from child welfare workers about investigated children and their families as they came into contact with child welfare authorities. While investigating alleged maltreatment is the core mandate for most child welfare authorities, situations that are considered to involve children at risk of maltreatment are also opened for preventive services. One of the main tasks of the study research team is to reclassify and evaluate these cases that are opened to participating agencies in different ways, some counting children, some counting families, some cases opened for child behaviour problems. For jurisdictions using family-based case counts, a final case selection stage is required to identify the specific children who had been investigated.

A significant challenge for the study is to overcome the variations in the definitions of maltreatment used in different jurisdictions. Investigating workers are trained by the study team to include investigations that using a single set of definitions corresponding to standard research classification schemes. For example, in jurisdictions that do not investigate allegations of educational neglect, workers are asked to include children in the CIS who were the subject of an educational neglect investigation. Conversely, if a child was investigated because of a behavioural concern and not maltreatment concern, workers are trained not to include that child in the study. Each investigation has a minimum of one and a maximum of three identified forms of maltreatment. Most child welfare authorities do not have a systematic mechanism for tracking new allegations on open cases and therefore new allegations on already open cases are not included.

Two sets of weights are applied to derive national annual incidence estimates. First, results are annualized to estimate the volume of cases investigated by each study site over the whole year. To account for the non-proportional sampling design, regional weights are then applied to reflect the size of each site relative to the child population in the region from which the site was sampled. CIS estimates cannot be unduplicated because annualization weights are based on unduplicated service statistics provided by the study sites. Therefore, estimates for the CIS refer to child maltreatment investigations.

An estimated 217,319 child maltreatment investigations were conducted in Canada in 2003 (excluding Québec). Forty-seven percent of these investigations were substantiated, involving an estimated 103,298 investigated children, for an incidence rate of 21.71 substantiated investigations per 1,000 children. In a further 13% of investigations there was insufficient evidence to substantiate maltreatment; however, maltreatment remained suspected by the investigating worker. Forty percent of investigations were unsubstantiated. This percentage of unsubstantiated cases is similar to or lower than the percentage of unsubstantiated cases reported in most jurisdictions and reflects laws that require the public and professionals to report all cases of suspected maltreatment. Most unsubstantiated cases are indeed reports made in good faith; only 5% of reports tracked by the CIS-2003 were considered to have been made with malicious intent (see Table 8-2 in the CIS-2003 Major Findings Report).

Nearly one third (30%) of all substantiated investigations involved neglect as the primary category of maltreatment, an estimated 30,366 neglect investigations at a rate of 6.38 substantiated investigations per 1,000 children. Exposure to domestic violence was the second most frequently substantiated category of maltreatment (an estimated 29,370 substantiated investigations for a rate of 6.17 per 1,000 children), followed closely by physical abuse (an estimated 25,257 substantiated investigations, a rate of 5.31 per 1,000 children). Emotional maltreatment was the primary category of substantiated maltreatment in 15% of cases (an estimated 15,369 substantiated investigations, a rate of 3.23 per 1,000 children) while sexual abuse cases represented 3% of all substantiated investigations (an estimated 2,935 substantiated investigations, a rate of 0.62 per 1,000 children).

2.2.2 National Incidence Study (NIS)

There have been four cycles of the National Incidence Study (NIS) conducted in the United States: NIS-1 (1979–1980); NIS-2 (1986–1987); NIS-3 (1993–1995) and NIS-4 (2004–2006) (results for the NIS-4 were not available at the time this chapter was written). The NIS includes children who were investigated by child welfare service agencies. The NIS employs the same methodology as the CIS, selecting a nationally representative sample of counties and a three month data collection period. The child protection agency in the sampled county is a key participant, providing basic demographic data on all the children who are reported and investigated during the three-month study period. Unlike the CIS, the NIS also surveys a representative sample of community professionals serving children and families who are likely to come into contact with maltreated children such as police and sheriffs' departments, public schools, day care centres, hospitals, voluntary social service agencies, mental health agencies, and the county juvenile probation and public health departments. Duplicate forms are unduplicated so that each child is included in the database only once. Finally, the data are weighted to represent the total number of children maltreated in the United States and annualized to transform the information from the 3-month data period into estimates reflecting a full year. Including children known to community professionals provides a more complete picture of the scope of child abuse and neglect.

Children identified to the study by non-child welfare sentinels and those who were investigated by a child welfare service professional are evaluated according to two sets of definitional standards: the Harm Standard and the Endangerment Standard. The Harm Standard was developed for the NIS-1, and has been used in all subsequent studies. It requires that an act or omission result in demonstrable harm in order to be classified as abuse or neglect. It is strongly objective in definition but sometimes excludes children whose maltreatment was substantiated as abuse or neglect by a child welfare professional. The Endangerment Standard allows children who were not yet harmed by maltreatment to be counted in the abused and neglected estimates if either a non–child welfare professional considered them to be endangered by maltreatment or if their maltreatment was substantiated by a child welfare professional.

Results from the first three NIS studies conducted in 1976, 1986, and 1993 consistently pointed to significant underdetection of cases of maltreatment known to professionals working with children. The 1993 study found that only one third of cases countable under the study Endangerment Standard had been investigated by child protective services (CPS; Sedlak & Broadhurst, 1996). An estimated 1,553,800 children experienced some form of maltreatment under the Harm Standard during 1993 (23.1 children per 1,000 children), which was a 67% increase from 1986 and a 149% increase from 1980. Using the Harm Standard, in 1993, 13.1 children per 1,000 (an estimated 879,000) were neglected; 5.7 children per 1,000 (an estimated 381,700) experienced physical abuse; 3.2 children per 1,000 (an estimated 217,700) were sexually abused; and 3.0 children per 1,000 (an estimated 204,500) suffered emotional abuse.

2.2.3 National Child Abuse and Neglect Data System (NCANDS)

In the United States, annual maltreatment statistics are reported by the National Child Abuse and Neglect Data System, which is a dataset resulting from the aggregation of state administrative child maltreatment data voluntarily provided by states. The dataset was created in response to requirements of the federal *Child Abuse and Prevention Treatment Act* (CAPTA) legislation in 1988. The stated purpose of NCANDS is to collect and analyze data on child abuse and neglect known to child protective services agencies (U.S. Department of Health and Human Services, 2008).

During the early years, states provided aggregated data on key indicators of child protective services but as of the 1993 data year states began to voluntarily submit case-level data (U.S. Department of Health and Human Services, 2008). As of 2000, the reported data comes from an aggregated data file, which results from the merging of three data sources: the Child File (i.e., case-level data), the Agency File, and the Summary Data Component (SDC). Each state maps data from its own child maltreatment information system to a standard NCANDS layout using supplied guidelines and with technical assistance from the project staff. All investigations or assessments of alleged maltreatment that receive a disposition in the given year are included in the case-level data collection component. The case-level data is structured into a unit of analysis that contains a unique identifier for each child and report, referred to as a report-child pair, which, among other advantages, permits longitudinal analysis of repeat events (Fluke, Shusterman, Hollinshead, & Yuan, 2008). Data are evaluated and validated through both qualitative analysis of items for compatibility and a set of rules used to assess data consistency and evaluate data ranges for accuracy, missingness, and cross-submission reliability. Information collected includes report sources, demographics of the children and the perpetrators, maltreatment types, dispositions of the assessment or investigation, worker and supervisor IDs, risk factors, and services and placements that result from the investigation. In addition, an ID linkage is provided to case-level data on children who are included in data submissions to the federal Adoption and Foster Care Analysis and Reporting System (AFCARS). Data in the Agency File are aggregated and include information regarding children and family funding sources, screened-out referrals, the Child Protection Service workforce, and additional information on child victims and child fatalities (U.S. Department of Health and Human Services, 2008). The NCANDS findings are published annually in a report series titled *Child Maltreatment*. Beginning in 2003 the data were submitted for the U.S. federal fiscal year. The annual *Child Maltreatment* reports based on NCANDS represent the most comprehensive reporting on child protective services by the U.S. federal government. Fifty states, the District of Columbia, and the Commonwealth of Puerto Rico are eligible to contribute to NCANDS. For 2007, 48 jurisdictions provided case-level data, two jurisdictions did not report and two jurisdictions reported using the (U.S. Department of Health and Human Services, 2008).

In the United States, an estimated 3.5 million children were investigated or assessed by CPS agencies in 2007, of which an estimated 794,000 children were determined to have been abused or neglected based on a victim rate of 10.6 per 1,000 children (U.S. Department of Health and Human Services, 2009). Approximately 60% of investigations involved child neglect (436,944 children) or medical neglect (6,759 children). Neglect continues to be the dominant form of maltreatment investigated by CPS in the United States. Physical abuse was noted in 10.8% of cases and sexual abuse in 7.6% (U.S. Department of Health and Human Services, 2009). A relatively large proportion of cases (13.1%) were labelled in a new category, multiple maltreatments, defined as two or more types of maltreatment reported (only those states that reported multiple maltreatment types are included in this analysis).

3 Component Comparisons

Table 1 presents a summary of the key components of the three North American surveillance systems. The purpose of this comparison is to assist researchers and policy analysts with interpreting data from these studies as well as to help officials from other countries in developing surveillance systems that are appropriately adapted to their needs. There are various infrastructure requirements for the CIS, NIS, and NCANDS. The three systems require considerable cooperation and participation on the part of their jurisdictions, agencies, and associated personnel. All three also require federal support in the form of mandates for data collection and financial support. A range of authorities involved with children including any kind of protection service.

The NIS sentinel methodology could be utilized in regions that do not have a formal child protection system in order to derive estimates of child maltreatment known to the social service sector. However, the sentinel methodology has enormous costs associated with the design and data collection phases of the study. The NIS is a congressionally mandated, periodic effort of what is now the Children's Bureau (CB), a unit within the Administration on Children, Youth, and Families (ACYF), within the Administration for Children and Families (ACF) in the U.S. Department of Health and Human Services. It requires not only the efforts of the child protection agency sampled within a jurisdiction, but also the enlistment of schools, police, hospitals, and community agencies. All four iterations of the NIS have been conducted under contract to Westat, whose headquarters is in Rockville, Maryland.

The CIS does not require a well-developed information system as specific details about the child maltreatment investigation are gathered directly from investigating workers. This methodology would also be appropriate for jurisdictions with formal child protection systems but not accompanying information systems. The Public Health Agency of Canada (Government of Canada) provides the majority of the funding for the cyclical data collection with additional support from all provinces and territories in the form of in-kind contributions of agency workers and administrative time and, if desired, oversampling contributions. University-based

Table 1 North American child maltreatment data collection systems

Descriptors	CIS-2003	NIS-3	NCANDS
Methodology	•Survey	•Survey, nationally representative sample	•Extracts from automated information systems
Coded by	•Investigating worker	•Submitted by CPS workers, child welfare sentinel and recoded by evaluative coders	•CPS workers
Level of measurement	•Investigations	•Child	•Investigations of reports •Child-report pair •Child
Number of forms of maltreatment	•Multiple forms, standardized	•Multiple forms, standardized	•Multiple forms; local definitions mapped to standard definitions
Type of maltreatment	•CIS: (5 main types) •Physical abuse (5 subtypes), sexual abuse (8 subtypes), emotional maltreatment (3 subtypes), neglect (8 subtypes), exposure to domestic violence	•Physical abuse, sexual abuse (3 forms), emotional abuse (4 forms), neglect (3 subtypes: physical neglect, emotional neglect, educational neglect), and other	•Neglect, physical abuse, medical neglect, sexual abuse, psychological maltreatment, and other
Child demographics	•Age, sex, Aboriginal status, living arrangements	•Age, sex, race, living arrangements	•Age, sex, race/ethnicity, living arrangements
Levels of substantiation/ disposition	•3 levels defined by study	•2 standards: harm standard and endangerment standard, then cases substantiated/indicated	•Substantiated, indicated, alternative response-victim, alternative response non-victim, unsubstantiated; intentionally false; unknown, closed without a finding; determined by case worker
Severity of harm	•Type of injury, chronicity, need for treatment for emotional and physical harm	•Severity of injury	•Fatalities only
Report makers	•Multiple reporting sources allowed	•Multiple reporting sources allowed; variety of sentinels included	•Professional and non-professional reporters to public child welfare agencies

Table 1 (continued)

Descriptors	CIS-2003	NIS-3	NCANDS
Child functioning	•22 functioning issues captured for all investigated children •Prior reports	•9 child functioning issues for substantiated victims •Prior reports	•Disability, risk factors, prior reports
Parent/caregiver risk factors	•Income, 9 parent factors; also household risks	•Income, 4 concerns for substantiated perpetrators, family structure, family size, residence in a metropolitan vs. rural area	•Risk factors including caregiver disabilities and other risk factors
Perpetrators	•Caregiver or other relationship to child; for non-parent perpetrators know only age and relationship	•Relationship to child, including non-parents, age, sex, employment status	•Age, sex, relationship to child
Receipt of services	•Court, ongoing care, Out-of-home care, referrals made on family behalf, criminal court	•Court, criminal court, service referrals	•Foster care, ongoing services, in-home services, court action
Duplication	•Partially unduplicated, cannot unduplicate annualization	•Each child included only once	•Duplicates included
Agency data	•Size, location, annual caseload, screening practices etc.	•Size, location, annual caseload, screening practices, etc.	•Available on state-by-state basis, number CPS workers, funding sources, preventive services; additional data on fatalities
Number of workers in study	•Yes, also age, education, job status, caseload levels, years experience	•Yes	•Yes
Agency location	•Yes	•Yes	•State and county identified

researchers in collaboration with Government of Canada personnel generate the major findings of the study and conduct secondary analyses.

NCANDS relies upon State departments of child welfare to extract data to a common electronic record format and submit data on each child who has been the subject of an investigation or assessment of alleged maltreatment. Jurisdictions that do not have sufficient person power to develop extracts or who do not have automated information systems provide data through the Summary Data Component in aggregate. NCANDS is federally sponsored by the Children's Bureau in the Administration of Children, Youth and Families (ACYF) in the Administration for Children and Families (ACF) in the U.S. Department of Health and Human Services, and receives technical support from Walter R. McDonald & Associates, Inc., with assistance from the American Humane Association.

3.1 Quality of Information

The CIS and NIS collect cross-sectional data that does not control for the passage of time. There is an unmeasured heterogeneity between samples because the children and families are selected from agencies that are different in each study cycle (Walkup & Yanos, 2005). Caution should be used when comparing changes in rates of reported maltreatment, as there may be important population differences or events that impact the each study cycle. However, the trend data obtained from these surveillance systems reveal important information about the epidemiology of reported child maltreatment without the enormous expense associated with longitudinal data collection. Both the NIS and the CIS demonstrate excellent reliability for whether an investigation was included in the sample or not (Sedlak & Broadhurst, 1996; Trocmé et al., 2005). However, data collected in the three North American surveillance systems are not independently verified.

The CIS collects the most detailed information about the investigated child including information about up to three forms of investigated maltreatment and 22 possible child-functioning concerns. The CIS, NIS and NCANDS gather detailed information about the demographics of the caregivers and possible risk factors. Similarly, the CIS and the NIS collect information about injuries, although both studies do not make estimates about fatalities given their relatively small sample sizes. The CIS documents the type of injury and whether medical treatment was required; the NIS documents the severity of the injury. NCANDS collects information only on fatalities.

NCANDS allows for children to be identified across multiple investigation events both within and across submission years, although only within a state's data rather than across states, and allows for linkages to more detailed placement data available for placed children in the U.S. AFCARS data program. Despite the collection of such detailed information by the CIS and NCANDS, it is important to note that the decision as to whether or not a case meets CIS or NCANDS definitions of abuse is subjectively determined by investigating workers.

3.2 Timely Access to Data

The surveillance systems reviewed in this paper have become integral to providing important context for child protection service provision and monitoring rates of reported child abuse and neglect. The timeliness of the data is an important consideration as the demands on the data from stakeholders are vast. The CIS requires two years from the start of data collection before data are available. Funding of the NIS does not permit regular cycles of data collection. Data for the first three cycles of the NIS study have been available the year after data collection is completed. Annual NCANDS data, which is published in a yearly report entitled *Child Maltreatment*, are available eighteen months after the close of the data collection year.

3.3 Usefulness of Data

Each of the three data collection efforts makes unique and important contributions in describing child maltreatment. The CIS provides an opportunity to examine trends in child maltreatment investigations and changes in child welfare services at a national level and to analyze them in more detail than is possible using current provincial and territorial administrative information systems. Comparisons between 1998 and 2003 data demonstrate the importance of public health datasets like the CIS, as findings from these studies have contributed to policy changes in several Canadian jurisdictions. For example, the findings from the CIS-2003 were used to inform the Children's Aid Society of Toronto's policy concerning children exposed to domestic violence. The CIS-2003 data was also used to inform the "Child Welfare Transformation" in Ontario when the child welfare sector moved to a differential response model. CIS data also supports provincial and territorial efforts to integrate their administrative systems to better learn from the diverse policies and programs that have been developed. Finally, the CIS datasets provide researchers across the country opportunities to examine in more detail the factors underlying changes in reported and substantiated maltreatment (Trocmé et al., 2005). The NIS has similar applicability within a U.S. context as the CIS does in Canada, but is also a somewhat richer dataset in that it includes children known to community professionals who may be experiencing maltreatment but have not come into contact with child welfare services. The large sample size included in the NCANDS dataset and its continuous census collection allows researchers to explore substantive issues, such as what leads to a recurrence of child abuse/neglect and factors that influence access to services, as well as providing data on trends. In addition, the annual report based on NCANDS data is a critical source of information for many activities of the federal government and is used to help assess the performance of several Children's Bureau programs (U.S. Department of Health and Human Services, 2008).

4 Discussion

Our concern with child abuse and neglect, and most research on the problems, derives from cases that have come to light through the existing social agencies. In focusing our attention only on those children readily accessible to study, we are working within a very narrow frame and within entirely too limited a population (Newberger, 1977).

Although Newberger's quotation is 30 years old, it highlights the need to be clear about the limitations of any measurement approach taken to describe maltreated children—the surveillance measurement systems described in this article reflect only child maltreatment identified to the community. One of the challenges in measuring the extent of child abuse and neglect is that the constructs underpinning child maltreatment are constantly evolving. The roots of child welfare can be traced to the enactment of the English Poor Law of 1601 (McGowan, 1983; Schene, 1998; Otto & Melton, 1990; Costin, 1985). This law acknowledged that the public had a responsibility to assist with the care of people who could not care for themselves (McGowan, 1983; Schene, 1998). Any intervention regarding children was limited to the poorest families who were given assistance by the state (Otto & Melton, 1990). A landmark point for increasing societal awareness about child abuse and neglect was the XIV Congress of Forensic Medicine in 1929, during which, Parisot and Caussade presented a paper entitled *On Abusing the Child* (Parisot, 1929). The discovery of child abuse through radiological identification of patterns of injuries in 1946, brought further societal attention to the issue of child abuse (Caffey, 1946). Following the report and publication of radiological evidence of child abuse, Kempe and Steele made their first presentation about battered child syndrome in Chicago in 1961 (as cited in Kempe, Silverman, Steele, Droegemuller, & Silver, 1962). The definition of maltreatment now includes sexual abuse (Tutty, 1993; Wurtele & Miller-Perrin, 1992), neglect (De Francis, 1956; Lapp, 1983; Martin & Walters, 1982), and emotional maltreatment (Brassard, Germain, & Hart, 1987; Thompson & Kaplan, 1993). Most recently, in some North American jurisdictions, the child welfare system has been investigating unprecedented reports of children being exposed to domestic violence (Trocmé et al., 2005).

Given the evolving nature of the identification, detection, and response to child maltreatment, no existing data collection system can represent all maltreated children. The commonalities and differences in the detection and classification capabilities of the three North American surveillance systems are illustrated in Fig. 1. The NIS is able to detect children not reported to a child protection service for abuse or neglect because it includes reports from sentinels. Both NCANDS and the CIS include a "suspected" level of verification, including children whose maltreatment has not been verified but remains a concern.

Although the rate of victimization is considerably higher in Canada than the United States, this difference reflects several important distinctions in the mandate and scope of the two countries. First, the rate of case substantiation is much higher in Canada compared to the United States. Only one quarter (24.9%) of reports were substantiated in the United States in 2005, with maltreatment remaining suspected ("indicated") in another 3% of cases (U.S. Department of Health and Human Services—Administration on Children, 2006), whereas 47% of investigations were substantiated in Canada in 2003, with maltreatment remaining suspected in another 13% of cases (Trocmé et al., 2005). A second and related point is that the rate of

Reported to CPS: Not reported to CPS:

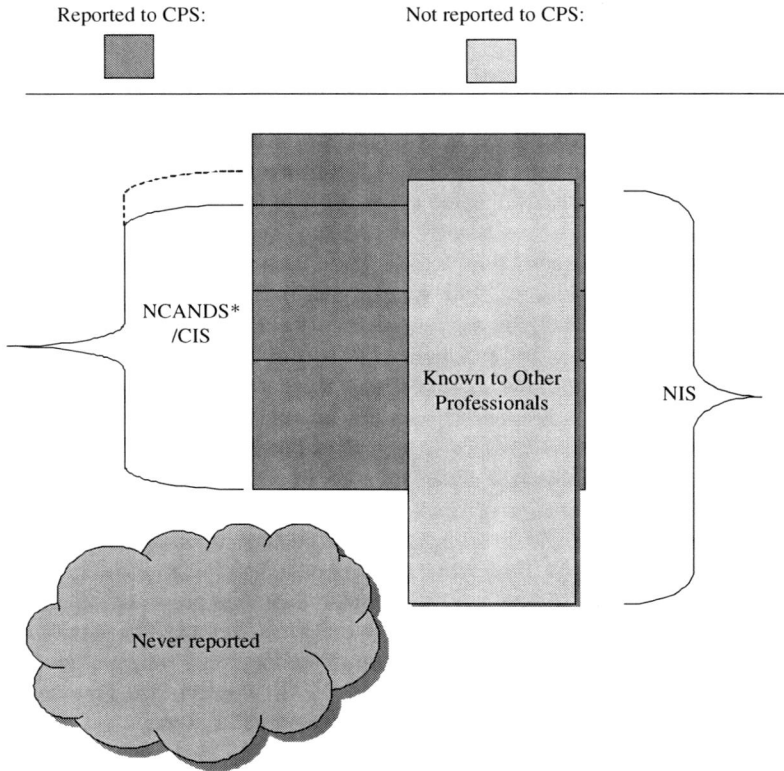

Fig. 1 Comparing North American child maltreatment data collection studies. Adapted from Fluke et al. *NCANDS collects data about screened out cases at an aggregate level

substantiated physical abuse is two and half times higher in Canada, a difference most likely associated with differences in standards with respect to acceptability of the use of corporal punishment. Three quarters of substantiated physical abuse cases in Canada involved inappropriate use of physical punishment (Durrant, Trocmé, Fallon, Milne, & Black, 2009). Third, there has been a major expansion across Canada in cases of exposure to domestic violence and, to a lesser extent, in cases of emotional maltreatment. As a result, the rate of victimization attributed to exposure to domestic violence is nearly as high as the rate of neglect, and the rate of emotional maltreatment is nearly as high as the rate of physical abuse.

5 Conclusion

The purpose of a child maltreatment surveillance system is to provide data on a timely basis in order to inform all interested stakeholders about trends and risks impacting children and families. An effective identification system provides the ability to develop the tools to make strategic funding decisions and target interventions (Wolfe & Yuan, 2001). This paper reviewed three surveillance methods in order to provide sufficient detail to compare their data as well as to highlight the strengths and limitations of each approach for jurisdictions trying to develop a surveillance system best suited to their capabilities. The NIS and the CIS use serial cross-sectional surveys of professionals to estimate the number of children maltreated in the year. NCANDS extracts administrative data on a yearly basis from state information systems. Each approach provides insight into the extent and nature of child maltreatment, which is the foundation for prevention of child maltreatment.

References

Bolen, R. M., & Scannapieco, M. (1999). Prevalence of child sexual abuse: A corrective meta-analysis. *Social Service Review, 73*(3), 281–313.

Brassard, M., Germain, R., & Hart, S. (1987). *Psychological maltreatment of children and youth.* Elmsford, NY: Pergamon.

Cicchetti, D., & Carlson, V. (1989). *Child maltreatment: Theory and research on the causes and consequences of child abuse and neglect.* New York: Cambridge University Press.

Caffey, J. (1946). Multiple fractures in the long bones of infants suffering from chronic subdural hematoma. *American Journal of Roentgenology* 56, pp. 163–173.

Costin, L. B. (1985). The historical context of child welfare. In J. Laird & A. Hartman (Eds.), *A handbook of child welfare* (pp. 34–60). New York: Free Press.

De Francis, V. (1956). Child protective service in the United States: Reporting a nationwide survey. Denver, CO: American Humane Association.

Durrant, J., Trocmé, N., Fallon, B., Milne, C., & Black, T. (2009). Protection of children from physical maltreatment in Canada: An evaluation of the Supreme Court's definition of Reasonable Force. *Journal of Aggression, Maltreatment & Trauma, 18*(1),64–87.

English, D., Upadhyaya, M., Litrowink, A., Marshall, J., Runyan, D., Graham, C. & Dubowitz, H. (2005). Maltreatment's wake: The relationship of maltreatment dimensions to child outcomes. *Child Abuse & Neglect, 29,* 597–619.

Fallon, B. (2005). Unpublished data on seasonal variation and child maltreatment typologies.

Finkelhor, D., Ormrod, R., Turner, H., & Hamby, S. L. (2005). The victimization of children and youth: A comprehensive, national survey. *Child Maltreatment, 10*(1), 5–25.

Fluke, J., Shusterman, G., Hollinshead, D., & Yuan, Y. T. (2008). Longitudinal analysis of repeated child abuse reporting and victimization: multistate analysis of associated factors. *Child Maltreatment, 13*(1), 76–88.

Kempe, C., Silverman, F., Steele, B., Droegemuller, W., & Silver, H. (1962). The battered child syndrome. *Journal of the American Medical Association, 18,* 17–24.

Lapp, J. (1983). A profile of officially reported child neglect. In C. Trainor (Ed.), *The dilemma of child neglect.* Denver, CO: American Human Association.

MacMillan, H. L., Fleming, J. E., Trocmé, N., Boyle, M. H., Wong, M., Racine, Y. A., Beardslee, W. R., & Offord, D. R. (1997). Prevalence of child physical and sexual abuse in the community: Results from the Ontario Health Supplement. *JAMA, 278*(2), 131–135.

MacMillan, H. L., Jamieson, E., & Walsh, C. A. (2003). Reported contact with child protection services among those reporting child physical and sexual abuse: Results from a community survey. *Child Abuse and Neglect, 27,* 1397–1408.

Martin, M., & Walters, J. (1982). Familial correlates of selected types of child abuse and neglect. *Journal of Marriage and the Family, 44,* 267–276.

McGowan, B. G. (1983). Historical evolution of child welfare services: An examination of the sources of current problems and dilemmas. In B. G. McGowan & W. Meezen (Ed.), *Child welfare: current dilemmas – future directions* (pp. 45–90). Itasca, IL: F. E. Peacock.

Newberger, E. H. (1977). Child abuse and neglect: Toward a firmer foundation for practice and policy. *American Journal of Orthopsychiatry, 47*(3), 374–376.

Otto, R., & Melton, G. (1990). Trends in legislation and case law in child abuse and neglect. In R. Ammerman & M. Hersen (Eds.), *Children at risk: An evaluation of factors contributing to child abuse and neglect* (pp. 55–83). New York: Plenum.

Parisot P., & Caussade L. (1929). Les sévices envers les enfants, *Annales de Médecine Légale 9*, pp. 398–426.

Runyan, D. K., Cox, C. E., Dubowitz, H., Newton, R. R., Upadhyaya, M., Kotch, J. B., Leeb, R. T., Everson, M. D., & Knight, E. D. (2005). Describing child maltreatment: Do child protective service reports and research definitions agree? *Child Abuse & Neglect, 29*(5), 461–477.

Schene, P.A. (1998). Past Present and Future Roles of Child Protective Services. *Future of Children*, 8(1), pp. 23–38.

Sedlak, A. (1991). *National incidence study and prevalence of child abuse and neglect: 1988* (rev. ed). Rockville, MD: Westat.

Sedlak, A. (2001). A history of the national incidence study of child abuse and neglect. Retrieved March 27, 2009, from Fourth National Incidence Study on Child Abuse and Neglect web site: https://www.nis4.org/nis3.asp

Sedlak A, J., & Broadhurst, D. D. (1996). *Third national incidence study of child abuse and neglect. Executive summary.* Washington, DC: U.S. Department of Health and Human Services.

Thompson, A. E., & Kaplan, C. (1993). Childhood emotional abuse. *British Journal of Psychiatry, 168*, 143–148.

Trocmé, N., Fallon, B., MacLaurin, B., Daciuk, J., Felstiner, C., Black, T., Tnmyr, L., Blackstock, C., Barter, K., & Cloutier, R. (2005). *Canadian incidence study of reported child abuse and neglect – 2003: Major findings.* Ottawa, Canada: Minister of Public Works and Government Service.

Trocmé, N., MacLaurin, B., Fallon, B., Daciuk, J., Billingsley, D., Tourigny, M., Mayer, M., Wright, J., Barter, K., Burford, G., Hornick, J., Sullivan, R., & McKenzie, B. (2001). *Canadian incidence study of reported child abuse and neglect: Final report.* Ottawa, Canada: Health Canada.

Tutty, L. M. (1993). Parent's perceptions of their child's knowledge of sexual abuse prevention concepts. *Journal of Child Sexual Abuse, 2*, 83–103.

U.S. Department of Health and Human Services, Administration for Children & Families. (2000). The National Child Abuse and Neglect Data System (NCANDS) The Detailed Case Data Component (DCDC) Agency File Record Layout. Accessed March 27, 2009, http://www.acf.hhs.gov/programs/cb/systems/ncands/ncands98/record/record.htm

U.S. Department of Health and Human Services, Administration on Children, Youth and Families. (2007). *Child maltreatment 2005.* Washington, DC: U.S. Government Printing Office.

U.S. Department of Health and Human Services, Administration on Children, Youth and Families. (2008). *Child maltreatment 2006.* Washington, DC: U.S. Government Printing Office.

Walkup, J., & Yanos, P. (2005). Psychological research with administrative datasets: An under-utilized strategy for mental health services research. *Professional Psychology, Research and Practice, 36*(3), 551–557.

Wolfe, D., & Yuan, L. (2001). A conceptual and epidemiological framework for child maltreatment surveillance. In L. Tonmyr & G. Phaneuf (Eds.), *A conceptual and epidemiological framework for child maltreatment surveillance.* Ottawa, ON: Health Canada.

Wurtele, S. K., & Miller-Perrin, C. L. (1992). *Preventing child sexual abuse: Sharing the responsibility.* Lincoln: University of Nebraska Press.

Fact-Based Child Advocacy: The Convergence of Analysis, Practice, and Politics in New York City

Gail B. Nayowith

1 Context

Petitioning one's government for relief, redress or action is as American as apple pie. A government "of the people, by the people and for the people" is at work every day in the nation's Capitol and in State Houses and Town Halls throughout the United States (Lincoln, 1863). Constituents of all sorts take their varied interests to these seats of power in the hope of securing attention and finding solutions to problems that are too big, too vexing or too complex for them to solve alone. State, county and municipal governments make policy on a broad array of issues from taxation and land use to education and public health. This multi-jurisdictional policymaking environment and the amount of policymaking that takes place locally, distinguishes the United States from many other countries.

There are several ways to weigh in on the issues and shape the outcomes of policy decisions in an American democracy. Americans express their preferences by voting with their feet, their wallets and through the ballot. Another way is by engaging in advocacy where Americans rally around causes or issues of concern and hold their elected officials accountable for producing results. On matters of policy and because of the many levels of government acting on policy matters, many Americans do more than vote in elections (National Conference Citizenship, 2009). They find common cause with others and join grassroots and elite civic organizations, action campaigns and movements designed to inform, influence and engage elected officials and government agency staffs as they consider and develop policy, program and budget priorities (Reid, 1999). Our kind of participatory democracy works best when the foot soldiers and the organizations representing them, are organized to act and respond (Cox, 1977).

Children as a demographic are unable to represent their interests directly (Minnow & Weissbourd, 1993). They have neither, direct representation in government as voters do, or a deep-pocket lobby to represent their interests as do large corporations and businesses. While children are the focus and intended recipients of many

G.B. Nayowith (✉)
Laurie M. Tisch Illumination Fund, New York, NY, USA

S.B. Kamerman et al. (eds.), *From Child Welfare to Child Well-Being*, Children's Well-Being: Indicators and Research 1, DOI 10.1007/978-90-481-3377-2_6, government policies, they are not usually the first priority when it comes to budget and rule-making and it often seems as if their best interest and well-being is used as a wedge in debates about national goals and spending (CCC, 2007). As a constituency, children fare poorly when competing for limited resources against other better organized, more active and more capable constituencies (Imig, 1996; Imig & Bryant, 1997).

Parents who might be expected to take a more direct role with government on their children's behalf are stretched, managing duties at home and at work with little opportunity to engage in civic life or the intense participation necessary to influence elected and government officials. Not surprisingly, the business of democracy takes a great deal of time; the one thing most parents do not have. Complicating matters, many parents are unfamiliar with and intimidated by the size and complexity of government and fear government interference or intrusion in family life. The sad reality for most American children is that neither they nor their parents are in a position to voice their concerns about the issues that most affect their lives and well-being: standard of living, health and development, education and safety and security (Kahn & Kamerman, 2002). To combat this lack of representation, voice and influence, concerned individuals have banded together to establish non-profit, independent child advocacy organizations in all 50 states and in a handful of big cities (Voices for America's Children, 2009).

Varying in size, scope of work, reach and influence these children's advocacy organizations have much in common. The most important feature is their singular focus on children's issues and sole commitment to improving child well-being through action that affects policymaking. Other characteristics include being nonpartisan and independent of government funding and free of any constraints that would prevent speaking out on matters of public policy, service delivery or reform. These organizations are governed by Boards of Directors and run by a paid professional staff or paid professional staff in conjunction with volunteers who hold no position or interest in the public, private or non-profit sector that would compromise the organization's ability to be an independent voice in policymaking or in the design, development or implementation of legislation, regulations, programs, budgets or policies for children. By design, independent child advocacy organizations do not provide services directly to children, youth or families, nor are they trade or membership associations. They focus their resources and competencies on state, local or national policy reform in the areas of: family economic security, early care and education, child welfare, k-12 education, physical and mental health/nutrition, juvenile justice/youth development, and child safety (Voices for America's Children, 2009).

This chapter will focus on the experiences of one child advocacy organization, Citizens' Committee for Children of New York, Inc. (CCC), arguably the oldest independent, multi-issue child advocacy organization in the United States, and its efforts to use facts and analysis, education and action in the service of making policies and developing programs and budgets that produce results for children (Citizens' Committee for Children of New York, 2008). In this chapter we will also examine the ways in which two important child policies have been developed, advanced and implemented in New York City—New York City Earned Income Tax Credit and a healthy food supply innovation called the NYC Green Carts. We will focus on the nexus between research and practice and the bridge that connects and reinforces facts, analysis and proposed solutions on one side and advocacy practice, implementation and politics on the other.

2 Why a Focus on Citizens' Committee for Children of New York

What makes CCC's work relevant to this volume is its long association with Dr. Alfred J. Kahn and the role it played in his professional life and development. Dr. Kahn served as Research Director and consultant to Citizens' Committee for Children of New York for 24 years from 1948 to 1972. During his long tenure at CCC, Dr Kahn completed his doctoral studies, was awarded the first social welfare doctorate in New York State and CCC became the most effective child advocacy and policy organization in the United States. His early research on Children's Courts was both the basis for his dissertation and the subject of his first academic writings.

During this period Dr Kahn was resident full-time at the Columbia University School of Social Work (CUSSW) where his seminal work in American and cross-national comparative social policy was focusing his attention on a geography far broader than that afforded by the five boroughs of New York City. Kahn's attempts to resign from CCC to devote himself to his broader interests were repeatedly refused, making him the most reluctant and longest serving staff member in the organization's history. He found himself repeatedly pulled back and lured in by projects that sought improvements in services and opportunities for New York City children. Such is the tension for people like Kahn, advocates by temperament and study, who are tempted by opportunity and drawn to results.

Finally in 1972 Dr. Kahn launched his final attempt to step away from CCC to focus full-time on his work at Columbia. His January 18, 1972 letter of resignation describes his long association and deep affection for CCC. "... I have felt for some time and for many reasons that my activity as a CCC staff member ... should end". He wrote of being "... urged ... to continue in connection with one activity or another ..." and he did so, agreeing even in this letter of resignation to continue with work on the Child Welfare Task Force and the Institutional Advocacy Project. His final paragraph expresses the strong hold that CCC continued to have on him after a two decades long association, "I have at various times and in many places in the past expressed my debts to CCC members and staff and my appreciation of what the CCC experience has meant for my professional and personal life. I shall not even attempt to put any of this in writing in this letter ..." (Kahn, 1972).

CCC's response to his letter of resignation acknowledged the role Kahn played as having "... certainly been a major factor in the success of the organization ..." and offered a humorous and light-hearted but still open-ended conclusion to this productive decades long association: "... We are too appreciative ... to permit anything as formal as a resignation to take place. Let's say, then, that we are in a period of transition ... and who knows what the future shall bring? Que Sera, Sera." (Beck, 1972).

In the years that followed, Dr. Kahn's influence could still be felt at CCC where 20 years later his student would become Executive Director, a position I held from 1992 to 2007. This chapter is about policy and advocacy efforts first undertaken by CCC at that time.

3 Facts and Analysis

3.1 Facts Matter

Strong child indicators have the power to convey the conditions of children's lives with precision and accuracy. The data stand in for the unique experiences of individual children. When aggregated into an index or placed in a ranking, child indicator data burst with new meaning, revealing trends, suggesting causation and showing impact. It is impossible for policymakers to imagine the varied and diverse life circumstances of the almost two million children and youth who live in New York City. Yet, this information is exactly what they need when the time comes to makes budgets, design programs or conduct oversight activities. This underscores the need for a reliable dataset organized into a rich narrative of facts that is presented in a way that is easy to understand and use. Reliable, easy-to-understand and use data demonstrates need, tracks progress made and foreshadows challenges ahead. Data is the starting point for making a case about where children stand and what children need.

A credible base of facts is the underpinning of any articulation or identification of a problem, for understanding the genesis of a problem and for proposing solutions (Imig, 1996). Credible data sources are trusted, reliable, accurate, and recurring and they are used by policymakers to improve child well-being. The field of child indicators has exploded, making it more possible than ever to measure and track child and youth well-being. And The Organization for Economic Cooperation and Development (OECD) has launched an initiative to promote the development and use of social, environmental and economic indicators in order to promote evidence-based decision-making through its "Measuring the Progress of Societies" global initiative (Child Trends, 2008). Child Trends reports 37 data and resource sources for child and youth indicators (Reidy & Winje, 2002; Brown, Hashim, & Marin, 2008; Burd-Sharps, Lewis, & Borges Martins, 2008).

Facts do matter, but facts alone are rarely enough to focus policymaker attention or guarantee a policy result. Data, regardless of its potency, doesn't normally galvanize political will or move policymakers to action, rather, constituents and influential people do. It is highly unusual in policymaking circles to be in a situation where facts about child well-being speak loudly enough to be heard over the din of competing information and other distractions. All day, every day, policymakers and their staffs sift through vast and seemingly endless amounts of information streaming in from all quarters and on all subjects imaginable. For policymakers especially, child data must have a practical use to be effective (Nayowith, 1993). This utility can range from pinpointing need among constituent families and identifying service gaps, to assisting with program planning and targeting resources. The strongest child indicators facilitate an obvious match between need and resources. The best child indicators should guide public policy in ways that make life better for every child (Kusek and Rist, 2004).

3.2 Keeping Track of New York City's Children

Citizens' Committee for Children of New York Inc. (CCC) has been keeping data since its founding in 1944. *Keeping Track of New York City's Children* was the natural outgrowth of efforts begun in the 1970s that produced the first *State of the Child* reports in New York City (Lash, 1976). But it wasn't until the late 1980s with the advent of easy-to-use software and affordable computer technology that CCC began building its child well-being indicator database in earnest. The first print edition of CCC's data-book on child well-being, called *Keeping Track of New York City's Children* (Keeping Track) was released in 1993 (Citizens' Committee for Children of New York, 1993). And it wasn't until 2006 that CCC was able to make a printed and an on-line searchable database version of *Keeping Track* available to policymakers and the public.

The more than 400 child and family indicators in Keeping Track are organized around the developmental needs of children. The chapters and on-line version provide data in eight broad categories: basic demographics; health; economic conditions; early care, education and out-of-school time; housing and community life; youth; and, child safety and family support; and is organized geographically by neighborhood (community district, school district, citywide, borough). The data is presented as charts, graphs, tables, rankings, indices and maps to make it easy to understand and use. This format is highly visual and relies on little text or narrative interpretation. Keeping Track reads like a graphic novel with pictures telling the story of progress, risk and vulnerability, disparities, challenges and trends (Gross & McDermott, 2009). An updated version of Keeping Track is released every two years to provide a regular and up-to-date source of data on child well-being. Keeping Track creates a record of fact, measuring over time, the quality of life for New York City children.

Keeping Track follows an open-source format so the formulae and individual indicators used in the calculations as well as the data sources are available in data tables organized by neighborhood. This invites replication, validation and improvement. Keeping Track also includes children's program data on service capacity and utilization and it includes detail on government expenditures for various children's services.

Keeping Track concludes with a unique feature that links problems and solutions. The final chapter offers various community assessment tools including: the return on investment of various preventive services; the elements of effective programs; a fill-in-the-blank graphic on risks to child well-being; a checklist of essential services needed for healthy development and well-being; a guide for assessing the capacity of children's programs to respond to community need; a ranking of communities on a continuum from those with most to those with fewest assets; a checklist of quality standards for child and youth programs; a listing of accredited programs; and, voting data on party registration and voter turnout by community (Citizens' Committee for Children of New York, 2005).

By synthesizing large data sets into basic indicators of social and economic well-being and tracking conditions for children by neighborhood, Citizens' Committee for Children of New York makes it possible for policymakers to locate their constituents and find their own place in the city as a whole. Arranging data geographically makes it possible to show the distribution of risk and opportunities for healthy development.

Keeping Track was intended to serve as the first step in an overall advocacy strategy to increase awareness about the needs of New York City children and to improve accountability among policymakers for progress or failure to improve child well-being. Keeping Track begins policymaking conversations with an accounting of facts on the ground and, because it also tracks expenditures on children's services, it becomes an opener for high-level conversations with policymakers about the relationship between needs and policies, programs and budgets for children.

Harnessing the power of information to propose fact-based solutions and good policy ideas can reduce risks to child well-being caused by poverty, poor health, housing instability, and other threats to child development (United Nations, 2000 and UNICEF, 2007). Data can be used to think big and as a rationale to advance plans for structural and lasting improvements. Keeping Track is used to identify priorities; to frame, motivate and guide policy and service system reform and improvement activities; and, it serves as an evidence base to support budget and policymaking efforts. When used intentionally and with these goals in mind, the data can prompt a rich dialogue about children and about public priorities.

Child indicators like the kind collected in Keeping Track are one way of documenting the facts and conditions in which children live. So too are vignettes; analyses of administrative data on service availability, accessibility, utilization and quality; surveys; focus groups; monitoring reports; photographs and videos; and, fact-finding field research projects. There are many techniques and tactics in the child advocacy arsenal and while good child advocacy always starts from a base of fact, children's interests are rarely advanced with facts alone.

Among the more effective advocacy practices, mass communications has emerged as a predominate form (Greenberg & Weber, 2008). Online communication through viral marketing via direct e-mail and social networks to send alerts, postcards, letters and petitions as well as targeted use of paid advertising and no-cost, earned media coverage enables a farther reach and triggers greater participation in a shorter period of time than more traditional means. Still popular and effective are participatory campaigns and fulfillment strategies that allow individuals to take action and "do something" with other like-minded people whether it's signing a petition, attending a rally or demonstration, testifying at a public hearing, acquiring knowledge at a briefing session, or meeting with and lobbying elected officials and other policymakers (Devane, 2008; Bobo et al., 2001b).

Taken together these two approaches: the use of child indicators and fact-based analysis; combined with effective advocacy practice that informs the public, builds public will and mobilizes public support to influence policymaker priorities, is what is necessary to improve child well-being.

3.3 Politics

Policymakers have come to rely on the data amassed by advocacy and policy organizations to do the research and analysis they haven't the time or expert staff to perform. Policymakers use trusted child advocacy organizations as a go-to resource for the facts and use these channels to gain perspective and points of view that amplify or are different from those customarily offered by service providing organizations, trade groups, labor unions, community, business, faith groups or professional associations. The politics of child advocacy as practiced in city halls, county seats, state capitols and in the nation's capitol, takes various forms but effective child advocacy always emanates from a strong base of data and fact. Using knowledge in the service of making policy means having the facts and understanding how to use them.

But facts are just a starting point in the practice of child advocacy. In order to make, shape or influence policy, the facts have to frame a problem cogently and then must provide a compelling rationale for and route to a solution that is advanced by advocates and implemented by policymakers. The practice of child advocacy marries fact, practical solutions and politics in the service of children and child well-being (Anello, 2005).

Understanding the political process and knowing how to pull the levers of democracy are necessary companions to facts and proposed solutions in any effort to improve child well-being. All policymaking occurs in a political environment and effective advocacy means knowing the shortest distance between the problem and the desired solution and developing a strategy for how to get there (Nayowith, 2007). The policymaking environment offers many opportunities for participation and influence. Effective advocates know how to use and create these opportunities for public participation to advance solutions to the problems that affect child well-being. Strategic approaches include tactics like knowing how to mobilize the community or a constituent group; knowing when and how to engage the media; knowing how to get a public hearing on an issue and using public hearings effectively; understanding how to advance a policy idea through legislation, regulation or litigation. It also means understanding the power of relationships and knowing which policymakers to go to when advancing a children's policy agenda and how to identify, create alliances with and support policymakers willing to champion children. Politics is about relationships, power and compromise. Achieving success for children in the public policy arena is done through the strategic use of community, social and political networks.

Ranking New York City's Communities by Risks to Child Well-Being

POVERTY	WEALTH	HEALTH	YOUTH
Percent of Children Receiving Public Assistance Percent of Children Living Below the Poverty Level Percent of Families with Income below $15,000	Bank Deposits Per Capita Percent of Home Ownership Percent of Luxury Rentals Median Household Income Percent of Families at Self-Sufficiency Standard	Infant Mortality per 1,000 Births Percent of Infants at Low Birthweight Percent of Mothers with Late or No Prenatal Care	Percent of Births to Teens (15-19 Years) Percent 16-19 Years Not in School and Not High School Graduate Youth Arrests for Felonies and Misdemeanors (20 Years and under)
Better since 2003 Worse since 2003	Better since 2003 Worse since 2003	Better since 2001 Worse since 2001	Better since 2002 Worse since 2002

Lowest Risk → Highest Risk

COMMUNITY LIFE	SAFETY	ENVIRONMENT	EDUCATION
Felony Reports per 1,000 Residents / Percent Clean Streets	Consolidated Investigations of Abuse and Neglect per 1,000 Children / Reported Violent Felonies per 1,000 Children	Lead Paint Violations per 1,000 Children (1-4 Years) / Facilities per Square Mile Storing >10,000 lbs. of Hazardous Materials	Percent of Students in Grades 3 Through 8 Who Meet State and City Reading and Math Standards

Better since 2003 / Worse since 2003 (Community Life, Safety); **Better since 2003 / Worse since 2003** (Environment); **Better since 2001 / Worse since 2001** (Education)

COMMUNITY LIFE

Bayside (Q11); East New York (K05); Flushing (Q07); Queens Village (Q13); Rego Park/Forest Hills (Q06);

Riverdale (B08); South Beach (S02); Throgs Neck (B10); Tottenville (S03);

Bay Ridge (K10); Brownsville (K16); Fresh Meadows/Briarwood (Q08); Howard Beach (Q10); Pelham Parkway (B11); Ridgewood/Glendale (Q05);

Sheepshead Bay (K15); The Rockaways (Q14); Upper East Side (M08); Willowbrook (S01);

Astoria/Long Island City (Q01); Battery Park/Tribeca (M01); Brownsville (K11); Canarsie (K12); East Flatbush (K17);

Elmhurst/Corona (Q04); Jackson Heights (Q03); Jamaica/St. Albans (Q12); Sunnyside/Woodside (Q02); Williamsbridge (B12); Woodhaven (Q09);

Chelsea/Clinton (M04); Concourse/Highbridge (B04); Coney Island (K13); Crown Heights South (K09); East Tremont (B06); Flatbush/Midwood (K14); Fordham (B07); Fort Greene/Brooklyn Hts (K22);

Greenwich Village (M02); Lower East Side (M03); Midtown Business District (M05); Murray Hill/Stuyvesant (M06); Sunset Park (K07); Unionport/Soundview (B09); Washington Heights (M12); Williamsburg/Greenpoint (K01);

Bedford Stuyvesant (K03); Bushwick (K04); Central Harlem (M10); Crown Heights North (K08); East Harlem (M11); Hunts Point (B02);

Marine Park/etc. (M09); Morrisania (B03); Mott Haven (B01); Park Slope (K05); University Heights (B05);

SAFETY

Sheepshead Bay (K15); South Beach (S02); Tottenville (S03); Upper East Side (M08);

Canarsie (K18); Elmhurst/Corona (Q04); Howard Beach (Q10); Queens Village (Q13); Ridgewood/Glendale (Q05); Riverdale (B09);

Jackson Heights (Q03); Murray Hill/Stuyvesant (M06); Pelham Parkway (B11); The Rockaways (Q14); Washington Heights (M12); Willowbrook (S01); Woodhaven (Q09);

Fort Greene/Brooklyn Hts (K22); Lower East Side (M03); Unionport/Soundview (B09); Williamsbridge (B12);

ENVIRONMENT

Bayside (Q11); Fresh Meadows/Briarwood (Q08); Howard Beach (Q10); Rego Park/Forest Hills (Q06);

South Beach (S02); The Rockaways (Q14); Tottenville (S03); Woodhaven (Q09);

Bay Ridge (K10); Borough Park (K12); Canarsie (K18); Flushing (Q07);

Queens Village (Q13); Sheepshead Bay (K15); Throgs Neck (B10); Willowbrook (S01);

Battery Park/Tribeca (M01); Bensonhurst (K11); Brownsville (K16); Flatbush/Midwood (K14);

Jackson Heights (Q03); Jamaica/St. Albans (Q12); Morrisania (B03); Rego Park/Glendale (Q05); Williamsburg (B12);

Astoria/Long Island City (Q01); Bedford Stuyvesant (K03); Bushwick (K04); Central Harlem (M10); East Flatbush (K17); East Harlem (M11); Greenwich Village (M02); Lower East Side (M03); Midtown Business District (M05);

Murray Hill/Stuyvesant (M06); Park Slope (K06); Pelham Parkway (B11); Riverdale (B08); Sunnyside/Woodside (Q02); Sunset Park (K07); Unionport/Soundview (B09); University Heights (B05); Upper East Side (M08); Upper West Side (M07); Williamsburg/Greenpoint (K01);

Chelsea/Clinton (M04); Crown Heights North (K08); Crown Heights South (K09); East Tremont (B06); Fordham (B07);

Fort Greene/Brooklyn Hts (K22); Hunts Point (B02); Manhattanville (M09); Morrisania (B03); Mott Haven (B01); Washington Heights (M12);

EDUCATION

Bay Ridge, Bensonhurst (20); Bayside, Douglaston, Little Neck (26); Flatbush, Midwood, Sheepshead Bay (22); Flushing, Whitestone (25); Gravesend, Coney Island (21); Jamaica, Forest Hills (28); Jamaica, Howard Beach, Rockaways (27);

Long Island City, Astoria (30); Queens Village, Rosedale, Holis (29); S. Brooklyn, Park Slope, Sunset Park (15); Staten Island (31); Stuyvesant Town, Upper E. Side (2); Upper West Side (3);

Brooklyn Hts, Downtown, Brooklyn (13); Bushwick (32); East Flatbush, Canarsie (18); Eastchester, Baychester, Co-op City (11); Lower East Side (1); Sunnyside, Woodside, Jackson Hts (24); Williamsburg, Greenpoint (14);

Bedford Stuyvesant (16); Brownsville, Ocean Hill (23); Central Harlem (5); Corona Park, Morrisania, Melrose (12); Crown Heights (17); East Harlem (4); East New York (19); East Tremont, Morris Heights (9); Hunts Point, Port Morris (8); Mott Haven (7); Riverdale, Kingsbridge, Fordham (10); Washington Heights (6);

Policy advocacy is an experiential practice that occurs in real time in the context of a policymaking calendar and processes that are outside of the advocate's control. Good advocates are experiential learners comfortable with risk. They are practitioners who possess a hearty appetite for action and results. Good advocates enjoy the rough and tumble world of policy and politics and the intersection between politics, policy and community needs. Good advocates are steeped in data that they can communicate in ways that move people and policymakers to action. Because of their age and status, children must be represented by surrogates in the lobbies of power. When it comes time for big budget and policy actions, child advocates protect, preserve and advance children's interests.

4 Getting it Done

4.1 Child Advocacy

> ...Americans know that without advocacy, there is no change...Strong evidence supported by strong advocacy leads to good policy...this is not a new story...it is as old as democracy itself (Walker, 2008). For decades Citizens' Committee for Children of New York (CCC) has been at the front lines of advocacy...Before there was UNICEF, the Global Fund for Children or the Children's Defense Fund, There was CCC. CCC created the template for the high performing children's advocacy organization... (Walker, 2008).

Citizens' Committee for Children of New York developed the template for effective policy advocacy in the service of child well-being. Its methods: documenting the facts, educating the community and advocating for change, are now the sine qua non for organizations in the United States and around the world. This framework has three basic components: identify the causes and effects of disadvantage and the barriers to success, recommend solutions, and work to make policies, budgets, and services more responsive to children (Tropman, Lauffer, & Lawrence, 1977, Bobo et al., 2001a).

The organization's materials say it best:
> Since its founding in 1944, Citizens' Committee for Children of New York, Inc (CCC) has convened, informed and mobilized New Yorkers to work on issues affecting children and to serve as champions for children who cannot vote, lobby or advocate on their own behalf to secure the rights, protections and services they deserve. CCC uses a unique approach to child advocacy that marries a tradition of citizen-lead, fact-finding and professional data analysis with the best features of public policy advocacy and citizen action to identify the causes and effects of vulnerability and disadvantage, promote the development of services in the community and work to make public policy more responsive to children. CCC gets policymakers to listen and act (CCC, 2001).

> CCC mobilizes New Yorkers committed to making children a priority; advocates for children by promoting new ideas and offering new solutions; analyzes and monitors programs for children to find out what works and what does not; educates the public and the media about children's issues and reaches out to New Yorkers to raise awareness and capitalize on their desire to do something for children; provides opportunities for New Yorkers to get involved and support programs that reward families who are working hard to make a good life for their children as well as help children in families who cannot; builds networks among civic, religious, and community groups and individuals and organizations who are determined to improve the quality of life for children and families; and, prepares

young people and adults to be leaders and prepares them for volunteer service (Citizens' Committee for Children of New York, 2006).

5 Securing Every Child's Birthright—A Citizens' Committee for Children Campaign

5.1 Advocacy Campaign

Getting government to make big, new investments in the human capital of poor and vulnerable children is not a simple matter. While the data show the deleterious effects of poverty and the interactive effects of poverty and disadvantage, proposals to reduce poverty are often viewed as profligate, paternalistic, overly generous or ill-timed. The main challenge is not whether child poverty can or should be reduced but how to reduce it. There is no shortage of proposals to take on the scourge of child poverty but there had not been a concerted effort to reduce child poverty or increase child well-being in the United States in decades.

To commemorate sixty years of service to New York City children, CCC staff and volunteers spent a study year in 2004, researching innovative ways to reduce risks to children and increase opportunities for success. They sought expert counsel from the best and brightest thinkers in the U.S. and abroad to provide new thinking about poverty, disadvantage and well-being and to offer strategic guidance in an effort to think anew about policies, programs and budgets for children. Charged with thinking big about the issues facing New York City children, youth, and families, participants were asked to frame a 21st century approach to improved child well-being and develop a set of proposals that moved beyond known safety net and social insurance programs to advance structural and lasting improvements in the areas of economic, housing, and developmental security.

A new advocacy campaign emerged from this effort—*Securing Every Child's Birthright*—conceived to harness the power and commitment of New Yorkers and work to ensure that every child is healthy, housed, educated and safe (Citizens' Committee for Children of New York, 2005). The goal of the campaign was to take on the issue of child poverty directly and work aggressively to eliminate the barriers to economic, housing and developmental security that stood in the way of a productive future for all New York City children. Aptly named, *Securing Every Child's Birthright*, the campaign was a call to action to increase the prosperity, assets and capacity of all children; promote housing stability and affordability; and provide early developmental opportunities for young children to grow up healthy, strong and supported by a solid foundation for learning and achievement. To benchmark and track the campaign's impact, CCC committed to holding itself accountable by monitoring trends in child well-being and tracking the number of policy initiatives or reforms initiated or underway that increased the availability of services, supports and benefits for poor or disadvantaged children and improved the material conditions of children's lives.

Securing Every Child's Birthright was born at the intersection of child indicators, politics and advocacy. The data detailed in *Keeping Track*, showed New York

City children making steady progress toward better health, academic achievement and increased safety at home and in the community. It also noted the continuing need to accelerate and amplify this progress and more firmly root improvements in neighborhoods hard pressed by poverty, poor housing and a weak infrastructure of municipal services and supports because it was in these neighborhoods, that child well-being lagged and where the future seemed dimmer for far too many children. The vision behind the *Securing Every Child's Birthright* campaign was a bedrock conviction that a bright future was the birthright of every New York City child.

And because the data in *Keeping Track* was organized in such a way that made it possible to tell which children needed help, where they lived, the kinds of help they needed and what types of assistance was already available, it was easy to imagine building a new advocacy campaign around it. The Preface to the 7th edition of *Keeping Track* issued that year noted, "Harnessing the power of information, fact-based solutions and good ideas can reduce risks to child well-being caused by poverty, housing instability and other threats to child development. The data in *Keeping Track* can be used to think big and to advance plans for structural and lasting improvements in the areas of economic, housing and developmental security to support working families and reduce child poverty, eliminate family homelessness and housing instability, and ensure the healthy development of young children. *Keeping Track* can be used to identify public priorities; to frame, motivate and guide policy and service system reform and improvement activities; and as an evidence base for budget and policymaking efforts." (Citizens' Committee for Children of New York, 2005). CCC committed to using the data in *Keeping Track* "to encourage a rich public dialogue about children and to set new priorities and goals for children through its new campaign *Securing Every Child's Birthright* aimed at ensuring a life of security, opportunity and achievement for every child." (Citizens' Committee for Children of New York, 2005)

It is important to note that the *Securing Every Child's Birthright* effort was a practical and aspirational campaign that advanced a series of proposals and options. It contemplated a sweeping array of child policy and program options, fully aware that some could advance quickly in the rough and tumble arena of local politics, budgets and competing priorities, while others would have to wait and be positioned for later action.

Many notable policy successes emerged from CCC's *Securing Every Child's Birthright* campaign. The first was an early victory, the New York City Earned Income Tax Credit that occurred in 2005 and three years later came a win on food policy and access to nutritious, affordable food (Anello, 2005; CCC March–July 2008). Neither victory came easy. Both required significant effort, resources and each posed its own special challenges. The vignettes distill the experiences of both efforts.

5.2 New York City Earned Income Tax Credit (EITC)

The year 2004 coincided with the 60th anniversary of CCC's founding and the publication of the seventh edition of *Keeping Track*. This edition was released in a post 9/11 climate that found a stronger and more stable city with jobs and tax revenues growing, massive development of residential and commercial properties underway, a record drop in crime and continuing improvement in child well-being. It was against this backdrop—of a city on the move, resilient, expansive and with its eyes on the future-that CCC embarked on an expansive campaign called *Securing Every Child's Birthright* (CCC, 2006).

It was evident in 2005 that the city had come through the recession, had recovered from the cataclysm of the post 9/11 economy and was flush with revenue. It was also clear that a different public conversation was necessary to reflect the new reality of economic growth and the rising fortunes of more New York City households. To this end, CCC created a new wealth index in its data book *Keeping Track* to capture, for the first time, the assets held by New York City residents and provide a basis for comparing the distribution of wealth and concentration of poverty across New York City neighborhoods (Destin, 2009).

The data made it clear that city revenues were strong and this fact was echoed by elected officials who, decided that it was time to reduce the tax burden on New Yorkers. And true to his word Mayor Michael R. Bloomberg, was about to do a property tax reduction to lower the tax rates for individual homeowners and commercial property owners. The prospect of a significant tax cut for property owners opened up the possibility of an extension of tax relief to more New Yorkers, not only those who owned property. The New York City Council, who among other things is the legislative body responsible, with the Mayor, for making the annual budget for The City of New York, had long supported more progressive taxation. CCC mounted a vigorous campaign to champion tax relief and tax benefits for low-income families and worked alongside City Council staff, the city council Speaker Gifford Miller and members of the New York City Council as it countered the Mayor's tax policy proposal with one of its own—the creation of the first local earned income tax credit in the United States.

The idea of creating a local EITC had implications far greater than tax equity although the tax equity argument was very compelling to policymakers at that time. The experience of the federal and New York State EITC's as an effective anti-poverty strategy added to the appeal of a New York City EITC. The idea that a low-wage earning family could supplement their earnings with an annual tax refund was irresistible to policymakers in the City Council and Mayor's Office (New York Times, 2004).

"Every budget has its own narrative", but it's one that follows one simple plotline: "all budgets are the children of politics and the offspring of compromise" and every budget is a statement of public priorities and local conditions (Angelo, 2009; Nayowith, 2009). Never was this more true than in the case of Introductory Number 402, a piece of local legislation sponsored by City Council

Speaker Gifford Miller, along with Council Members Weprin, Martinez, Nelson, Clarke, Gennaro, Katz, Seabrook, Sears and Stewart.

Intro. 402 was introduced by the City Council to reduce personal income taxes by providing an Earned Income Tax Credit (EITC) for New York City residents. When it was adopted, the NYC-EITC was tied to the federal EITC so that when the federal EITC increased in the future, the value of the NYC-EITC would rise too. The NYC-EITC was set at a level ". . . equal to 5% of the Federal Earned Income Tax Credit" with a fixed cost adjustment built in pegged to the federal EITC (New York City Mayor's Office and New York City Council, 2005). In 2005, the NYC-EITC applied ". . . to approximately 700,000 households with incomes under $34,692. These hard working New Yorkers were to receive up to $215 as a result of this credit with 75% of the beneficiaries from households that earn less than $20,000 per year" (New York City Council, 2005).

In signing the legislation the Mayor and City Council noted the importance of the federal and state EITCs in reducing poverty and its deep pleasure ". . . that the City will soon offer this valuable tool in fighting poverty. It is especially helpful to families making the transition from welfare to work. Studies showed that families use this credit for some of their most vital needs. Whether it is used to pay rent and utilities or used to pay for college tuition or job training, the earned income tax credit has helped lift people out of poverty" (New York City Mayor's Office, 2005).

There was one final hurdle once Intro. 402 was approved by the City Council and signed it into law by the Mayor, it had to be approved by the New York State Legislature and Governor before it could be enacted (Kahn & Kamerman, 1998). The Mayor and City Council described this process as follows: " As with the property tax rebate, this local law requires legislative approval from Albany before it can be implemented. By signing this bill today, we ensure that, when Albany does act, the credit will still be available for this tax year." The Mayor, City Council, and Citizens' Committee for Children of New York mounted a campaign that secured approval of its tax package of property tax relief and the NYC-EITC in 2005.

Today more than 800,000 low-wage earning households receive NYC-EITC tax refunds in amounts ranging from $591 annually for individuals to $$6,512 annually for households with more than one child. And these refunds serve the dual purpose of incentivizing work effort by making work pay and increasing household income that improves the material conditions in which children grow up.

5.3 Food Policy and Access to Nutritious, Affordable Food

CCC launched its *Securing Every Child's Birthright* campaign in 2005 to ensure economic, housing and developmental security for all New York City children. By 2006 the campaign had already produced some important results—the nation's first local earned income tax credit NYC-EITC, a child and dependent care tax credit

NYC-CCTC, and the Newborn Home Visiting program reaching 10,000 newborns annually. Three important goals accomplished in as many years. In 2007, CCC chose to move on another element in its *Securing Every Child's Birthright* campaign— policies to improve children's access to healthy, affordable food—a core policy priority in the campaign's developmental security platform.

First, CCC had to "sell the problem and then, it had to sell the solution" (Peterson, 2009). By increasing the availability of nutritious, affordable food in every New York City neighborhood and by promoting better food choices, CCC argued that New York City would be building a strong foundation for children's health, learning and development. CCC forged an alliance with the New York City Department of Health and together they spearheaded a sophisticated campaign to bring fresh produce to New York City neighborhoods known as food deserts— communities with limited or no access to fresh produce—through an innovative program called the Green Cart (New York City Department of Health and Mental Hygiene, 2007). NYC Green Carts capitalized on New Yorkers' familiarity and comfort with street vending as a convenient retail outlet for purchasing food. The idea was to promote this indigenous business model that would add 1,000 fresh produce vendors to sidewalks in the city's most disadvantaged communities that had few grocery stores, farmers markets or other retail outlets for purchasing fresh produce.

CCC completed an extensive review of U.S. food policy initiatives. It conducted community focus groups in Brooklyn and the Bronx to measure consumer demand, surveyed the availability of fresh foods, and tested preliminary policy recommenda- tions. CCC also held a focus group with produce vendors working in more affluent neighborhoods to understand the business model and purchasing, distribution, and licensing constraints, as well as possible incentives that might make it attractive for vendors to sell in less affluent food desert neighborhoods.

CCC mounted an inside/outside advocacy campaign to get the NYC Green Carts on the street. CCC worked inside with the Deputy Mayor for Health and Human Services, Mayor's Food Policy Coordinator, New York City Department of Health and Mental Hygiene and City Council Speaker to introduce legislation to lift the

Table 1 Earned income tax credit eligibility requirements and credit amounts tax year 2008 returns

	Maximum combined credit ($)	Maximum federal credit ($)	Maximum state credit ($)	Maximum city credit ($)	Maximum income ($)
Families with more than one qualifying child	6,512	4,824	1,447	241	38,646 (41,646 MFJ*)
Families with one qualifying child	3,937	2,917	875	146	33,995 (36,995 MFJ*)
Individuals	591	438	131	22	12,880 (15,880 MFJ*)

MFJ: Married Filing Jointly (NYC Department of Consumer Affairs, 2009)

cap on street vendor permits and create a new class of NYC Green Cart vendors who would be licensed and receive permits for the sale of fresh produce solely in food desert communities. And CCC worked outside too, organizing and mobilizing a coalition of over 100 health, housing, anti-hunger, community development, social service and advocacy organizations to support the introduction of NYC Green Carts in needy communities. CCC's coalition held a press conference on the steps of City Hall; engaged and connected thousands of New Yorkers through e-advocacy with elected officials who would be voting on NYC Green Cart legislation; persuaded editorial boards of major newspapers to write editorials in support of NYC Green Carts; and generated dozens of print, radio and television news stories (New York Daily News, 2008).

The major political challenge to overcome came as established food retail interests and trade organizations worried about competition organized and pushed back with a well-financed opposition campaign to defeat the legislation. It also came from City Council members running for office who counted on food retailers to make large contributions to their re-election campaigns. Despite some unpleasantness, CCC and its allies stood strong buoyed by conviction and research evidence that showed the lifelong benefit of good nutrition. CCC and its allies convinced the public, the media and worried Council members that nutrition affects children's growth and development and their ability to learn in school. They succeeded in convincing policymakers that far too many children were deprived of fresh produce and healthy food in a city where everyone should be able to purchase fresh fruit and vegetables.

Working alongside the New York City Department of Health and Mental Hygiene, CCC made the health research and indicator data available in easy-to-understand and use formats (New York City Department of Health and Mental Hygiene, 2008). It showed that poor access to healthy foods was a contributing factor in the growing obesity epidemic and that diet-related health problems disproportionately affected low-income children and families. The data showed that limited access to nutritious, affordable food contributed to growing rates of childhood obesity in New York City and placed approximately 500,000 children at risk of developing significant health problems as adults. Community-level data showed that supermarkets were non-existent or not in walking distance in many low-income communities and that many neighborhoods had few healthy food retail outlets, forcing residents to rely on fast-food restaurants and corner stores with limited food inventory and unreasonably high prices." Data comparing the communities of Harlem and the Upper East Side found that supermarkets in Harlem were 30% less common, and that only 3% of bodegas in Harlem carried leafy green vegetables as compared to 20% on the Upper East Side. The NYC Green Cart legislation would create produce pushcart vending opportunities in neighborhoods where at least 12% of adults reported, to the Health Department, that they did not eat any fruits or vegetables on the previous day' (New York City Department of Health and Mental Hygiene, 2007).

CCC and its allies argued that in food desert neighborhoods ". . . for these children, healthy eating was not solely a matter of personal responsibility or individual taste, nor is a better diet achieved simply by increasing access to emergency food programs or expanding enrollment in government benefits programs. It was a matter of making healthy, affordable foods easily available. In many neighborhoods, purchasing healthy, affordable food requires time-consuming and costly trips—to other neighborhoods. Not surprisingly then, children and families often go without healthy foods—and suffer devastating consequences. Soaring obesity rates, heart disease, and diabetes disproportionately plague residents living in 'food deserts.' " (New York City Department of Health and Mental Hygiene, 2007).

On December 18, 2007, Mayor Michael R. Bloomberg and City Council Speaker Christine C. Quinn proposed NYC Green Cart legislation (Local Law 9) to improve access to fresh fruits and vegetables in neighborhoods with the greatest need. The Mayor and City Council Speaker proposed legislation that would increase the number of food vendor carts that would sell fresh fruits and vegetables only. The carts would be located in neighborhoods throughout the five boroughs of New York City where access to fresh fruit and vegetables was limited. Cart permits would be issued for vendors in specific areas throughout the five boroughs where fruit and vegetable consumption was low. Supported by Council Members Comrie, Rivera, Speaker Quinn, Brewer, Fidler, Gerson, James, Koppell, Palma, Recchia Jr., Seabrook, Stewart, Weprin, Arroyo, Vann, Mendez, Barron, Jackson, Mark-Viverito and White Jr., the NYC Green Cart legislation, called for 1,000 permits to be phased in over two years, and required vendors to operate in designated neighborhoods with the Bronx and Brooklyn getting 500 permits; Queens receiving 250 permits; Manhattan 200, and Staten Island receiving 50 permits. The NYC Green Cart legislation passed in the City Council in March 2008 (New York City Mayor's Office, 2008a and New York City Council, 2008b).

6 Conclusion

The challenge of this chapter was to bridge the divide between data, advocacy practice and policy outcomes in the service of improved child well-being. It traced the efforts of one child advocacy organization Citizens' Committee for Children of New York as it developed a successful advocacy campaign—*Securing Every Child's Birthright*—that used a strong base of facts to identify problems and generate promising policy solutions. It detailed a campaign that coupled analysis and policy development with strategic advocacy to secure legislation and resources. And, it described two significant outcomes of this campaign to improve child well-being: increased access to healthy, nutritious food through the NYC Green Cart initiative and tax policy changes that increased household earned income through the NYC Earned Income Tax Credit.

Although this review strips out much color and detail, it does offer some insight into the relationship between data, advocacy and politics in the service of improving child well-being. Three broad lessons emerge: pick your battles, accept that the perfect is the enemy of the good, and understand what success is (Voltaire, 1764; Patton, 1970; Angelo, 2009). The data describe the conditions in which children live and the totality of their needs. The policy arena never provides ample space for child advocates to take holistic action on all of the facts or issues of concern. In the world of policy and politics, the facts about children bang up harshly against other interests and the full range of policy options, no matter how innovative or laudable, are never given complete consideration. Advocates must consider atmospherics and context as they identify and select policy proposals most likely to succeed and base their work on securing the biggest gains possible for children. It is this in this place where fact, analysis, practice and politics converge.

References

Anello, R. (Personal Communication, February 2005).

Angelo, L. (Personal Communication, March 2009).

Beck, Bertram correspondence with Alfred J. Kahn (Personal Communication, January 18, 1972 and January 31, 1972) 1972.

Bobo, K. A., Kendall, J., & Max, S. (2001a). Organizing models: The underlying structure of organizations. In K. Bobo, J. Kendall, & S. Max (Ed.), *Organizing for social change Midwest Academy Manual for activists* (3rd ed., pp. 62–69). California: Seven Locks Press.

Bobo, K. A., Kendall, J., & Max, S. (2001b). A guide to tactics. In K. Bobo, J. Kendall, & S. Max (Ed.), *Organizing for social change Midwest Academy Manual for activists* (3rd ed., pp. 48–61). California: Seven Locks Press.

Brown, B., Hashim, K., & Marin, P. (2008, November). *A guide to resources for creating, locating, and using child and youth indicator Data.* Child Trends & Kids Count.

Burd-Sharps, S., Lewis, K., & Borges Martins, E. (2008). *The measure of America.* American Human Development Report 2008–2009.

Citizens' Committee for Children of New York, Inc. (2001–2007). *Budget impact analysis.* http://www.cccnewyork.org/publications. Accessed 4 May, 2009,

Citizens' Committee for Children of New York, Inc. (2001–2008). Annual reports. http://wwwcccnewyork.org/publications. Accessed 4 May, 2009.

Citizens' Committee for Children of New York, Inc. (1993–2008). *Keeping track of New York City's children* (Editions 1–8). New York: Citizens's Committee for Children of New York, Inc.

Cox, F. M. (1977). Exercising influence. In F. M. Cox, J. L. Erlich, J. Rothman, & J. E. Tropman (Eds.), *Tactics and techniques of community practice* (pp.195–198). Itasca, IL: Peacock.

Destin, M. (2009). *Assets, inequality, and the transition to adulthood: An analysis of the Panel Study of income dynamics.* The Aspen Institute Initiative on Financial Security Issue Brief, March 2009.

Devane, T. (2008). High-leverage ideas and actions you can use to shape the future. In P. Holman, T. Devane, & S. Cady (Eds.), *The change handbook: The definitive resource on today's best methods for engaging whole systems* (pp. 620–632). San Francisco: Berret-Koehler Publishers.

Greenberg, E. H., & Weber, K. (2008). *Generation we: how millennial youth are taking over America and changing our world forever.* Accessed fall, 2008, http://gen-we.com.Pdf

Gross, K. S., & McDermott, P. A. (2009). Use of city archival data to inform dimensional structure of neighborhoods. *Journal of Urban Health, Bulletin of the New Academy of Medicine, 86*(2),161–182.

Kusek, J. Z., & Rist, R. C. (2004). *Ten steps to results-based monitoring and evaluation systems.* The World Bank 2004.

Imig, D. (1996). Advocacy by proxy: The children's lobby in American politics. *Journal of Children and Poverty, 2*(1), 31–49.

Imig, D., & Bryant, K. (1997). The Children's crusaders: Public interest advocacy and policy agendas for children. *Presentation annual meeting of the American Political Science Association.* Washington DC, August 28–31.

Kahn, A. J., & Kamerman, S. B. (2002). *Beyond child poverty: The social exclusion of children.* New York: The Institute for Child and Family Policy at Columbia University.

Kahn, A. J., & Kamerman, S. B. (1998). *Big cities in the welfare transition.* New York: Cross-National Studies in Research Program Columbia University School of Social Work.

Lash, T. (1976/1980). *State of the child New York City I and II.* New York: Foundation for Child Development.

Lincoln, A. (1863). *The Gettysburg Address.* November 19, 1863.

Minnow, M., & Weissbourd, R. (1993). Social movements for children. *Daedalus: Journal of the American Academy of Arts and Sciences, 122*(1) pp. 1–23.

National Conference on Citizenship in association with CIRCLE and Seguaro Seminar (2006). *America's Civic Health Index: Broken engagement.* http://www.ncoc.net/index. php?tray=content&tid=top5&cid=279. Accessed 4 May 2009.

Nayowith, G.B. (Personal Communication, June 1993).

New York City Mayor's Office and New York City Council, Press Release, June 2005.

New York City Department of Health and Mental Hygiene. (2007).

New York City Mayor's Office. NYC Green Carts. (2008a). http://www.nyc.gov/html/doh/ html/cdp/cdp_pan_green_carts.shtml

New York City Council. NYC Green Carts. (2008b). http://www.council.nyc.gov/html/releases/ 011_022708_prestated_greencarts.shtml. Release 011-2008.

New York Daily News. (2008).

New York City Department of Consumer Affairs Office of Financial Empowerment. (2009). New York City Earned Income Tax Credit. http://www.nyc.gov/html/ofe/html/ poverty/taxcredit.shtml

New York City Department of Health and Mental Hygiene (2008). Green Carts. http://www. nyc.gov/html/doh/html/cdp/cdp_pan_green_carts.shtml

New York Times. (2004). Mike McIntyle & Jennifer Steinhauer. Budge Deal Gives City HomeOwner, Tax Rebate, June 22.

Patton, C. V. (1970). Being roughly right rather than precisely wrong: Teaching quick analysis in planning curricula. In J. Rothman, J. L. Ehrlich, & J. E. Tropman, (Eds.), *Strategies of community intervention* (pp. 297–307). Itasca, IL: Peacock.

Peterson, P. (2009). *Common Sense California.* In an e-mail communication 1/6/09 to NCDD-Discussion ListServ.

Reid, E. (1999, December 13–14). Perspectives on child advocacy. *The roles of Child Advocacy Organizations in addressing policy issues conference papers.* Washington DC: The Urban Institute.

Reidy, M., & Winje, C. (2002). *Youth indicator initiatives in states.* Chicago: Chapin Hall Center for Children at the University of Chicago.

The Child Indicator: The Child, Youth and Families Indicators Newsletter (2008, Spring). OECD's "Measuring the progress of societies" global project. *The Child Indicator.* Publication # 2008–17, Vol. 8, Issue No. 1, Vol. 8. 9(1).

Tropman, J. E., Lauffer A., & Lawrence, W. (1977). A guide to advocacy. In F. M. Cox, J. L. Erlich, J. Rothman, & J. E. Tropman (Eds.), *Tactics and techniques of community practice* (pp. 199–207). Itasca IL: Peacock.

United Nations. (2000). *Millennium development goals UN millennium summit.* http://www. endpoverty2015.org/goals. Accessed 9 May, 2008.

UNICEF. (2007). Progress for children. *A World Fit for Children Statistical Review,* Number 6 December.

Voices for America's Children. (2009). http://wwww.voices.org

Voltaire (*François-Marie Arouet* 1764). (Le Mieux est l'ennemidu bien) http://en.wikiquote. org/wiki/Voltaire

Walker, D. (2008, October 21). *Inaugural Gail B. Nayowith Lecture.* Celebration Breakfast Citizens' Committee for Children of New York, Inc.

Using Early Childhood Wellbeing Indicators to Influence Local Policy and Services

Claudia J. Coulton and Robert L. Fischer

Indicators are measures of the condition or status of populations or institutions that can be compared over time or between places and groups. In recent years, there has been growing interest in developing indicators at the local level that can reflect on the well being of children and their families in communities. Rather than being seen as the content of government reports, local indicators are typically used as tools for action and important drivers of local policy and programs. Given that much civic action and involvement are local, there is the need to bring the idea of child well being indicators down to the community level that can support civic engagement and child advocacy. Moreover, child policy manifests itself in large part locally through programs, services and institutions. Local indicators can help to shape this policy implementation toward greater effectiveness and equity.

This chapter focuses on the development and application of child well being indicators at the local level, with a focus mainly on the USA context. By local, we are referring to sub-state geographic areas or political jurisdictions such as regions, counties, cities, towns or neighborhoods. Local indicators are also variously referred to as community indicators and neighborhood indicators. The chapter begins with background information on the importance of local context for children and the relationship of community indicators to concerns about child wellbeing within a local context. Next, the chapter reviews a number of methodological issues and challenges that characterize local indicators work. Third, the chapter discusses the infrastructure that is needed to sustain local indicators work, including both producing child wellbeing indicators and seeing to it that they are used to address policy and program. Finally, we provide several case studies that demonstrate how child wellbeing indicators have been developed and applied in selected locales.

C.J. Coulton (✉)
Center on Urban Poverty and Community Development, Mandel School of Applied Social Sciences, Case Western Reserve University, Cleveland, OH, USA
e-mail: claudia.coulton@case.edu

S.B. Kamerman et al. (eds.), *From Child Welfare to Child Well-Being*, Children's Well-Being: Indicators and Research 1, DOI 10.1007/978-90-481-3377-2_7, © Springer Science+Business Media B.V. 2010

1 Rationale for Local Indicators

Local indicators are necessary because there is considerable variation in child well-being depending on where children live. National or state level indicators mask these differences. Indicators in selected locations can reveal groups of children in great distress even when things are generally improving for children overall. Indeed, the existence of inequality of child wellbeing is often starkly revealed when indicators in one community are compared with another or with national or statewide averages. Such differences often provide justification for changes in public policy, program delivery or distribution of resources. Disparities in child wellbeing can guide efforts to mobilize communities to act on improving conditions for children. And local indicators that reveal pockets of concern about child wellbeing can be used to target resources to areas where they are needed most.

The recognition that place matters for child wellbeing has received increased attention in the scientific literature in recent years. Many studies demonstrate that disadvantaged places have higher rates of negative outcomes for children that are of societal concern such as poor school performance, anti-social behavior, health problems and victimization (Coulton & Korbin, 1995; Ellen & Turner, 1997; Leventhal & Brooks-Gunn, 2000). The mechanisms that are responsible for these place-based disparities in child indicators are the subject of a large amount of research and scientific debate (Duncan, Magnuson, & Ludwig, 2004; Entwisle, 2007; Friedrichs, Galster, & Musterd, 2003; Kling, Liebman, & Katz, 2007; Sampson, Morenoff, & Gannon-Rowley, 2002; Shinn & Toohey, 2003). Yet all of the studies point to the fact that child wellbeing cannot be assumed to be uniform and indeed is likely to vary systematically within nations, states and regions.

There are many reasons that child wellbeing may differ by place and these distinctions have implications for the interpretation of local indicators. One possibility is commonly referred to as *selection*, meaning that households with particular characteristics related to child wellbeing either choose or are forced into particular locations (Duncan et al., 2004). An illustration of selection is when families who are constrained by limited economic resources or personal problems locate in distressed neighborhoods. But if selection is the explanation, it is the clustering of these households, rather than the place itself, that is responsible for place based differences in child indicators. Nevertheless, if selection results in differential location of children and families who are at risk, local indicators can be useful in pinpointing those geographic areas of greatest need so that programs and services can be targeted accordingly.

An alternative to the selection explanation is that there are *contextual* effects of place that are responsible for local variations in child wellbeing that are over and above that which can be explained by characteristics of the individual families. For instance, the concentration of poor and minority households has been linked to various community social processes that are deleterious to children. Among these are the lack of mainstream socialization influences, exposure to disorder and crime and low levels of collective efficacy in the community (Elliott et al., 1996; Leventhal & Brooks-Gunn, 2000; Sampson et al., 2002; Wilson, 1987, 1996). The possibility of contextual effects suggests that local indicators of child wellbeing would also include markers for the relevant social processes that have been found to be harmful to child wellbeing. These types of indicators could be used to address policy toward negative community social conditions rather than the children or families themselves.

Places also differ in their *institutional and political resources*. The structure of local governments and jurisdictions are intertwined with power and wealth differentials that favor some locations over others (Dreier, Mollenkopf, & Swanstrom, 2001). In particular, processes of economic and racial segregation deprive low income children and children of color of opportunities because fewer resources flow to the places where they live (Altshuler, Morrill, & Mitchell, 1999; Sampson & Sharkey, 2008). Differences in the quality of public schools, child care centers, youth development programs and other child serving institutions are all markers of place based inequalities in child wellbeing. Thus, indicators related to the effectiveness of child serving institutions become relevant to improving child wellbeing at the local level.

Another reason for place-based differences in child wellbeing relates to variation in the *built environment*. Deteriorated housing, which tends to be concentrated in specific locations, has been linked to poor health and educational outcomes for children (Mueller & Tighe, 2007). Thus, indicators of housing quality and exposure to lead, mold or other signs that child wellbeing may be compromised are useful locally. Aspects of healthy living, such as physical activity and healthy eating, are also influenced by the built environment (Burdette & Hill, 2008; Burdette & Whitaker, 2004; Fein, Plotnikoff, Wild, & Spence, 2004). Locations of playgrounds, parks and safe places to walk can contribute to local variation in indicators of child wellbeing. Similarly, the presence of fast food restaurants and alcohol outlets are aspects of the built environment that have negative effects on measures of child health and development (Burdette & Whitaker, 2004; Theall et al., 2009). Local indicators pertaining to the built environment are useful in addressing these types of influences on child wellbeing.

Finally, the *spatial proximity* of a place to opportunities can be an important factor contributing to disparities in child wellbeing. For example, locations of job opportunities are not uniform, and spatial mismatch diminishes employment success especially for inner city youth who live far away from jobs in the suburbs (Houston, 2005; Howell-Moroney, 2005). Similarly, the distance of children's and families' residences from social services can be a barrier to utilization (Allard, Rosen, & Tolman, 2003; Joassart-Marcelli & Giordano, 2006). Another illustration is the negative effects on health that have been attributed to the lack of grocery stores that carry fresh foods in some low income neighborhoods (Larson, Story, & Nelson, 2009; Rundle et al., 2009). Local indicators of spatial access to resources and services are potentially useful in measuring this aspect of child wellbeing.

2 Conceptual Framework for Local Indicators

The preceding discussion serves to broaden the basis for child indicators at the local
level to not only include direct markers of the health and development of children
and families but also measures of disparities in local context and environment.
This broader view is represented in the diagram in Fig. 1. At the center of the
diagram is the individual child. Local indicator work frequently attempts to measure aspects of health and development for the child population within local areas.
Examples of indicators of this type include measures of school achievement, health
status and health care utilization, youth development, and victimization (Coulton &
Korbin, 2007).

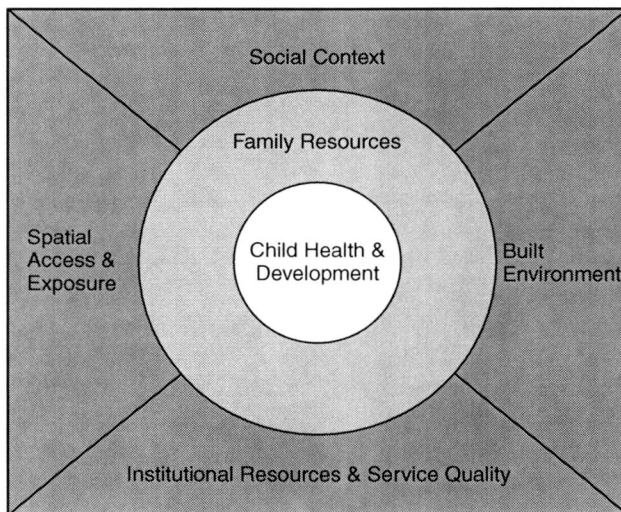

Fig. 1 Schematic for local child well being indicators

Additionally, as shown in the circle surrounding the child, household and family
resources pertinent to child wellbeing are also frequent targets of local indicators
development. Family composition, parental employment status, parent educational
attainment, and poverty status of families, are illustrations of the many indicators
used at the local level. Additionally, indicators of families' involvement with their
children (e.g. daily reading to young children, family meal times) and participation
in the community have been examined in some locales.

As shown in the outer layer of Fig. 1, other aspects of place that directly or
indirectly influence the wellbeing of the child and family are also targets for local
indicator development. At the top of the diagram are measures of the social context in which children live and the resulting influences to which they are exposed.
Examples of local indicators that tap into social context are measures of community violence levels on the negative side and civic participation rates as a sign of

community organization on the positive side. Local indices of the economic or racial segregation of children are markers of potential isolation from the mainstream opportunity structure.

With respect to the built environment, areas where children live can be characterized on the degree to which they promote healthy activities and exposure. Measures of the extent of walkability of the streets or proximity to parks and playground areas are increasingly of interest. The quality of parks and playgrounds are additional aspects of the built environment that should be taken into account (Colabianchi, Kinsella, Coulton, & Moore, 2009). Another measure gaining increased attention is the proximity to food markets with healthy and affordable food (Odoms-Young, Zenk, & Mason, 2009). Environmental hazards, particularly exposure to lead or mold, are additional child wellbeing indicators related to the built environment that are often tracked by local indicators (Edwards, Triantafyllidou, & Best, 2009; Renner, 2009).

Indicators related to institutional and service quality are also important to a broad understanding of child wellbeing at a local level. Sometimes the focus is on inputs, such as per capita expenditures on children's services or teacher student ratios. Other times the focus is disparities in outcome indicators of service quality, such as passage rates on proficiency tests or rates of successful program completion. Equity of access to quality services is also a frequent focus of local indicator work (Hallam, Rous, Grove, & LoBianco, 2009)

Finally, the relative advantage or disadvantage conferred by the spatial locations of children is a relatively novel area for indicator development. However, geographic information systems now make it possible to develop measures based on child weighted distances to important resources such as stores with healthy foods or health clinics, or to potentially negative influences such as alcohol outlets or pollution sites (Freisthler, Gruenewald, Remer, Lery, & Needell, 2007). Such spatial measures promise to provide a more realistic appraisal of how the geographic distribution of children, families, resources and dangers affect child wellbeing within local areas.

3 Methodological Issues

While there is growing interest and utilization of local indicators of child wellbeing, there are a number of methodological challenges that arise in this work. These generally have to do with the fact that local indicators are based on small geographic units and require different data sources than are typically used for national and state level indicators (Coulton & Korbin, 2008; Sawicki & Flynn, 1996).

3.1 Local Area Boundaries and Population

There are 3 types of geographic units that are commonly used for local indicators: Political jurisdictions such as cities, towns or wards; Service catchment areas such as school zones or health districts; or Statistical units such as census tracts or postal codes. In order to track change over time in child wellbeing, or to compare child wellbeing indicators among local areas it is important that these units be stable, mutually exclusive and have sufficient population to support reliable measurement.

One concern at a practical level is that local boundaries may be overlapping or changed over time. For example, the government redefines census geography periodically. School boards change attendance zones as needed. Moreover some statistical units do not have clear or non-overlapping geographic designations. For example, postal codes are for the purpose of delivering mail and do not necessarily have a clear or constant spatial demarcation nor comport with other jurisdictions. The methods for addressing these problems of changing or overlapping geography differ depending on the type of geographic identifiers that are available in the data that are being used to generate the indicators. If the data contain street addresses or latitude and longitude codes, the analyst can hold boundaries constant despite changing or overlapping definitions imposed externally. However, if the data source does not include such detailed geography, but only a census tract or postal code, then an estimation method is needed. For example, if a census tract is divided into two, which is not uncommon in areas where population is growing, the original data from one tract can be apportioned based on the relative sizes of the area to the two new tracts. Nevertheless, it must be remembered that any such estimation methods introduces error.

A second concern is that local units can be of various sizes, but unit size can affect results. This problem is recognized by geographers as the modifiable areal unit (MAUP) problem (Anselin, 1988; Heywood, Cornelius, & Carver, 1998). The MAUP derives from the fact that if the size or number of geographic units is changed, the relationships among indicators measured on the areal units may also change. For example, the correlations between child poverty and infant mortality will differ depending upon whether census tracts, cities or postal codes are used as the units of analysis.

A final limitation affecting local indicators is the problem of small populations and low rates of rare events. Low numbers children in small areas can lead to unreliable estimates. For example, in a given year there will be very few incidents of rare events such as infant deaths in a neighborhood or town. A change in even one death can raise the infant mortality rate markedly without reflecting a true change in health status of the population. A related problem is that population estimates for small areas have less reliability than for large areas. Population estimates often serve as the denominator for local indicators that are expressed as rates. For example, the teen birth rate is typically the number of births to teens per 1,000 females ages 15–19. For rare events, local indicators need to use multiyear averages or groupings of jurisdictions to achieve a large enough numbers so that there is confidence in the estimates. Additionally, various types of shrinkage estimates are possible (Bradshaw et al., 2009).

3.2 Data Sources

While national child wellbeing indicators often come from repeated surveys, data used to craft local indicators have largely come from administrative agencies

(Coulton, 2008). This is due to the fact that surveys seldom have sufficient sample size or are repeated too infrequently to be useful for tracking child wellbeing locally. Examples of administrative records that are used for child indicators include birth and death certificates, child abuse and neglect reports, public assistance records, juvenile court filings, child care records, school records, tax filings, 911 and 211 calls, crime reports, property records and many more. The application of geographic information system (GIS) technology to these administrative records makes it feasible to calculate many indicators for small areas and to display them in ways that are practically useful. However, the use of administrative records data presents some special problems that differ from those familiar to researchers who use national survey data.

Confidentiality: At the national level, government surveys on the status of children are typically released without individual identifying information, making breaches of confidentiality very unlikely. However, local indicators require data sources that contain geographic identifiers, such as the home address or some other precise locational information. Many administrative data sources contain such individual information, but the privacy of the records is protected either by law or custom. Therefore, individuals using administrative records for local indicators need to enter into confidentiality protection agreements with the agencies supplying the data and implement strong safeguards for data security. In addition, care must be taken to prevent indicators that are crafted from these data being used to identify individuals. This can be avoided by requiring minimum cell sizes so that breakdowns by age, race, sex, gender or other identifying information do not inadvertently breech confidentiality within small areas.

Data accuracy: Records from agencies are typically collected by program staff, not researchers. When these records are used to develop child wellbeing indicators, it is important to check with the agency about each data element to make a judgment about accuracy. There may be important sources of variation between agencies or between staff members that need to be taken into account. Moreover, reporting bias is an additional problem in using administrative records data. This arises in situations where an event must be reported in order for an administrative record to be generated. For example, crimes are known to be underreported to the police, and law enforcement jurisdictions differ in their response to crime reports. These two factors can affect whether a crime record is generated and how the crime is classified. Child abuse and neglect reports are vulnerable to similar problems resulting from the biases in reporting and agency response.

Record selection: A complicating factor in using administrative data is ensuring that the correct records have been extracted for the indicator that is desired. Although not always explicit, most measures require that decisions be made about (1) a window of time; (2) whether persons or events are the unit; (3) whether all cases or just new cases should be counted; and (4) how to handle duplicates. For example, a child maltreatment report is an event that involves one or more children. In a given year, the same child may be reported multiple times. Further, a single event may yield several reports. Child maltreatment cases may be carried as open records in the child welfare agency database over several months or years. Such data make it possible to use several different counts for local indicators.

Among the possibilities are: (1) the total number of maltreatment reports in a year; (2) the number of individual children who were reported as maltreated at least once in a year; (3) the total number of maltreatment cases served by the agency at a point in time during the year; and (4) the total number of maltreated children ever served during the year by the agency. In these respects, users need to be clear about exactly how their calculations are made and what the resulting measures mean.

Administrative data are often organized by month, quarter, or year. Most are event driven, generating a record, for example, when a person is eligible for a program, a crime is reported, or a child is born. However, communities may require some measures that reflect the fact that these events happen over time to children or families. For example, birth cohorts can be tracked to determine the proportion that experience a child maltreatment report by a particular age, but this requires matching child maltreatment events across years and merging in birth certificates (Sabol, Coulton, & Korbin, 2004). Probabilistic matching techniques have been successfully used to link records in this way in order to craft local child indicators based on combinations of administrative data sources (Goerge, Van Voorhis, & Lee, 1994).

4 Building Capacity for Local Indicators Work

As the above discussion suggests, it takes considerable investment and effort to develop and implement indicators of child wellbeing at the local level. The necessary data tend to come from a variety of agencies, all of which must be engaged in the process. The records that are used for the indicators often require special preparation and analysis. Because indicators are most useful when they can be compared across time and place, the collection of indicator data and preparation of indicator results has to be sustained and is often at a relatively large scale. It cannot be done effectively without building strong local capacity to collect, manage and analyze the necessary data and interpret the resulting indicators for action.

The National Neighborhood Indicators Partnership (NNIP) is a program that fosters this type of capacity building in the USA. NNIP partners have all built the capacity to use local indicators to address issues of significant social policy concern (Howell, Pettit, Ormond, & Kingsley, 2003). The Cleveland and Des Moines examples provided in the section below come from NNIP partners' work. These organizations work in collaboration with community collaborators to identify key issues of concern. They then craft indicators that enable the community to assess the patterns and take action to address the issues. The indicators become tools to understand the issues, shape the action, advocate for program or policy change and evaluate the success. NNIP organizations serve as information intermediaries in their local communities, where they have built the infrastructure to track social indicators across a variety of domains on an ongoing basis. Nearly all partners include indicators of child wellbeing in some aspect of their work. Information about all of the partners and their work can be found at http://www.urban.org/nnip.

Another fruitful approach to promoting local indicator capacity is the initiation of nationwide collaborative efforts to produce indicators that can be applied to small areas, such as neighborhoods and towns. An example of this being done for early childhood development comes from the Human Early Learning Partnership in Canada (Hertzman, McLean, Kohen, Dunn, & Evans, 2002). This coalition of faculty in universities throughout Canada has collaborated with provincial and local governments to implement early child development measurement on a massive scale so that it can be mapped and tracked by community. A cornerstone of their work is the Early Development Indicator (EDI), applied to the population of kindergarten children. The investments made in the scientific development of this indicator, and the uniform application of it in many schools has enabled communities to take a careful look at this key marker and where they stand relative to other communities or where there are pockets of inequality within their local areas. The indicators have been widely use to address local concerns, advocate for program improvements and expansion, and monitor the results of these actions.

Another nationwide example that is important to highlight is the development of a child wellbeing index for small geographic areas throughout England (Bradshaw et al., 2009). The index covers multiple domains including income, health, education, housing, environment, crime and children in need. Because there are no national surveys that can supply these data for small areas, the index relies primarily on administrative records data. For example, the index for income uses counts of children in households that claim various benefits such as income supports or tax credits. The health indicator combines rates of hospital admissions and disability allowances. Most of the rates are standardized by population estimates for the small areas. The researchers invested considerable effort in determining for each domain the most valid methods for combining the separate measures. Applying these methods, indices for the 7 domains are calculated for small areas in England known as Local Super Output Areas (LSOA), of approximately 1,500 population. Maps reveal that there are concentrations of children at risk in particular cities and regions that sometimes defy the overall national pattern. These indices now have the potential to be used by local governments and organizations to address concerns in their areas.

In addition to building the capacity to generate local indicators, it is necessary to also assure that they will be used in the development of local policies and programs for children. This raises the question as to the degree of readiness among local policy makers and program directors to become more evidence based. Even though national governments and agencies in many parts of the world have begun to mandate an evidenced based approach, this capacity is uneven at the local level. Thus, in addition to seeking specific policies to improve the lives of children, advocates need to include requirements that local indicators be generated to show that the policies are working. To make such promises real, the resources to produce the indicators need to be earmarked and used to build the local capacity to provide this evidence using rigorous and unbiased methods. In this way, child wellbeing indicators become a tool for assuring that local policies to promote child wellbeing are continuously evaluated and improved.

5 Application of Local Indicators to Policy and Program

Despite these challenges, the development and application of local indicators has grown rapidly, in particular since the widespread availability of geographic information system (GIS) tools which have made it possible to manage, analyze and display data for small geographic areas. Local indicators are often key ingredients in shaping the policy debate in cities, counties and states. Constituencies use local indicators to educate their representatives in government about conditions affecting children in their communities. Program directors use local indicators to craft services so that they are responsive to local needs. Advocacy groups use local indicators to mobilize political action around children's issues. And local officials use indicators to inform voters about the value and importance of supporting public spending on systems serving children. In fact, local indicators when broadly endorsed can bring disparate groups together with a common focus on doing what is necessary to move the indicators in a positive direction.

In this section we provide a few examples demonstrating how local child wellbeing indicators are being used to influence policies and programs affecting children and families in their communities. One of the challenges of selecting examples is that much of this work is not captured in the scientific literature or published in widely available reports. Instead it is disseminated in memos, presentations, advocacy briefs, web postings and other report formats that can be produced quickly and targeted directly to the local action agenda. There are undoubtedly many similar applications to the ones we cover here taking place in cities, towns and regions around the world. These two cases were chosen because they were locally generated efforts that have already had clear policy impacts in their communities.

5.1 Towards Medical Homes for Children in Cleveland

A public/private partnership in Cuyahoga County (Cleveland), Ohio, has fielded a set of community strategies targeting the needs of young children and their families. Initiated in 1999, the project (now called Invest in Children) has consciously linked its strategies to a set of child-focused indicators (e.g., child maltreatment rates, health insurance coverage, child care and preschool enrollment) and used these to gauge its progress and modify the efforts of the initiative (Fischer et al., 2008a). As part of this project, the partners sought to ensure health care insurance coverage for all children as well as effective use of health care services including preventive care. The project adopted the term "medical home" to describe it goal. Though it was originally developed specific to children with special heath care needs, it has been expanded to all children (American Academy of Pediatrics, 2007). The medical home reflects a sustained relationship between a family and a primary care physician, so that care has continuity and maximizes the value of preventive care and consultation with a physician (i.e., anticipatory guidance).

An initial set of studies used indicators of health insurance coverage and continuous enrollment in Medicaid/Healthy Start as signs of a medical home. Health insurance coverage was calculated at the percent of children with health insurance coverage based on data from the Ohio Family Health Survey. The sample design of this survey allowed estimates at the local level and, because it was a repeated survey, these estimates could be compared over time. Continuous enrollment in Medicaid was measured by average spell length for children enrolled by year. Medicaid enrollment records served as the data source for this indicator. Tracking of these tow indicators showed that excellent progress was being made on enrolling eligible families and helping them to avoid unnecessary disruptions in their coverage. Cuyahoga County compared favorably with similar counties in the region, and coverage was quite uniform across all neighborhoods and municipalities within the County (Koroukian, Polousky, Fischer, & Coulton, 2005).

However, beyond coverage and enrollment, another indicator of whether young children have a medical home is that they receive the recommended number of comprehensive preventive visits (CPV) with a pediatrician. In order to calculate this indicator, claims and encounter data on the utilization of health care services by children enrolled in the Healthy Start/Medicaid program were obtained from the Ohio Department of Job and Family Services. The claims and encounter records carry diagnosis and procedure codes that make it possible to identify CPVs (also known as well child care). This made it possible to calculate the proportion of newborns continuously enrolled in Medicaid who received the recommended number of well-child visits during their first year of life.

The analysis of utilization of preventive care showed increasing proportions of newborns on Medicaid in Cuyahoga County receiving the recommended number of well-child visits in the first year of life. However, county-wide the rate of success advanced only from 22% of children born in 1999 to 39% in 2003, so even with the progress the majority of newborns were not getting the full number of recommended visits. Data were also examined at the neighborhood level and differential rates of success were apparent based on where children lived.

These findings resulted in two initiatives to increase the prevalence of medical homes among Medicaid children. One effort involved enhanced messaging to parents about the importance of preventive care for newborns. This messaging was comprehensive and coordinated through a range of the service strategies to parenting families, so that parents would receive a consistently reinforced message about the importance of these visits. So, for example, medical home materials were distributed directly to parents by their Medicaid managed care organization, through home visiting programs, as well to parents through regulated child care providers (centers and home-based settings).

A second effort involved exploring tactics for identifying and engaging families before they had gotten off track with their use of preventive care for their infant. During 2006–2007, exploratory work was conducted about programmatic approaches to the issue. Analyses showed that among Medicaid families where the newborn had received no well-child visit in the first four months of the infant's life, 34% were engaged with other community-based services during that same time. This suggested that it would be possible to develop an early warning system so that families that missed a visit could be identified quickly and engaged through an existing relationship of a community agency. Though the concept had merit, it was ultimately determined to be unworkable due to the inability to secure the essential data on well child visits in time to intervene with families.

Another concept that developed in these discussions involved the notion of using dedicated staff to assist parents of newborns in navigating the health care system and maintaining the schedule of needed well-baby visits, immunizations, etc. This resulted in a Medical Home pilot program launched at two clinic locations. The pilot assigned a family liaison to each site to recruit families into the project and to work with them to effectively use preventive and other necessary health care services for their newborn and their family. Further tracking of indicators demonstrated that parents improved their appointment keeping and children received more preventive services, compared to historical controls.

This example shows how indicators selected by community partners can be used not only to monitor change over time but can also lead to the development of new program efforts. Furthermore, the continued tracking of these key indicators lets the partners know if their efforts to improve child wellbeing, in this case defined as having a medical home, actually makes a difference. The identification of key indicators as well as the securing of essential data on selected indicators can be a resource and time-intensive undertaking. Despite this, indicator data can be quite influential in formative decision making at the community level.

5.2 Addressing Lead Exposure in Des Moines

There is clear and convincing evidence that lead poisoning in children has profoundly negative influences on development. Even though this has been recognized for many years and there are successful methods of lead abatement that could nearly eliminate this exposure, many children continue to be exposed to lead in their home environments. Exposure tends to concentrate in neighborhoods built before the prohibition against lead in paint and where the housing is in disrepair. Despite this scientific understanding, many children continue to experience lead poisoning suggesting that policy and program changes are needed at the local level to address this significant problem.

Recognizing that lead was a key factor in disparities in the development of young children The Child and Family Policy Center in Des Moines analyzed indicators of lead exposure among young children in all of that city's neighborhoods (Bruner, 2007). They did this work in collaboration with a consortium of organizations concerned about the fact that many children in Des Moines entered kindergarten at a disadvantage because they were not ready for school.

Two indicators were chosen for this work:

$$Positive\ lead\ screening\ rate = \text{number of positive screenings (in excess of}$$
$$10\,\mu g/dL)/\text{number of children screened}$$
$$Lead\ testing\ rate = \text{number of lead screening tests/population}$$
$$\text{of children 0–5}$$

Data on lead screening results were obtained from the county health department. They were geocoded and analyzed by census tract.

The Child and Family Policy Center produced maps and tables showing the census tracts with highest rates of lead exposure as indicated by positive lead screening rates. These high risk tracts were then compared with one another and with low rate tracts to determine the percentage of children in these tracts that had been screened. They found that testing rates varied considerably and that many tracts that had high positive lead screening rates had relatively low lead testing rates. Even in the census tract with the highest proportion of positive lead screens, only 30% of the child population had been tested. This documented the fact that many children with lead exposure were being missed by the policies and programs that were currently in place. Further investigation showed that simply outreaching to areas with the oldest housing and only testing children that were thought to be at risk by health care providers was missing many children who might be exposed.

The indicators related to lead exposure and testing of Des Moines children were shared with the county health department's lead poisoning prevention coalition. This coalition was made up of a number of groups that had responsibilities related to one or more aspects of the problem, ranging from housing and environmental groups to health care providers to early education advocates. The coalition was convinced by the indicators that the coverage of lead testing was quite uneven, and many high risk children in high risk neighborhoods were not getting tested. Coalition members acted upon the indicators to conduct further investigation of the problem, including identification of some of the barriers to the expansion of testing, treatment, prevention and lead abatement.

Using the indicators related to lead in children, coalition members advocated for several policy changes in Iowa. The fact that the indicators showed problematic disparities in access to lead screening in some of the highest lead poisoning neighborhoods was particularly important in how the policy was shaped. One policy result was that the state legislature passed legislation requiring that all children show evidence of lead screening at the time of kindergarten entry. This now insures that there are full population based indicators of lead poisoning available to monitor the situation and identify areas of concern. Additionally, the department of public health in Des Moines used the local indicators to obtain funding for an ongoing lead screening and abatement campaign focused on the youngest children in the neighborhoods that the indicators showed to be at high risk. By continuing to track these indicators, the community has been able to monitor the impact of these policy changes. Thus far, it is clear that more children are being screened, resulting in early identification and treatment. The increase in the lead abatement programs is resulting in fewer children experiencing lead poisoning.

6 Conclusion

The fact that local areas are unequal along many dimensions raises the possibility that child wellbeing differs markedly by place of residence. Indeed, in many nations or regions there are concentrated pockets of child disadvantage even though on the average child wellbeing in the population as a whole shows positive trends. In order to identify and monitor disparities in child wellbeing, it is necessary to craft indicators that can be practically and accurately applied to small areas. These local indicators for children need to tap the various aspects of inequality such as disparities in social and economic composition of the residents, differential access to resources and amenities, and disproportionate exposure to dangers in the environment.

A local child wellbeing indicator is a measure that stands for something of value. It is not the value or goal itself, but a proxy or sign. Indicators are calculated for multiple points in time and multiple locations so that comparisons can be made. To be useful in local policy and program, indicators need to have some relationship to the perceptions and aspirations of community residents and organizations and to be revealing of where the community stands relative to itself and other communities. Indicators have to be practical. This means that the data needed to calculate the indicator must be available at a reasonable cost and, on an ongoing basis. The indicator itself has to be able to be calculated with reasonable accuracy, although parties within the community may debate the interpretation or meaning. Also, indicators should have implications for action, either to drive change or preserve the status quo.

The use of local indicators for monitoring conditions for children is a major undertaking that promises to have substantial benefits for the communities involved. Such sets of indicators can be crafted to the needs of the local decision makers and augmented over times as new strategies and needs arise. After the initial upfront investment of time and resources in the creation of such capacity, the efforts required to maintain them are proportionally less. This article has illustrated the ways in which specific indicator data related to child well-being have been used by local decision makers to change policies, design programs, monitor progress and enhance community service strategies.

References

Allard, S. W., Rosen, D., & Tolman, R. M. (2003). Access to mental health and substance abuse services among women receiving welfare in Detroit. *Urban Affairs Review, 38*(6), 787.

Altshuler, A., Morrill, W., & Mitchell, F. (1999). *Governance and opportunity in metropolitan America*. Washington, DC: National Academy Press.

American Academy of Pediatrics. (2007). *Joint principles of the patient-centered medical home*. Available at http://www.medicalhomeinfo.org/. Accessed April 25, 2009.

Anselin, Luc. (1988). *Spatial econometrics: Methods and models*. Boston: Kluwer Academic.

Bradshaw, J., Noble, M., Bloor, K., Huby, M., McLennan, D., Rhodes, D., et al. (2009). A child well-being index at small area level in England. *Child Indicators Research, 2*(2), 201–219.

Bruner, C. (2007). *School readiness resource guide and tool kit*. Washington, DC: The Urban Institute.

Burdette, A. M., & Hill, T. D. (2008). An examination of processes linking perceived neighborhood disorder and obesity. *Social Science & Medicine, 67*(1), 38–46.

Burdette, H. L., & Whitaker, R. C. (2004). Neighborhood playgrounds, fast food restaurants, and crime: Relationships to overweight in low-income preschool children. *Preventive Medicine, 38*(1), 57.

Colabianchi, N., Kinsella, A. E., Coulton, C. J., & Moore, S. M. (2009). Utilization and physical activity levels at renovated and unrenovated school playgrounds. *Preventive Medicine, 48*(2), 140–143.

Coulton, C. J. (2008, January). *Catalog of administrative data sources for neighborhood indicators.* Washington, DC: The Urban Institute.

Coulton, C. J., & Korbin, J. E. (1995). Community level factors and child maltreatment rates. *Child Development, 66*(5), 1262–1276.

Coulton, C. J., & Korbin, J. E. (2007). Indicators of child well-being through a neighborhood lens. *Social Indicators Research, 84*(3), 349–361.

Dreier, P., Mollenkopf, J. S., & T. Swanstrom (2001). *Place matters: Metropolitics for the twenty-first century.* Lawrence, Kansas: University Press of Kansas.

Duncan, G. J., Magnuson, K. A., & Ludwig, J. (2004). The endogeneity problem in developmental studies. *Research in Human Development, 1*(1), 59–80.

Edwards, M., Triantafyllidou, S., & Best, D. (2009). Elevated blood lead in young children due to lead-contaminated drinking water: Washington, DC, 2001–2004. *Environmental Science & Technology, 43*(5), 6118–6123.

Ellen, I. G., & Turner, M. A. (1997). Does neighborhood matter: Assessing recent evidence. *Housing Policy Debate, 8*(4), 833–866.

Elliott, D. S., Wilson, W. J., Huizinga, D., Sampson, R. J., Elliott, A., & Rankin, B. (1996). The effects of neighborhood disadvantage on adolescent development. *Journal of Research in Crime & Delinquency, 33*(4), 389–426.

Entwisle, B. (2007). Putting people into place. *Demography, 44*(4), 687–703.

Fein, A. J., Plotnikoff, R. C., Wild, T. C., & Spence, J. C. (2004). Perceived environment and physical activity in youth. *International Journal of Behavioral Medicine, 11*(3), 135–142.

Fischer, R. L., Lalich, N., & Coulton, C. (2008a). Taking it to scale: Evaluating the scope and reach of a community-wide initiative on early childhood. *Evaluation and Program Planning, 31*, 199–208.

Fischer, R. L., Nelson, L., Mikelbank, K., & Coulton, C. (2008b). Space to learn and grow: Assessing early childhood and education in a large urban county. *Child and Youth Care Forum, 37*(2), 75–86.

Freisthler, B., Gruenewald, P. J., Remer, L. G., Lery, B., & Needell, B. (2007). Exploring the spatial dynamics of alcohol outlets and child protective services referrals, substantiations, and foster care entries. *Child Maltreatment, 12*(2), 114–124.

Friedrichs, J., Galster, G., & Musterd, S. (2003). *Neighbourhood effects on social opportunities: The European and American research and policy context,* Routledge.

Goerge, R., Van Voorhis, J., & Lee, B. J. (1994). Illinois longitudinal and relational child and family research database. *Social Science Computer Review, 12,* 351–365.

Hallam, R. A., Rous, B., Grove, J., & LoBianco, T. (2009). Level and intensity of early intervention services for infants and toddlers with disabilities. *Journal of Early Intervention, 31*(2), 179–196.

Hertzman, C., McLean, S. A., Kohen, D. E., Dunn, J., & Evans, T. (2002). *Early development in Vancouver: Report of the community asset mapping project.* Ottawa: Canadian Institute for Health Information.

Heywood, I., Cornelius, S., & Carver, S. (1998). *Introduction to geographical information systems.* New York: Addison Wesley Longman.

Houston, D. (2005). Employability, skills mismatch and spatial mismatch in metropolitan labour markets. *Urban Studies, 42*(2), 221–243.

Howell, E. M., Pettit, K. L. S., Ormond, B. A., & Kingsley, G. T. (2003). Using the national neighborhood indicators partnership to improve public health. *Journal of Public Health Management and Practice, 9*(3), 235–242.

Howell-Moroney, M. (2005). The geography of opportunity and unemployment: An integrated model of residential segregation and spatial mismatch. *Journal of Urban Affairs, 27*(4), 353–377.

Joassart-Marcelli, P., & Giordano, A. (2006). Does local access to employment services reduce unemployment? A GIS analysis of one-stop career centers. *Policy Sciences, 39*(4), 335–359.

Kling, J. R., Liebman, J. B., & Katz, L. F. (2007). Experimental analysis of neighborhood effects. *Econometrica, 75*(1), 83–119.

Koroukian, S., Polousky, E., Fischer, R, & Coulton, C. (2005). Medicaid enrollment and utilization in Cuyahoga County: Evaluating the early childhood initiative amid other health systems changes. *Cuyahoga County early childhood initiative evaluation: Phase II final report.* Cleveland, OH: Mandel School of Applied Social Sciences, Case Western Reserve University.

Larson, N. I., Story, M. T., & Nelson, M. C. (2009). Neighborhood environments: Disparities in access to healthy foods in the U.S. *American Journal of Preventive Medicine, 36*(1), 74–81.

Leventhal, T., & Brooks-Gunn, J. (2000). The neighborhoods they live in: The effects of neighborhood residence on child and adolescent. *Psychological Bulletin, 126*(2), 309.

Mueller, E. J., & Tighe, J. R. (2007). Making the case for affordable housing: Connecting housing with health and education outcomes. *Journal of Planning Literature, 21*(4), 371–385.

Odoms-Young, A., Zenk, S., & Mason, M. (2009). Measuring food availability and access in African-American communities: Implications for intervention and policy. *American Journal of Preventive Medicine, 36*(4), S145–S150.

Renner, R. (2009). Mapping out lead's legacy. *Environmental Science & Technology, 43*(6), 1655–1658.

Rundle, A., Neckerman, K. M., Freeman, L., Lovasi, G. S., Purciel, M., Quinn, J., et al. (2009). Neighborhood food environment and walkability predict obesity in New York City. *Environmental Health Perspectives, 117*(3), 442–447.

Sabol, W. J., Coulton, C. J., & Korbin, J. E. (2004). Building community capacity for violence prevention. *Journal of Interpersonal Violence, 19*(3), 322–340.

Sampson, R. J., Morenoff, J. D., & Gannon-Rowley, T. (2002). Assessing neighborhood effects: Social processes and new directions in research. *Annual Review of Sociology, 28*(1), 443–478.

Sampson, R. J., & Sharkey, P. (2008). Neighborhood selection and the social reproduction of concentrated racial inequality. *Demography, 45*(1), 1–29.

Sawicki, D. S., & Flynn, P. (1996). Neighborhood indicators: A review of the literature and an assessment of conceptual and methodological issues. *Journal of the American Planning Association, 62*(2), 165–183.

Shinn, M., & Toohey, S. M. (2003). Community contexts of human welfare. *Annual Review of Psychology, 54*(1), 427.

Theall, K. P., Scribner, R., Cohen, D., Bluthenthal, R. N., Schonlau, M., & Farley, T. A. (2009). Social capital and the neighborhood alcohol environment. *Health & Place, 15*(1), 323–332.

Wilson, W. J. (1987). *The truly disadvantaged: The inner city, the underclass, and public policy.* Chicago: University of Chicago Press.

Wilson, W. J. (1996). *When work disappears.* Chicago: University of Chicago Press.

Social Policy and the Transition to Adulthood for Foster Youth in the US

Mark E. Courtney

Judging by the amount of attention they have drawn in recent decades, foster youth appear to be an important target of social policy in the U.S.; three times since the late 1980s the Social Security Act has been amended to try to better support the transition to adulthood for foster youth. The most recent amendment, the Fostering Connections to Success and Increasing Adoptions Act of 2008, will provide federal financial support to states that choose to continue to parent young people will into the transition to adulthood. This evolution over time in federal policy arguably reflects a fundamental rethinking of the relationship between the state and the children of the state as they approach adulthood.

In this essay, I briefly describe the U.S. child welfare system in order to put into context the experiences of youth in out-of-home care. I then summarize what the available research says about outcomes for young people making the transition to adulthood from foster care in the U.S., pointing out that the research helps make a compelling case for a policy focus on this population. I describe the evolution of U.S. policy towards foster youth making the transition to adulthood, showing that policy has evolved substantially over the years, and arguing that recent policy developments provide an excellent opportunity to improve transition outcomes for foster youth. Lastly, I comment on the ways in which Alfred J. Kahn's work has influenced and should continue to influence policy and practice directed towards this population.

1 Overview of the U.S. Child Welfare System

According to federal estimates, 510,000 children lived in out-of-home care in the U.S. on September 30, 2006 (U.S. DHHS, 2008a). About half (46%) of these children lived with non-relative foster parents (traditional family foster care), 24% lived

M.E. Courtney (✉)
School of Social Work, University of Washington, Seattle, WA, USA
e-mail: markec@u.washington.edu

Portions of this paper were excerpted from "The Difficult Transition to Adulthood for Foster Youth in the US: Implications for Public Policy," *Social Policy Report*, December 2008.

in foster care with relatives, 17% lived in group homes or other children's institutions, 3% in a pre-adoptive home, 5% were on a trial home visit, 2% had run away from care but were still legally the responsibility of the child welfare agency, and 1% were living in a supervised independent living setting.

Public child welfare programs are operated under the legal framework provided by Titles IV-E and IV-B of the Social Security Act, with Title IV-E providing states with federal reimbursement for a large part of the costs of foster care for children through age 18.[1] Children enter foster care when a public child welfare agency, with the review and supervision of the juvenile or family court, determines that they should be removed from their home in order to protect them from maltreatment and/or dependency. Courts require child welfare agencies to make "reasonable efforts" to prevent placement of children in out-of-home care, such efforts generally consisting of social services provided to the child's family. When the agency and court deem these efforts unsuccessful and the child enters foster care, the court must approve a "permanency plan" for the child according to provisions provided in federal law. The most common initial plan is for the child to return to the care of parents or other family members and the court generally requires the child welfare agency to make reasonable efforts to preserve the child's family of origin by providing services intended to help reunite the child with the family. Often children and youth cannot return home, leading the child welfare agency to attempt to find another permanent home for the child through adoption or legal guardianship.

The vast majority of children in out-of-home exit to what are considered "permanent" placements; of the estimated 289,000 children who left out-of-home care in the U.S. during FY 2006, 86% went to live with family, were adopted, or were placed in the home of a legal guardian (U.S. DHHS, 2008a). A few (2%) were transferred to another public agency such as a probation or mental health department and a few (2%) ran away and were discharged from care.

In spite of state efforts to find permanent homes for children and youth in care, some adolescents reach the point where they are discharged to "independent living," usually due to reaching the age of majority or upon graduation from high school. This is often referred to as aging out of the foster care system since few states allow youth to remain in care much past their eighteenth birthday (Bussey et al., 2000). According to federal government data, 26,517 youth exited care via legal emancipation in 2006, though the data do not distinguish the youth who chose to do so when given the opportunity from those involuntarily discharged due to their age (U.S. DHHS, 2008a). These statistics also do not accurately count the number of young people who leave foster care without the permission of the child welfare agency and court as they approach the age of majority; some youth who are categorized as runaways leave care for this reason and some young people go to live with their family of origin as they approach the age of majority and end up being counted as reunified with their family as opposed to having aged out of care.

---

[1] States are reimbursed for a portion of their foster care maintenance payments (i.e., payments to foster care providers) and allowable administrative costs of the foster care program.

It is worth noting that few young people who make the transition to adulthood from foster care spent the bulk of their childhood in care. A study of youth in care on their sixteenth birthday found that most had entered care since their fifteenth birthday and only one-in-ten had entered care as preteens (i.e., twelve or younger) (Wulczyn & Brunner Hislop, 2001). Nearly half (47%) of these youth were returned to their families at discharge from the child welfare system and more youth experienced "other" exits (21%, mainly transfers to other child serving systems such as the juvenile justice system) or ran away from care (19%) than were emancipated (12%). In short, most teens in out-of-home care enter care during their adolescence and relatively few remain in care until they age out. This means that for most youth transitioning to adulthood from foster care much water had gone under the bridge before they entered care; they generally had spent many years in troubled homes, yet they maintain strong relations with members of their family of origin (Courtney & Dworsky, 2006).

2 Research on the Transition to Adulthood for Foster Youth

A number of studies over the years have tried to assess outcomes for foster youth making the transition to adulthood in the U.S. While this research literature is limited in a number of ways, calling for caution in interpretation (for a discussion of these limitations, see Courtney & Hughes-Heuring, 2005), the findings of these studies suggest that the transition is difficult, to say the least. On average, young people transitioning from care in the U.S. have had poor educational experiences, leaving them with very limited human capital upon which to build a career or economic assets (Barth, 1990; Cook, Fleischman, & Grimes, 1991; Courtney, Piliavin, Grogan-Kaylor, & Nesmith, 2001; Courtney et al., 2005; Festinger, 1983; Frost & Jurich, 1983; Jones & Moses, 1984; Pecora et al., 2005; Zimmerman, 1982). They often suffer from mental and behavioral health problems that can negatively affect other aspects of well-being and these problems are less likely to be treated once they leave state care (Barth, 1990; Cook, 1992; Cook et al., 1991; Courtney et al., 2005a; Fanshel, Finch, & Grundy, 1990; Festinger, 1983; Jones & Moses, 1984; McDonald, Allen, Westerfelt, & Piliavin, 1996; McMillen et al., 2005; Pecora et al., 2005; Zimmerman, 1982). They often engage in crime and become involved with the justice and corrections systems after aging out of foster care (Barth, 1990; Courtney et al., 2001, 2005; Fanshel et al., 1990; Frost & Jurich, 1983; Jones & Moses, 1984; J. McCord, McCord, & Thurber, 1960; Zimmerman, 1982). Their employment prospects are bleak and most live in poverty during the transition (Barth, 1990; Cook et al., 1991; Courtney et al., 2001, 2005; Dworsky & Courtney, 2000; Festinger, 1983; Goerge et al., 2002; Jones & Moses, 1984; Macomber et al., 2008; Pecora et al., 2005; Pettiford, 1981; Zimmerman, 1982). Too many former foster youth experience homelessness and housing instability after leaving care (Cook et al., 1991; Courtney et al., 2001, 2005; Fanshel et al., 1990; Jones & Moses, 1984; Mangine, Royse, Wiehe, & Nietzel, 1990; Pecora et al., 2005;

Sosin, Coulson, & Grossman, 1988; Sosin, Piliavin, & Westerfelt, 1990; Susser, Lin, Conover, & Streuning, 1991). Former foster youth have higher rates of single parenting than their peers (Meier, 1965; Festinger, 1983; Cook et al., 1991; Courtney et al., 2005). Recent research suggests that transition outcomes between ages 17 and 21 are more problematic for males than for females in terms of employment, higher education, and criminal justice system involvement (Courtney et al., 2007a). Interestingly, in spite of separation from their families, usually for many years, most former foster youth rely on their families to some extent during the transition to adulthood, though this is not always without risk (Barth, 1990; Cook et al., 1991; Courtney et al., 2001, 2005; Festinger, 1983; Frost & Jurich, 1983; Harari, 1980; Jones & Moses, 1984; Zimmerman, 1982).

3 The Transition to Adulthood in the US: Implications for Child Welfare Policy

One criterion by which to judge child welfare policy is the extent to which it leads to child welfare practice that is consistent with normative supports provided by parents to their children. By this measure, public policy directed towards assisting foster youth making the transition to adulthood should take into account the kinds of support that young people generally receive during the transition. Researchers have provided evidence that traditional markers of the transition to adulthood, such as living apart from one's parents, completion of education, family formation and financial independence, are all happening later in life than was the case for much of the 20th Century (Settersten, Furstenberg, & Rumbaut, 2005). In general, most young people today do not experience these transitions until their mid to late "20s and many not until their 30s." These developments are associated with an extension of the period during which children are dependent upon their parents for significant care and support. For example, in 2001 approximately 63% of men between 18 and 24 years old and 51% of women in that age range were living with one or both of their parents (U.S. Census Bureau, 2001). Young adults also rely heavily on their parents for material assistance during the transition to adulthood with parents in the U.S. providing roughly $38,000 for food, housing, education, or direct cash assistance from 18–34 (Schoeni & Ross, 2004). Arnett (2004) coined the term "emerging adulthood" to describe the period extending from the late teens through the twenties in which young people engage in self-focused exploration of different possibilities in love and work, though he acknowledges that disadvantaged young people often face challenges during the transition to adulthood that make this experimentation difficult.

Given the extended normative transition to adulthood, U.S. social policy directed towards assisting foster youth in transition arguably should provide states with the ability to continue to serve as parent for foster youth well into their 20s in order to provide support during the transition period. The limited research pertinent to this topic points to the potential benefits of extended support. For example, research indicates that discontinuities in health insurance caused when youth age out of foster care contribute to decreases in health and mental health services utilization (Courtney et al., 2005; Kushel et al., 2007; McMillen & Raghavan, 2009). Research comparing outcomes between young people allowed to remain under the care and supervision of child welfare authorities past age 18 and those that left care earlier provides some evidence that extending care results in improved outcomes in the areas of educational attainment, earnings, pregnancy, and receipt of transition services (Courtney et al., 2007a, 2005). Similarly, a study of alumni of Casey Family Services, a private child welfare agency, that compared young adult outcomes between program alumni that were adopted, exited care prior to age 19, or exited care after age 19, found that extending services past age 19 was associated with better self-sufficiency and well-being (Kerman et al., 2002). Despite the fact that young people in the U.S. are not generally abandoned by their parents at age 18, and the body of research on the potential benefits of extending foster care into early adulthood, states still routinely discharge youth from care at age 18.

4 The Evolution of U.S. Child Welfare Policy Regarding the Transition to Adulthood

In the 1980s child welfare advocates began to push for funding directed towards helping foster youth prepare for adulthood. In 1985, the Independent Living Initiative (Public Law 99-272) provided federal funds to states under Title IV of the Social Security Act to help foster youth prepare for independent living. Funding for the Independent Living Program (ILP) was reauthorized indefinitely in 1993 (Public Law 103-66). The ILP gave states great flexibility in terms of what kinds of services they could provide to Title IV-E eligible youth who were at least sixteen and no more than twenty-one years old, including: outreach programs to attract eligible youth, training in daily living skills, education and employment assistance, counseling, case management, and transitional independent living plans. ILP funds could not, however, be used for room and board. The federal government required very little reporting from states about the ILP beyond creation of state ILP plans (U.S. GAO, 1999). A study by the General Accounting Office found that about 60% of all eligible youth received some type of independent living service in 1998 (U.S. GAO, 1999).

The Foster Care Independence Act (FCIA) of 1999 (Public Law 106-169) amended Title IV-E to give states more funding and greater flexibility in operating independent living programs. The FCIA doubled federal independent living services funding to $140 million per year, allowed states to use up to 30% of these funds for room and board, enabled states to assist young adults 18–21 years old who have left foster care, and permitted states to extend Medicaid eligibility to former foster children up to age 21. An amendment to the law allows Congress to appropriate $60 million per year for education and training vouchers of up to $5,000 per year for youth up to 23 years old.

State performance is a much higher priority under the FCIA than under earlier iterations of Federal policy in this area. The Department of Health and Human Services (HHS) is required to develop a set of outcome measures to assess state performance in managing independent living programs and states will be required to collect data on these outcomes; HHS issued regulations to implement these provisions of the law in 2007. The data requirements include collecting information on transition outcomes from cohorts of foster youth in each state at age 17, 19 and 21. Over time this could potentially build a nationwide longitudinal database on the transition to adulthood, at least through age 21, for foster youth in the U.S. In addition, the FCIA requires that 1.5% of funding under the statute be set aside for rigorous evaluations of promising independent living programs (i.e., using random-assignment evaluation designs whenever possible). The program created by the FCIA is named the Chafee Foster Care Independence Program (the "Chafee Program") after the late Senator John Chafee.

The Independent Living Initiative and Foster Care Independence Act exhibit characteristics that exemplify the philosophy guiding U.S. policy towards foster youth making the transition to adulthood for more than two decades. First, both the names of the laws and their provisions make clear that the primary purpose of federal policy is to render foster youth "independent" or, in other words, to end their dependence on the state. Both laws emphasize what might be called soft services intended to help young people become self-sufficient but prohibit or severely limit the kinds of concrete support for basic needs often provided by families for their adult children; the 1985 law did not allow states to use program funds for room and board and the 1999 law's provision allowing states to use up to 30% of funds for room and board barely scratched the surface of the need for such support (Courtney & Hughes-Heuring, 2005). Second, neither of these laws fundamentally altered the fact that U.S. policy, by ending funding for the foster care program at age 18, encourages states to abdicate their parenting role when young people reach the age of majority. The Title IV-E entitlement to reimbursement of foster care maintenance and administration costs is by far the greatest source of federal funding for foster care; in the absence of IV-E reimbursement beyond age 18 only a handful of child welfare jurisdictions have extended foster care past 18. Once a young person has been discharged from foster care, the state no longer has any legal responsibility to provide the young person with help.

Given this lack of accountability, it is not surprising that significant gaps remain in the safety net for foster youth making the transition to adulthood. Youth aging out of foster care continue to receive relatively little in the way of transition services despite the available research suggesting that many have needs across all of the domains of functioning targeted by independent living programs. Prior to the increase in funding provided by the 1999 law, U.S. government estimates suggested that two-fifths of eligible foster youth did not receive any independent living services (U.S. GAO, 1999). Although the situation appears to have improved somewhat in the wake of increased federal funding, a GAO survey of state independent living coordinators found that large percentages of older youth—up to 90%

in some states—still do not receive many of the services called for in the law (U.S. GAO, 2004). Several years after the new funds became available Courtney et al., (2004) asked 17–18 year old foster youth in three Midwestern states to report on whether they had received support services or training in the areas of educational support, employment/vocational support, budget and financial management, housing, and health education. Depending on service domain, between one-third and one-half of youth reported that they had not received any service in a given domain. The likelihood of service receipt declined significantly after age 18 for those young people who had left care (Courtney et al., 2007a).

That former foster youth often lose access to health insurance at 18 is particularly problematic given their relatively high need for services, particularly mental health services. Perhaps because so few of them retain responsibility for youth over age 18, most states have not taken up the option of extending Medicaid to former foster youth through age 21 (Patel & Roherty, 2007). It appears that in states where the Medicaid extension does not exist most youth exiting foster care find themselves without health insurance (Courtney et al., 2001, 2005). Recent research has shown a relationship between exiting foster care, loss of health insurance, and reductions in health and mental health services utilization (Courtney et al., 2001, 2005; Kushel, Yen, Gee, & Courtney, 2007; McMillen & Raghavan, 2009).

Fortunately, recent developments in federal child welfare policy lay the groundwork for significant improvement in the state's role as surrogate parent for youth making the transition to adulthood from foster care. The Fostering Connections to Success and Increasing Adoptions Act (Public Law 110-351), hereafter referred to as the "Fostering Connections Act", unanimously passed by both houses of Congress and signed into law on October 7, 2008, amends several elements of Title IV-E of the Social Security Act, some of which pertain to older youth. The Fostering Connections Act allows states, at their option, to provide care and support to youth in foster care until the age of 21 provided that the youth is either (1) completing high school or an equivalency program; (2) enrolled in post-secondary or vocational school; (3) participating in a program or activity designed to promote, or remove barriers to, employment; (4) employed for at least 80 hours per month; or (5) incapable of doing any of these activities due to a medical condition. The protections and requirements currently in place for younger children in foster care would continue to apply for youth ages 18–21. Youth ages 18–21 could be placed in a supervised setting in which they are living independently, as well as in a foster family home, kinship foster home, or group care facility. States could also extend adoption assistance and/or guardianship payments on behalf of youth through age 21 if the adoption or guardianship was arranged after the youth's 16th birthday. The Fostering Connections Act also requires child welfare agencies to help youth with the transition to adulthood by requiring, during the 90-day period immediately before a youth exits from care between ages 18 and 21, that the young person's caseworker, and other representatives as appropriate, helps the young person develop a personal transition plan. The plan must be as detailed as the youth chooses and include specific options on housing, health insurance, education, local opportunities for mentoring, continuing support services, workforce supports and employment services. The new law does not alter the Chafee Program, meaning that states can still use Chafee funds for a wide range of transition services.

I now turn to an examination of the opportunities presented by the Fostering Connections Act and limitations of U.S. policy that will need to be addressed if the new policy framework is to realize its full promise.

5 Opportunities and Lingering Challenges

The Fostering Connections Act is a fundamental reform of U.S. child welfare policy directed towards the transition to adulthood for foster youth. It marks a philosophical shift towards acknowledging continuing state responsibility for parenting of foster youth into early adulthood; Title IV-E is the policy and fiscal backbone of the U.S. foster care system and providing IV-E support to age 21 represents a fundamental shift away from the idea that state responsibility for the wellbeing of foster youth ends at the age of majority. The title of the law suggests a move away from an exclusive focus on encouraging youth to be "independent" towards efforts to help youth make the *connections* they will need to be successful during the transition. The law's provisions clearly convey the idea that state-supervised out-of-home care for young adults ought to differ in significant ways from care provided to minors; in order to claim IV-E finding for youth over 18, states will need to engage these young adults in activities that are developmentally appropriate (e.g., higher education and employment) and HHS is required to develop regulations that will allow states to create more developmentally-appropriate care settings for young adults (e.g., supervised independent living arrangements).

Second, in giving states entitlement funding for providing transition-age youth with basic necessities and case management services, the law provides a foundation upon which states can better array a range of services and supports for these youth. While many states at least on paper have policies that call for provision of independent living services through age 21 (e.g., state independent living plans), the poor economic circumstances of youth who leave care and resulting instability of their living arrangements arguably undermine efforts to engage these young people in services. This might explain why Courtney and colleagues (2007) found that foster youth in Illinois, which allows youth to remain in care to age 21, were much more likely than their peers in Iowa and Wisconsin, who were generally discharged at 18, to have received a variety of transition services between 19 and 21. The ability to use IV-E funds to stably house foster youth between 18 and 21 may allow states to better engage youth in Chafee Program-funded services. Giving state child welfare agencies IV-E funding to continue providing case management beyond age 18 may also help these agencies play the kind of coordinating role that is necessary to help young people navigate the various public institutions that should also be engaged in the parenting role (i.e., post-secondary education; workforce development; health and mental health services; housing).

While the Fostering Connections Act creates a Federal policy framework that gives state child welfare agencies the tools to fundamentally change the way that the U.S. supports foster youth in transition to adulthood, several challenges remain in the way of significant progress, including: the probability that many states will not take up the option of extending foster care past age 18; a poor knowledge base regarding the effectiveness of independent living and other transition services; the lack of established and well-evaluated models of coordination between child welfare agencies and other public institutions in providing support to foster youth; the complexities of maximizing "permanency" for foster youth in transition; and, the fact that the law's eligibility requirements still exclude important high-risk populations. In addition, several lines of research will be needed along the way if states are to have the knowledge base to seriously address these challenges.

5.1 Continuing Ambivalence of States Towards Parenting Young Adults

Although the Fostering Connections Act gives states the option of using Title IV-E funds to provide care and supervision to young people to age 21, it is far from clear that many states will take up the option. Continuing concern in Congress that young people allowed to remain in foster care past 18 would simply remain "dependent" on the state and not engage in the kinds of activities needed to make a successful transition from care is reflected in the provisions of the Fostering Connections Act regarding requiring youths' participation in such activities. Similar concern at the state level could block passage of enabling legislation. The fact that many states have yet to take up the option to extend Medicaid to former foster youth through age 21 should temper optimism about quick action by states to extend their foster care programs beyond age 18.

Stronger empirical evidence of the benefits of extended care to young people in terms of their wellbeing and the benefits to taxpayers of preventing costly negative outcomes would help convince state-level policymakers to extend care (e.g., early or unwanted pregnancy; crime; dependence on other forms of government assistance). While there is some evidence to support extended care as a protective factor during the transition to adulthood for foster youth (Courtney et al., 2007b; Kerman et al., 2002), this evidence is far from definitive. Moreover, it remains unclear exactly what aspects of extended support are most important in helping foster youth to experience successful transitions.

Fortunately, the implementation of the National Youth in Transition Database (NYTD) provisions requiring states to track transition outcomes for foster youth between ages 17 and 21 can provide the kind of information necessary to assess how between-state variation in state policy and service provision influences transition outcomes. The American Public Human Services Association and the Chapin Hall Center for Children at the University of Chicago have formed a partnership to engage states in planning for the NYTD. A major focus of this effort is to ensure that data elements will go beyond the outcomes called for in federal law to include data on the kinds of services and supports provided to youth regardless of whether they are still in care or not. Policymakers at the state level may find it easier to support extending care past age 18 if analysis of between-state differences in outcomes for foster youth in transition provides additional evidence in support of extending care.

5.2 Lack of Knowledge Regarding the Effectiveness of Services

Another challenge to improving policy and practice directed towards foster youth transitions to adulthood is the lack of evidence in support of existing interventions. Policymakers and practitioners want to know "what works" in helping foster youth successfully transition to adulthood, but sound empirical evidence is not yet available. The field of youth services has developed in recent years general youth development principles, but little empirical evidence exists to support particular independent living and transition services. A review of evaluation research on the effectiveness of independent living services found no experimental evaluations of independent living programs (Montgomery et al., 2006). While the authors of the study reviewed eight non-randomized controlled studies and found some evidence that some programs may have protective effects, they conclude that the weak methodological quality of the evidence tempers the validity of those findings. Recently, as part of the federally-funded program of evaluation research on independent living programs, HHS released the findings of experimental evaluations of a life skills training program and a tutoring-mentoring program in Los Angeles County, California (U.S. DHHS 2008b, 2008c). Neither of the interventions demonstrated an effect on any of the outcomes the programs were intended to improve.

The dearth of studies that evaluate the effectiveness of independent living programs and the numerous methodological limitations of nearly all those that do exist means that no definitive statement can be made about program effectiveness. Only a focused and sustained program of rigorous evaluation research will remedy this situation. The research will need to involve experimental designs, larger samples than have been employed in the past, and better measurement of both the interventions and outcomes of interest. The program of evaluation research funded through the Chafee Program is a step in the right direction, but it will not be sufficient to move policy and practice forward on its own.

5.3 Poor Coordination of the Various "Arms" of the State

Poor integration and coordination of the efforts of the child welfare system with the efforts of other public institutions continues to limit the effectiveness of government efforts to support foster youth in transition to adulthood. Of course, current and former foster youth are generally eligible for whatever services exist in a given community for young adults that face challenges making the transition to adulthood (e.g., vocational rehabilitation services for persons with disabilities). In fact, in recent years Federal policy has evolved to make foster youth in transition a target population for federally- and state-funded educational, employment, and housing programs (Congressional Research Service, 2008). Moreover, growing out of the 2003 White House Task Force Report on Disadvantaged Youth, the U.S. Departments of Education, Health and Human Services, Justice and Labor have committed to a collaborative approach at the national, state, and local levels through an initiative called Shared Youth Vision to develop innovative programs, enhance the quality of services delivered, improve efficiencies, and improve the outcomes for the youth served by these agencies. Foster youth and former foster youth are one target of these coordination efforts at the Federal level and in the states participating in the initiative, though it is too soon to assess whether these efforts have been effective at improving services or youth outcomes.

While the relatively new focus in targeting federal programs towards foster youth and better coordinating the efforts of those programs is hopeful news, it remains to be seen if good will can overcome organizational obstacles to delivering support to foster youth. In many jurisdictions, child welfare agencies attempt to reinvent the wheel by providing services that are not within their primary realms of expertise. For example, many public agencies provide employment services for foster youth directly or through contracts instead of working with existing workforce development agencies that have experienced job developers and trainers and longstanding relationships with local employers. Similarly, the influx of Chafee Program funding for transitional housing has led some public child welfare agencies to attempt to develop new housing programs on their own or with traditional residential care providers, instead of working with existing providers of services to runaway and homeless youth; historically few child welfare agencies had funding for transitional housing, leaving runaway and homeless youth service providers to pioneer the creation of transitional housing programs serving foster youth.

The desire by child welfare agencies to go it alone may be at least partly a recognition that other public institutions are not always eager to assist the child welfare system in parenting the children of the state. For example, in an age of increased public accountability for achieving improvement in measurable outcomes related to their core missions, providers of educational and employment supports may be reluctant to engage foster youth given the many challenges they often bring with them.

At any rate, ensuring that foster youth have the range of services and supports at their disposal to maximize their potential for success will require more coordination and integration of services than currently takes place. State child welfare agencies that are able to provide ongoing case management past age 18 as a result of state legislative action to implement the Fostering Connection Act may be in an enhanced position to facilitate such coordination.

5.4 Making Sense of "Permanency" for Foster
Youth in Transition

In recent years policymakers and child advocates have called for greater efforts to ensure "permanency" for youth aging out of foster care, arguing that too often the foster care system allows young people to age out of care with no connection to a permanent family (Frey, Greenblatt, & Brown, 2007). The success of these advocacy efforts can be seen in the provisions of the Fostering Connections Act extending adoption and guardianship subsidies from 18 to 21, which reflect the concern that failing to do so would undermine the permanency of these family relationships. Advocates have also called for programmatic efforts to create and support foster youths' relationships with nonrelated adults, drawing upon research evidence regarding the importance of permanent supportive relationships and connections to an adult for the long- and short-term wellbeing of young people generally (Beam, Chen, & Greenberger, 2002), as well as research showing positive associations between informal mentoring relationships and adult outcomes for former foster youth (Ahrens, DuBois, Richardson, Fan, & Lozano, 2008).

While the interest in creating interventions to foster the development of lasting connections between foster youth and unrelated adults is understandable, it should be done with caution for at least two reasons. First, it is one thing to observe an association between positive youth-adult relationships and positive outcomes for youth but quite another to go about creating such relationships through social service programs. Scholarship on youth mentoring gives reason for caution in developing mentoring programs for vulnerable youth (Spencer, 2006). Moreover, these young people have generally experienced multiple failed relationships with adults who were supposed to care for them, including their parents and adults in failed foster care placements; the last thing they need is yet another failed relationship with an adult. Research is sorely needed on how natural mentoring relationships are formed and maintained by foster youth and emerging programs intended to create new supportive relationships for foster youth should be rigorously evaluated.

Second, recent research suggests that most foster youth making the transition to adulthood from foster care feel close to and are in regular contact with one or more members of their family of origin (Courtney et al., 2005, 2007a), though, not surprisingly, many of those relationships pose serious challenges for the young people (Courtney et al., 2001; Samuels, 2008; Samuels & Price, 2008). Unfortunately, the child welfare field continues to fail to take full account of the enduring relationships that the vast majority of foster youth maintain with their families. As states take up the option to continue to care for foster youth as young adults, it will be increasingly important for policymakers and practitioners to acknowledge that in most cases the state is actually *co-parenting* these young people. Research is needed to help child welfare authorities understand how to do this well.

5.5 Too Narrowly Defining the Population Needing Continued Parenting by the State

Perhaps the most important limitation of current policy, and the provisions of the new Fostering Connections Act, is the target population. As noted above, few youth actually age out of the child welfare system, yet this population remains the primary focus of federal law. By including youth that exit foster care after their 16th birthday to adoption or legal guardianship in the population eligible for continuing assistance, the Fostering Connections Act significantly expands the population that is likely to receive help from the child welfare system in making the transition to adulthood. However, a large number of young people who remain in state care late into adolescence but who exit prior to the age of majority are still left out.

Many foster youth, even those who have been in out-of-home care for some time, are discharged from care to a member of their family of origin. This group dwarfs in size the group that ages out of care (Wulczyn & Brunner Hislop, 2001). Child welfare services providers seldom reach out to these youth, even those that received independent living services while they were in care, both because they are generally not funded by government to do so and because they assume that the task of helping these young people manage the transition to adulthood has passed back to the family. Yet, at some point, generally not too far in the distant past, society forcibly separated these same families from their children. Moreover, research suggests that many of these familial relationships are tenuous at best and that many of these youth will find themselves in need of another place to live and other adults to rely on for advice before long (Cook et al., 1991; Courtney et al., 2001).

What of the children who run away from out-of-home care in the year or so before reaching the age of majority (Courtney et al., 2005b; Finkelstein, Wamsley, Currie, & Miranda, 2004)? These youth may be the most at-risk of poor adult outcomes and there are more of them than there are youth who age out of care. This group can be very difficult to engage in services, yet, as media reports point out, too often child welfare agencies make little or no effort to reconnect with these youth when they leave out-of-home care (Anderson, 2002; Kresnak, 2002).

The next round of federal child welfare reform legislation and state policy reform efforts should seriously consider the wisdom of excluding from ongoing support young people who return home to their families shortly before the age of majority and those who exit from care to runaway status. Moreover, Federal rulemaking in implementing the Foster Connections Act should consider the conditions under which young people who choose to exit care after age 18 may reenter care at a later date. Since it is quite normal for young people to try to go it alone as young adults only to need to return to the nest for some period if things get rough, policy should not constrain child welfare authorities from making provision for similar opportunities for foster youth in transition. One way to address the current arbitrariness of eligibility policy regarding the transition to adulthood for foster youth would be to make any young person who spent some minimum amount of time in state care after the age of 16 eligible to return to care through age 21.

U.S. social policy directed towards supporting the transition to adulthood for youth in state care has rapidly evolved over the past two decades. From a policy framework that did not acknowledge youths' transitions from care at all, to one that emphasized preparing foster youth for "independence" at the age of majority, the U.S. is now poised to make a major commitment to parenting the children of the state into early adulthood. While this latest shift makes sense in terms of what average parents do for their children these days, and the limited track record of states taking on this role provides grounds for optimism, it is likely that the next several years will see the rapid development of a wide range of state and local strategies for carrying out this new task of government. Policy and program development should actively involve the young adults who will be most affected by these experiments in state parenting. In addition, the government agencies and philanthropic entities involved in generating new ideas would be well advised to invest in the kinds of research and evaluation along the way that will be necessary for the new policy regime to be successful.

6 Conclusion: The Importance of the Work of Alfred J. Kahn

It makes perfect sense to attend to research and policy concerning the transition to adulthood for foster youth in a volume dedicated to Alfred J. Kahn. Some of the central concerns of his scholarship have influenced policy in this area and should continue to inform policy development going forward. Professor Kahn spent many years as a scholar, consultant to government and philanthropy, and advocate arguing for child and family policies focused on the developmental needs of children and youth. His influence in this regard is reflected in his tenure as Chairman during the early 1980s of the Committee on Child Development Research and Public Policy of the United States National Academy of Science. Professor Kahn was also long an advocate for a more universal approach to providing services to children and families than the categorical and residual approach favored in the U.S., believing that social services should be good enough for every American, not for the poor alone.

As a participant in debates over the future of child welfare policy directed towards foster youth, I can attest to the influence of Professor Kahn's ideas. The Fostering Connections Act is arguably one of the most developmentally appropriate policy changes in the history of U.S. child welfare policy, moving away from a narrow focus on preventing "dependency" on government towards recognition of government's responsibility to provide the adult children of the state with the same kinds of support provided to young people by the "average" family, directed towards the same ends. I suspect that Professor Kahn's response to the passage of the Fostering Connections Act might have been to rightly wonder why U.S. policy does not provide the kinds of supports funded through the Act to a much broader population of vulnerable young people in transition. Professor Kahn was also one of the first social welfare scholars to point out the need for social welfare institutions focused on distinct social needs or problems to better coordinate their efforts and he was instrumental in identifying models for collaboration and coordination. As I noted above, the success of the Fostering Connections Act will largely depend on whether institutions serving young people in transition can find better ways to work together.

Lastly, Professor Kahn spent much of the latter part of his career learning from cross-national study of social problems and institutions about how best to meet the needs of children and families. The transition to adulthood for children in state care is not a problem unique to the U.S.; there is now a burgeoning field of scholarship on the subject around the world (Stein & Munro, 2008) and an International Research Network on Transitions to Adulthood from Care. As the U.S. welfare state moves into the role of parenting young adults making the transition to adulthood, it would be wise for all concerned to follow Professor Kahn's lead and look abroad for new ideas.

References

Ahrens, K. R., DuBois, D. L., Richardson, L. P., Fan, M., & Lozano, P. (2008). Youth in foster care with adult mentors during adolescence have improved adult outcomes. *Pediatrics, 121*(2), 246–252.

Anderson, T. (2002, October 1). 500 Foster kids missing. *Los Angeles Daily News*. http://www.dailynews.com/Stories/0,1413,200 percent257E20954 percent257E896518,00. html. Accessed 27 October, 2002.

Arnett, J. J. (2004). *Emerging adulthood: The winding road from the late teens through the twenties*. Oxford: Oxford University Press.

Barth, R. (1990). On their own: The experiences of youth after foster care. *Child and Adolescent Social Work, 7*, 419–440.

Beam, M. R., Chen, C., & Greenberger, E. (2002). The nature of adolescents' relationships with "very important" nonparental adults. *American Journal of Community Psychology, 30*(2), 305–325.

Bussey, M., Feagans, L., Arnold, L., Wulczyn, F., Brunner, K., Nixon, R., et al. (2000). *Transition for foster care: A state-by-state data base analysis*. Seattle, WA: Casey Family Programs.

Congressional Research Service. (2008). *Youth transitioning from foster care: Background, federal programs, and issues for Congress*. Washington, DC: Author.

Cook, R., Fleischman, E., & Grimes, V. (1991). *A national evaluation of Title IV-E foster care independent living programs for youth in foster care: Phase 2, Final Report Volume 1*. Rockville, MD: Westat.

Cook, S. K. (1992). *Long term consequences of foster care for adult well-being* (Ph.D. dissertation, University of Nebraska, Lincoln).

Courtney, M. E., & Dworsky, A. (2006). Early outcomes for young adults transitioning from out-of-home care in the U.S.A. *Child and Family Social Work, 11*, 209–219.

Courtney, M. E., Dworsky, A., Cusick, G., Havlicek, J., Perez, A., & Keller, T. (2007a). *Midwest evaluation of the adult functioning of former foster youth: Outcomes at age 21*. Chicago: Chapin Hall Center for Children at the University of Chicago.

Courtney, M. E., Dworsky, A., & Pollack, H. (2007b). *When should the state cease parenting? Evidence from the Midwest Study*. Chicago: Chapin Hall Center for Children at the University of Chicago.

Courtney, M. E., Dworsky, A., Ruth, G., Keller, T., Havlicek, J., & Bost, N. (2005a). *Midwest evaluation of the adult functioning of former foster youth: Outcomes at age 19*. Chicago: Chapin Hall Center for Children at the University of Chicago.

Courtney, M. E., & Hughes-Heuring, D. (2005). The transition to adulthood for youth "aging out" of the foster care system. In W. Osgood, C. Flanagan, E. M. Foster, & G. Ruth (Eds.), *On your own without a net: The transition to adulthood for vulnerable populations* (pp. 27–67). Chicago: University of Chicago Press.

Courtney, M. E., Piliavin, I., Grogan-Kaylor, A., & Nesmith, A. (2001). Foster youth transitions to adulthood: A longitudinal view of youth leaving care. *Child Welfare, 6,* 685–717.

Courtney, M. E., Skyles, A., Samuels, G. M., Zinn, A., Howard, E., & Goerge, R. M. (2005b). *Youth who run away from substitute care.* Chicago, IL: Chapin Hall Center for Children at the University of Chicago.

Courtney, M. E., Terao, S., & Bost, N. (2004). *Midwest Evaluation Of The Adult Functioning Of Former Foster Youth: Conditions Of Youth Preparing To Leave State Care.* Chicago: Chapin Hall Center for Children at the University of Chicago.

Dworsky, A., & Courtney, M. E. (2000). *Self-sufficiency of former foster youth in Wisconsin: Analysis of unemployment insurance wage data and public assistance data.* Madison, WI: IRP. (found at http://aspe.os.dhhs.gov/hsp/fosteryouthW100/index.htm)

Fanshel, D., Finch, S. J., & Grundy, J. F. (1990). *Foster children in life course perspective.* New York: Columbia University.

Festinger, T. (1983). *No one ever asked us: A postscript to foster care.* New York: Columbia University.

Finkelstein, M., Wamsley, M., Currie, D., & Miranda, D. (2004). *Youth who chronically AWOL from foster care: Why they run, where they go, and what can be done.* New York: Vera Institute.

Frey, L. L., Greenblatt, S. B., & Brown, J. (2007). *A call to action: An integrated approach to youth permanency and preparation for adulthood.* Seattle, WA: Casey Family Programs.

Frost, S., & Jurich, A. P. (1983). *Follow-up study of children residing in the Villages* (unpublished report). Topeka, KS: The Villages.

Goerge, R., Bilaver, L., Joo Lee, B., Needell, B., Brookhart, A., & Jackman, W. (2002). *Employment outcomes for youth aging out of foster care.* Chicago: Chapin Hall Center for Children at the University of Chicago. (found at http://aspe.os.dhhs.gov/hsp/fostercare-agingout02/).

Harari, T. (1980). Teenagers exiting from family foster care: A retrospective look. (Ph.D. dissertation, University of California, Berkeley).

Jones, M. A., & Moses, B. (1984). *West Virginia's former foster children: Their experiences in care and their lives as young adults.* New York: CWLA.

Kerman, B., Wildfire, J., and Barth, R. P. (2002). Outcomes for young adults who experienced foster care. *Children and Youth Services Review 24*(5): 319–344.

Kresnak, J. (2002). *Photos of missing foster kids could go on state website.* Detroit Free Press, September 13, 2002, http://nl3.newsbank.com/nl-search/we/Archives?p_action=list&p_topdoc=11&p_maxdocs=210. Accessed 27 October, 2002.

Kushel, M., Yen, I., Gee, L., & Courtney, M. E. (2007). Homelessness and health care access after emancipation: Results from the Midwest Evaluation of Adult Functioning of Former Foster Youth. *Archives of Pediatrics & Adolescent Medicine, 61,* 927–1011.

Macomber, J. E., Cuccaro-Alamin, S., Duncan, D., Kuehn, D., McDaniel, M., Vericker, T., et al. (2008). *Coming of age: Employment outcomes for youth who age out of foster care through their middle twenties.* Washington, DC: The Urban Institute.

Mangine, S., Royse, D., Wiehe, V., & Nietzel, M. (1990). Homelessness among adults raised as foster children: A survey of drop-in center users. *Psychological Reports, 67,* 739–745.

McCord, J., McCord, W., & Thurber, E. (1960). The effects of foster home placement in the prevention of adult antisocial behavior. *Social Service Review, 34,* 415–419.

McDonald, T. P., Allen, R. I., Westerfelt, A., & Piliavin, I. (1996). *Assessing the long-term effects of foster care: A research synthesis.* Washington, DC: CWLA.

McMillen, J. C., & Raghavan, R. (2009). Pediatric to adult mental health service use of young people leaving the foster care system. *Journal of Adolescent Health, 44*(1): 7–13.

McMillen, J. C., Zima, B. T., Scott, L. D., Auslander, W. F., Munson, M. R., Ollie, M. T., et al. (2005). The prevalence of psychiatric disorders among older youths in the foster care system. *Journal of the American Academy of Child and Adolescent Psychiatry, 44,* 88–95.

Meier, E. G. (1965). Current circumstances of former foster children. *Child Welfare, 44*, 196–206.

Montgomery, P., Donkoh, C., and Underhill, K. (2006). Independent living programs for young people leaving the care system: The state of the evidence. *Children and Youth Services Review, 28*, 12, 1435–1448.

Patel, S., & Roherty, M. (2007). *Medicaid access for youth aging out of foster care*. Washington, DC: American Public Human Services Association.

Pecora, P. J., Kessler, R. C., Williams, J., Downs, A. C., English, D., White, J., et al. (2005). *Improving family foster care: Findings from the Northwest Alumni Study*. Seattle, Washington: Casey Family Programs.

Pettiford, P. (1981). *Foster care and welfare dependency: A research note*. New York: Human Resources Administration, Office of Policy and Program Development.

Samuels, G. M. (2008). *A reason, a season, and a lifetime: Relational permanence among young adults with foster care backgrounds*. Chicago, IL: Chapin Hall Center for Children at the University of Chicago.

Samuels, G. M., & Pryce, J. M. (2008). "What doesn't kill you makes you stronger": Survivalist self-reliance as a resilience and risk among young adults aging out of foster care. *Children and Youth Services Review, 30*(10): 1198–1210.

Schoeni, R., & Ross, K. (2004). *Family Support During The Transition to Adulthood*. Policy Brief #12. Philadelphia, PA: University of Pennsylvania, Dept. of Sociology.

Settersten, R., Furstenberg, F. F., & Rumbaut, R. G. (Eds.) (2005). *On the frontier of adulthood: Theory, research, and public policy*. Chicago: University of Chicago Press.

Sosin, M., Coulson, P., & Grossman, S. (1988). *Homelessness in Chicago: Poverty and pathology, social institutions, and social change*. Chicago: University of Chicago, Social Service Administration.

Sosin, M., Piliavin, I., & Westerfelt, H. (1990). Toward a longitudinal analysis of homelessness. *Journal of Social Issues, 46*(4), 157–174.

Spencer, R. (2006). Understanding the mentoring process between adolescents and adults. *Youth & Society, 37*(3), 287–315.

Stein, M., & Munro, E. R. (Eds.) (2008). *Young people's transitions from care to adulthood: International research and practice*. London: Jessica Kingsley Publishers.

Susser, E., Lin, S., Conover, S., & Streuning, E. (1991). Childhood antecedents of homelessness in psychiatric patients. *American Journal of Psychiatry, 148*, 1026–1030.

U.S. Census Bureau (2001). Survey of Income and Program Participation, 2001, Wave 2. Retrieved on August 30, 2006 From: http://www.census.gov/population/socdemo/child/sipp2001/tab04.xls

U.S. Department of Health and Human Services, Administration on Children, Youth and Families. (2008a). The AFCARS Report: Preliminary FY 2006 estimates as of January 2008 (14). http://www.acf.hhs.gov/programs/cb/stats_research/afcars/tar/report14.htm. Accessed 26 September, 2008.

U.S. Department of Health and Human Services, Administration for Children and Families. (2008b, July). *Evaluation of the early start to emancipation preparation tutoring program: Los Angeles County*. Washington, DC: Author.

U.S. Department of Health and Human Services, Administration for Children and Families. (2008c, July). *Evaluation of the life skills training program: Los Angeles County*. Washington, DC: Author.

United States General Accounting Office. (1999). *Foster care: Effectiveness of independent living services unknown* (Report no. GAO/HEHS-00-13). Washington, DC: U.S. General Accounting Office.

United States Government Accountability Office. (2004). *Foster youth: HHS actions could improve coordination of services and monitoring of states' independent living programs* (Report no. GAO-05-25). Washington, DC: U.S. Government Accountability Office.

Wulczyn, F., & Brunner Hislop, K. (2001). *Children in substitute care at age 16: Selected findings from the Multistate Data Archive*. Chicago: Chapin Hall Center for Children at the University of Chicago.

Zimmerman, R. B. (1982). Foster care in retrospect. *Tulane Studies in Social Welfare, 14*, 1–119.

Part III
Theoretical Perspectives

The Ecological Perspective on the Human Rights of Children

Edmund Bruyere and James Garbarino

All children need to grow up in a family environment where they are supported, loved and nurtured. Yet, poverty and its socially toxic correlates continue to influence the developmental outcomes of children living in the United States. But the effects of poverty and its correlates do not provide the complete picture. Research identifying 40 Developmental Assets and their relationship to child well-being is strongly suggesting a large percentage of kids from more affluent families, as well as kids living in poverty, are at-risk or vulnerable to the negative influence of surrounding environments. This chapter addresses the social environment influencing children and families and its influence on child well-being. Using an ecological perspective—which addresses the influence of risk and opportunity to child well-being—we analyze how ratification of the United Nations Convention on the Rights of the Child would improve the lives of millions of children and families struggling for survival in the United States.

1 An Ecological Perspective

We begin with an outline of an ecological perspective on child and adolescent development as a way of setting the stage for our analysis of how a human rights approach can provide the foundation for improving child well-being. Three principles underlie the ecology of human development. First, children are recognized as active participants who are influenced, not only by the perceived reality of others, but by their personal perception of events. Correspondingly, each subjectively perceived event creates personal meaning. Second, children, as well as adults and other elements of their environments, shape each other and adapt and respond accordingly to changes over time. Finally, a series of interconnected concentric structures—the micro-, meso-, exo- and macro-systems—directly and indirectly influence development,

E. Bruyere (✉)
Center for the Human Rights of Children,
Developmental Psychology Loyola University, Chicago, IL.
ebruyere@luc.edu

S.B. Kamerman et al. (eds.), *From Child Welfare to Child Well-Being*, Children's Well-Being: Indicators and Research 1, DOI 10.1007/978-90-481-3377-2_9, © Springer Science+Business Media B.V. 2010

with the child as a set of biological and psychological systems at the focal point of influence. These structures merge to make up the child's ecological perspective or social map of their world (Garbarino, 1992).

Two principles are vital to understanding the ecological perspective. First, it focuses on 'development in context, "in the sense that it attempts to describe and explain the interaction of biological and social forces through the direct and indirect influence of the concentric makeup of the micro-, meso-, exo- and macro-systems on the behavior and development of children. Second, it seeks to make the world a better place for everyone by focusing on strategies for dealing with the risks and opportunities which influence the social environment of children and families" (Garbarino, 1992).

As part of the ecological environment, the microsystem is the environment which has the most direct influence on child development (Bronfenbrenner, 1979). Within this system the child progressively engages in activities which become more complicated (e.g., drinking from a bottle filled with formula, crawling, walking, playing, attending school, etc.). In addition, as children mature they take on social roles which will affect competence, self-esteem and confidence. And of course, by engaging with others, they will form relationships with family members. Correspondingly, experiences in the microsystem will influence a child's perception of its environment and future interactions. Therefore, the risks as well as the opportunities available in the microsystem are vital to the developmental outcomes of children.

From infancy onward, reciprocal interactions occur between child and caregiver. The function of these interactions generally will lead to an attachment relationship which will be the building block for healthy (or unhealthy) human development (Ainsworth, 1978; Sroufe & colleagues, 2005). Ainsworth's (1978) classic study on attachment relationships in the *Strange Situation* identified three types of attachment relationships influenced by the type of care-giving infants and children receive. The most positive and developmentally appropriate relationship is *securely-attached*, which is achieved through accepting, sensitive, and responsive care-giving. "Normal" infants raised by this type of care-giver show considerably better social, emotional and psychological outcomes. In contrast, anxiously-attached relationships (*anxious-resistant* and *anxious-avoidant*) are distinct in that infants are raised by care-givers who are less attentive, sensitive and aware. As compared to their securely-attached peers, anxiously-attached infants display behaviors which are developmentally delayed and face developmental risk even though their behaviors are organized, expected and functional (Sroufe et al., 2005).

Main & Solomon (1990) identified a fourth attachment relationship category— the disorganized/disoriented attachment relationship. Parental behavior is characterized by chaotic routines, insensitive responsiveness and care, unavailability, physical, psychological and emotional maltreatment, and unpredictable affection. These behaviors are deleterious, and the life outcomes associated with children raised with a disorganized/disoriented relationship often result in psychopathology, failed relationships with significant others, poor educational attainment, and problems with the criminal justice system.

The fact that we can identify and classify infants and children based on the type of care they receive tells us much about the influence of the microsystem on human development. It reveals that the internal and external assets which affect parenting behavior will either expose children to risk or create opportunity (Garbarino, 1992). For example, investigating the influence of social and economic stress on rates of child maltreatment, Garbarino (1976) found that a significant amount of the variation in maltreatment of children was associated with inadequate social support and economic stress. These findings were substantiated by a 30 year longitudinal study conducted by Sroufe & colleagues (2005). In regards to "developmental opportunity," they identified a number of protective factors which influence parenting skills under levels of high stress. These factors include having a strong support system, knowledge and ability of parenting, and the ability to provide a stable home environment. It appears that at-risk children who are raised by caregivers who have others to help and assist them with the stressors of parenting, have the ability and knowledge to parent, and are able to provide a stable and nurturing home environment, show greater levels of competence and better behavior than children whose parents lack these assets.

The mesosystem—the relationship between two or more settings—also influences a developing child (Bronfenbrenner, 1979). A few examples of mesosystem structures include the relationship between a child's home and school environment, home and health and social service agencies, and home and religious institutions. For the purposes of this section, we will focus on the connection between a child's home and systems of parental support which are provided through social service agencies, including health services.

The extent to which children are influenced by mesosystem environments depends upon reciprocal transactions between settings (Bronfenbrenner, 1979). Therefore, development is not only influenced by the rate at which children and/or parents interact with the second environment, but also by the interaction of the second environment with the child and its parents. To illustrate, we know that healthy outcomes for children, whether physiologically, emotionally or psychologically, are associated with the extent to which they are engaged with community health experts from the time that most mothers learn that they are pregnant. That is, it is important that a developing fetus receives proper nutrition maternally, and mothers attend regular prenatal doctor visits as well as limit the amount of harmful toxins they ingest in their bodies (Shaffer, 2002). In this example, it is vital that mothers of developing fetuses take the initiative to seek medical help and assistance while pregnant. In turn, by forming relationships with medical professionals they make connections with vital resources which can help them deliver a child who has the ability to thrive as a newborn infant.

What are the roles of health care professionals in the connection between environments? If we change our focus from fetuses to children under the age of three we will discover that there is a dramatic difference in the way health care systems in Europe prioritize the health of children and caregivers as compared to the US system of health care (Goldhagen, 2003; Kamerman & Kahn, 2001).

The connection between the home of a child born in the US and nurses and pediatricians is unidirectional. In all but a few communities it is the responsibility of parents to seek out health care, not only for themselves but also for their children. Only when parents have arrived at the doctor's office are they given valuable health related information and treatment. While we agree this is still a reciprocal transaction between two settings, the level of outreach on the part of US health care professionals (and other formal institutions) is much different than their European counterparts (Bronfenbrenner, 2005; Kamerman & Kahn, 2001).

The philosophy behind child health care in European countries like Denmark, Great Britain, Sweden, and is one of outreach and prevention (Kamerman & Kahn, 1993). While not uniform in policy implementation, their goal is to reach out to children and families to prevent child health issues, assist with practical issues related to raising children, and to disseminate valuable information. Quite simply, the goals of the European *Home Health Visiting* program are to reduce risk and maximize opportunity as they relate to children and families.

We hope the distinction is clear. In the US health care system, the decision to seek medical assistance for children is the responsibility of the caregiver. Only when they contact medical professionals is it expected that medical professionals will communicate with parents. Once again, the level of outreach is unidirectional. In contrast, many European countries have added an important element of the mesosystem structure, that is, they seek to optimize *inter-setting communications* through a bidirectional connection which shares a common goal-the proactive protection of children and families. We will elaborate on how this difference in philosophies and dissemination of knowledge affects children and families at a later point.

1.1 Exosystem: Definition, Risk, and Opportunity

In contrast to the micro- and meso-systems, children have no direct participation and influence on decisions made in the exo-system (Bronfenbrenner, 1979). However, they are affected by the decisions, legislation and tenets made by policy-makers and bureaucratic administrators at multiple levels of government and private for-profit and non-profit organizations (corporations, city, state and national levels, hospitals, and social services). How does the exosystem affect children and families? Again we can look to the US as an exemplar in how policies from local government and/or decisions made by employers create risk and/or opportunity for children and families. We consider the influence of granting medical leave.

In 1993, after years of debate, the US Congress and President Clinton passed and signed the Family Medical Leave Act (FMLA). In brief, FMLA granted public employees (and private as well but with tighter provisions) a three month unpaid leave of absence to take care of an immediate family member who is sick, personal medical crisis newborns, and adoptees, as well as foster children. In addition, employees who had employer paid medical coverage will continue to have it during their absence.

Does FMLA go far enough in protecting children and families or does it create risk? From the viewpoint of the exosystem, employers as well as local governments have been given the opportunity to make decisions which will either increase benefits that lead to lower profit but increase opportunity for children and families, or to implement policies that do the bare minimum according to federal law and place children and families at risk.

Employers could choose to implement policies which grant paid medical leave (Kamerman & Kahn, 2001). Benevolent actions like this would help children and families during their darkest or brightest moments. Policies supporting paid leave would unburden families from financial stress which often leads to placing children at risk for malnourishment, maltreatment and poor educational and health outcomes.

There are other decisions which would create opportunity for children and families. Employers could choose to grant medical leave to employees who have no choice but to give a two weeks notice of absence. Additionally, they could adopt policies which do not require employees to use accrued sick and vacation pay before granting a medical leave of absence. Each of these benevolent decisions would benefit children and families by releasing them of unseen circumstances and needless stress (Frank & Zigler, 1996).

1.2 Macrosystem: Definition, Risk, and Opportunity

The macrosystem is a blueprint of how a society as a whole decides how it will live and what and who it will value (Bronfenbrenner, 1979). Within the structure of the macrosystem lies the micro-, meso-, and exo-systems, each of which is influenced by morals and values of a society (or global community). It is here where state and federal governments as well as international governmental bodies—like the United Nations—implement policies based on social consensus. It is these same policies which will have a significant influence on the developmental outcomes of children and families.

The United States, as well as other countries like Great Britain, have experienced periods of history where social policy has been influenced by social action and change oriented to special attention and priority for meeting the needs of children and families, particularly poor children and families. For example, the abolition of the slave trade in Great Britain did not begin with an out-cry of citizens against the trade of African slaves, but with the White, poor, and often homeless, Anglo-Saxon children who were kidnapped from English ports and then enslaved to serve in British-American colonies (Donoghue, 2008). Similarly, after years of accepting slavery as a necessity for economic development, the fledgling United States of America fought a bloody civil war from 1861 to 1865 over conflicting moral values and economic interests.

Leap ahead 100 years to 1965, and the US once again found itself in the midst of a number of social battles, including a fight for economic justice. President Johnson's *Great Society* declared war on poverty with dramatic results. From 1964–1973 Johnson's policies reduced the number of poor from 19 to 11%—a decrease of more than 40% (NY Times, 1992). Subsequently, well intended legislation brought temporary relief to millions of impoverished Americans, including minorities and the elderly, through increases in food stamp assistance, Medicare, early childhood education, and college tuition. It was clear that the policies of the 1960s were working, but was it enough to protect the children and families in poverty forever?

Of course, the answer to this question is "no." In the 1980s, President Reagan waged war on the economic and social policies of Presidents Franklin Roosevelt and Lyndon Johnson (Barlett & Steele, 1992). The Tax Reform Act of 1986 resulted in a major redistribution of wealth towards the upper income groups, and inevitable social and financial disaster for millions of children and families. Benefitting from this policy, top earners experienced a 22 point reduction in personal income tax (50–28%), while bottom earners—the ones who could least afford it—saw their tax liability increase from 11 to 15%. A major consequence of the loss in federal tax revenue meant financial responsibility for social programs like Medicaid, educational assistance, and Food Stamp entitlements shifted to individual states (O'Connor, 1998). As a consequence, the Tax Reform Act not only resulted in placing those at the bottom of the income ladder—the poor and working poor—with a more onerous increase in personal taxes but also placed three million American citizens-including children-at risk for adverse outcomes because they were cut off from vital social supports (Barlett & Steele, 1992).

What does British uproar over indentured slavery and kidnapping, the US Civil War and the subsequent freeing of human beings who were unjustly kidnapped from Africa, Johnson's War on Poverty, and Reagan's reduction in funding of social programs have to do with the macrosystem? During each of these periods of time, social consensus lead to policies which changed the way governments and people treated each other. These changes took place because the values and morals of a society had changed. In the case of British slavery policies, the US Civil War and Johnson's War on Poverty, the effect was profound for children and families. African American children and families, and the White enslaved British-American children, were set free and given the opportunity to experience freedom—of course we know freedom is not synonymous with justice. Similarly, Johnson's policies gave people living in poverty hope, financial freedom through education, and many elderly the right to live the rest of their lives with relative financial freedom and assistance with medical care.

Conversely, the policies of the Reagan era undermined the hard fought social and economic policies of the Roosevelt and Johnson eras (O'Connor, 1998). The corresponding negative effects of these egregious fiscal and social policies placed thousands of American children at risk for negative developmental outcomes. It was almost as if the social consensus of the 1980s said, "we care nothing about children and families," even as public declarations of "family values" were increasing—particularly among the very politicians who were leading the charge against the actual support systems for poor and minority families. The political rhetoric of the Republican Party in the 2008 national elections appears to mirror this pattern—indeed to be its culmination.

As an American society, part of a global community, do we overwhelmingly believe that children and families should suffer from social and economic injustice? If so, we should consider the long-term effects that await us as a nation. But if not, we should ask ourselves, "How can we permanently protect children and families from suffering social and economic injustice?" How do we reduce risk and create opportunity for children and families? We along with countless other child and family advocates living here and abroad believe the blueprint for structural change and the foundation for improving child well-being *begins* by ratifying the United Nation's Convention on the Rights of the Child which would serve as a permanent blueprint for protecting the human rights of children (Bedard, 2007; Goldhagen, 2003; Kamerman & Kahn, 2001; Limber & Flekkoy, 1995; Rutkow & Lozman, 2006).

2 The United States Child Welfare System: Children and Families

Three common issues evoke the child welfare system to intervene on behalf of children and families. The first is child maltreatment (sexual, emotional physical abuse) and/or neglect. Prevent Child Abuse of America (2008) reported that in 2006 there were 1 million substantiated cases of child maltreatment of which 1,530 children lost their precious lives. Thus, the child welfare system will get involved in known and reported situations of maltreatment and neglect and intervene to do what is in the best interest of the child (McCarthy et al., 2003). It is an unfortunate fact of life, given the nature of reported statistics, that we are never able to get an accurate count of how many children actually are maltreated and neglected each year because many cases go unreported.

The child welfare system may also get involved in the lives of children through voluntary or involuntary separation from parent(s). Through state mandate, the child welfare system has the power to intervene on behalf of the best interest of the child to assure that all children have a safe and secure place to live. Separation may occur for numerous reasons, including abuse and neglect, abandonment, and drug and alcohol addiction. Additionally, the death of one or both parents, or a voluntarily relinquishment of parental rights, may require child welfare to take custody of a child and facilitate placement in a safe and secure home (McCarthy et al., 2003).

The US foster care system is often the only choice for temporary placement. Approximately 500,000 children are placed in foster care in any one year, and as of 2001, 117,000 of these children were waiting for adoption (Adoption.com, 2008). For most children involuntarily separated from their parents, the end goal is always to reunite or connect them with a family who is able to provide a safe and secure environment.

The US Congress of Catholic Bishops (2008) reports that 7.7 million families and approximately 13 million children were impoverished in 2006, with roughly 52% of these children being raised by a single parent. When the realities of poverty—its causes and effects—are understood, it becomes clear that the most important reason child welfare intervenes on behalf of children is through the direct and indirect influence of poverty. Researchers have found strong correlations between ineffective parenting and maltreatment and neglect, on the one hand, and poverty, on the other.

For example, Watson, Kirby, Kelleher, & Bradley (1996) analyzed the effects of poverty on parenting and found that poverty affects multiple aspects of parenting, including being unable to provide a home conducive to learning and emotional development. Furthermore, Brooks-Gunn & Duncan (1997), and Brown, Cohen, Johnson, & Salzinger (1998) report that children from low income families experience higher rates of abuse and neglect than children from any other population. We must keep in mind that the influence of poverty is complex and a number of related factors may contribute to ineffective parenting, negative child outcomes and the intervention of the child welfare system. We must also be careful to avoid casting moral blame on parents who lack the skills and resources to be good parents because of their own life experience and situation in the socioeconomic order.

2.1 UN Convention on the Rights of the Child and Poverty

The United Nations Convention on the Rights of the Child (1989) takes a clear stand on issues of economic disparities as they relate to children and families with explicit and implicit language that developmental outcomes for children should not be highly correlated with parental income (Limber & Flekkoy, 1995). Language within the Convention challenges governments to take action in reducing economic disparities, and also implies that developmental outcomes for *all* children should not be influenced by the effects of adverse experiences. Moreover, the Convention recognizes that poor children should be afforded the same opportunities for optimal development as those from working, middle income and affluent families. To illustrate, Article 4 of the Convention is specific about the responsibilities of countries in addressing issues of poverty: "... With regard to economic, social and cultural rights, States Parties shall undertake such measures to the maximum extent of their available resources and, where needed, within the framework of international co-operation." And clearly the Convention also recognizes the role of the family in providing opportunity and healthy outcomes for children. Language from the Preamble asserts:

> ... Recognizing that the child ... should grow up in a family environment, in an atmosphere of happiness, love and understanding ... Recognizing that, in all countries in the world, there are children living in exceptionally difficult conditions, and that such children need special consideration ...

Furthermore, Article 19, sections 1-2 assert that countries have a responsibility to protect and reduce the effects of poverty, such as child maltreatment on the lives of children:

> States Parties shall ... protect the child from all forms of physical or mental violence, injury or abuse, neglect or negligent treatment, maltreatment or exploitation, including sexual abuse, while in the care of parent(s), legal guardian(s) or any other person who has the care of the child.

> Such protective measures should, as appropriate, include effective procedures for the establishment of social programmes to provide necessary support for the child and for those who have the care of the child ...

What can we take away from these Articles? One way to answer this question is to take a look at how the United Nations Children's Fund (UNICEF) has graded the US in terms of child well-being and where our children stand in experiences with developmental assets.

2.2 Child Well-Being in the United States

We begin this section by painting a brief portrait of the current state of child well-being in the US as measured by rates of poverty, access to educational resources, child health and safety, and developmental assets. Some 22% of children living in the US are relatively poor (UNICEF, 2007). That is, 22 out of every 100 children live in families making less than 50% of the national median income or $24,100 (US Census, 2007). Although the US is recognized as the eighth wealthiest nation in the world, it leads 24 of the world's wealthiest nations with the highest rate of children living in poverty (UNICEF, 2007). In comparison, Sweden, the seventeenth wealthiest nation in the world, has the least number (3%) of children living in poverty. Because children living in single parent households are more likely to be poor, we should mention that the US also leads with the highest number of 11, 13 and 15 year olds (the only ages reported from findings) living in single-parent households (28%; UNICEF, 2007).

According to UNICEF (2007), when considering economic deprivation we must account for the rate at which children are denied access to *educational resources* (e.g., desks, a quiet space to work at home, personal computers, dictionary, computer software, Internet access, calculator, and school texts). Twenty-five percent of US 15 year-olds report having six or fewer educational resources; in addition approximately 12% have less than 10 books in their homes.

The US ranks last among the world's 25 wealthiest countries in overall child health and safety as well (UNICEF, 2007). While there is no doubt great progress has been made in reducing the number of premature infant deaths, low-birth weight newborns, and unvaccinated children, 7:1000 infants born in the US today will die before age one; and 8:1000 newborns weigh less than five pounds. In addition, we have yet to achieve a 100% vaccination (measles, DPT, etc.) rate for children between the ages of 12–23 months (current level is 94%). Finally, among the world's 25 wealthiest nations, only New Zealand leads the US in the number of children and adolescents between ages 0–19 dying due to accident, murder, suicide or other forms of violence (22/100,000).

2.3 Developmental Assets

For over 50 years, the Search Institute in Minneapolis, Minnesota—a non-profit organization—has been conducting research evaluating child and adolescent development (Benson, 2007). This body of research has culminated into the development of an extensive array of peer-reviewed literature, educational materials and the identification of 40 Developmental Assets vital to optimal child and adolescent development. The Search Institute has surveyed approximately 2.5 million students in K-12 across the US. Subsequently, findings indicate there are 40 developmental assets vital to child well-being.

The assets are both external and internal. Twenty of the external assets fall under the categories of Support, Empowerment, Boundaries and Expectations, and Constructive Use of Time. The additional 20 internal assets are categorized under a Commitment to Learning, Positive Values, Social Competencies, and Positive Identity. The assets are not inherent in children but reflect their experience in the world they live in (Scales & Leffert, 2004).

Research has shown that the more assets a child experiences the greater likelihood they will thrive, be protected from risk, and succeed in life. Conversely, the fewer assets accumulated the more likely children are to do poorly. Based on an aggregate sample of 148,189, 6–12 grade students, the Search Institute found that 17% of youth experience 0–10 assets which place them at-risk for adverse outcomes; 42% are categorized as "vulnerable" with 11–20; 32% experience an adequate amount of assets with 21–30; and 8% are considered to be thriving with 31–40. If we look closely at these numbers we can conclude that approximately 50% of today's young people are at-risk or vulnerable to alcohol and drug use, academic failure, violence, and sexual activity (Benson, 2007).

In relation to poverty, family structure, educational resources, and child health and safety the Search Institute cites statistics which complement the research on child well-being conducted by UNICEF. Findings have shown that on average, children living in poverty experience three fewer assets (17 vs. 19.8) than those who are not living in poverty (Benson, 2007). Moreover, if we account for family structure, 22.1% of children being raised by a single parent experience 0–10 assets, and 45.9%, 11–20 assets. Compare these numbers with their peers who are raised in two-parent families and we see that 15.3% experience 0–10, and 40.4%, 11–20 assets. Clearly, income level and family structure affect the accumulation of developmental assets.

Next, if we take into account "parental involvement" and "exposure to creative activities," as educational resources, we will see there are a large percentage of children who are asset deficient in these areas as well (Benson, 2007). For example, only 29% of students surveyed reported that their parents were actively involved in helping them succeed in school; and 21% reported being involved in creative activities like music and theater. The data tells us that the correlation between economic prosperity and developmental assets is weak at best.

How do children fare in terms of perceived safety? Only 51% of children report feeling safe at home, school and in their neighborhood; 37% perceive neighbors as caring; 27% experience positive modeling of adult behavior; and 63% report having best friends who model responsible behavior (Benson, 2007).

3 United Nations Convention on the Rights of the Child

Being party to the United Nations Convention on the Rights of the Child requires two steps—signing and ratifying. By 1990, 100 countries had done so. The United

States was not one of them. It was signed in 1995 under the auspices of President Bill Clinton, but failed to achieve ratification in the US Senate (as is required by the Constitution for all international treaties). By 2008, some 191 countries had signed and ratified the UN Convention, with Somalia and the US the only hold outs (Limber & Flekkoy, 1995; Rutkow & Lozman, 2006). It appears that Somalia intends to ratify the UN Convention once that country has a stable centralized government in place (Bedard, 2007). But what about the United States? What is it about the Convention on the Rights of the Child that some in the US find so threatening and therefore refuse to take action to protect the inalienable and inherent rights of children?

This question was answered in part by a proposed resolution submitted by the late Senator Jesse Helms. On behalf of 26 other co-sponsors, the Republican Senator submitted a resolution to President Clinton which presented three reasons the US should not ratify the Convention. These included arguments that the treaty threatened parental rights, undermines and restricts Federal sovereignty and State authority, and that the US Constitution already serves as the protector of human rights for every American citizen (Rutkow & Lozman, 2006).

One of the greatest concerns of course—which is no doubt a misconception spread through conservative propaganda—has been on what the Convention would do to parental authority. Arguments have been made that the Convention places families at risk because it undermines parental authority by granting children the same rights as parents. Additionally, some argue that children would be allowed to divorce or sue parents, and be given the right to make decisions regarding such matters as abortion pornography, and religion (Fagan, 2001; Rutkow & Lozman, 2006). All of these issues have been addressed and dismissed as groundless by those familiar with both the Convention and the realities of children's lives in the US (Bedard, 2007).

4 An Ecological Perspective on the Human Rights of Children

One telling criterion of the worth of a society—a criterion that stands the test of history—is the concern of one generation for the next

Urie Bronfenbrenner

The right of a child to enjoy a supportive and nurturing family environment is the foundation of the Convention (Melton, 2005; preamble). Many leading "child rights" scholars agree that the microsystem of a child's home should include the following elements: a strong support system; competent, loving and nurturing parents; stability and structure; and the opportunity to thrive and grow to one's potential (Benson, 2007; Bronfenbrenner, 2005; Garbarino & Bedard, 2001; Kamerman & Kahn, 2001; Melton, 2005). How can we use the ecological perspective for setting the agenda for the human rights of children? Beyond the microsystem concerns, the real agenda for action and change lies in the social environment surrounding the microsystem which leads us to the macro-, exo- and meso-systems.

4.1 Macrosystem

We begin with an analysis of the macrosystem as it relates to the human rights of children and the creation of opportunity because this is where the flow of policy decisions based on social consensus ebb to reach social systems within the exosystem, mesosystem, and ultimately to the lives of millions of children living in families struggling for survival in the microsystem.

For change to occur and opportunity to increase in the lives of millions of children and families, a broad and sweeping consensus of social change needs to take place. What is required is a structural overhaul of policy and legislation (Benson, 2007; Bronfenbrenner, 2005; Garbarino, 1992; Kamerman & Kahn, 2001). These decisions should not only be guided by the Constitution of the United States but should also coordinate with the tenets set forth in the Convention. In reality, upon ratification of the Convention (an international treaty) the US Constitution mandates that federal legislation align with said treaties (Limber & Flekkoy, 1995).

To institute the structural overhaul of policy and legislation it is going to take a change in attitude about who is responsible for whom. The Convention is based on the guiding principle that, as a people, we have a responsibility not only for our own children and other family members, but also to children and families everywhere (Melton, 2005). This of course goes against the theoretical and economic foundation of our country which is based on the philosophy of individual and family independence, not interdependence (Garbarino, 1992). While there is no doubt that this philosophy has been at the core of our success as a nation, it has also contributed to the struggle of millions of our own citizens.

The importance of the Search Institute is perhaps one of the most vital links we have in reopening the dialogue regarding the importance of the Convention. The Search Institute is producing data which indicate that, not only are children from poor and disadvantaged groups of youth at-risk, but so are children from more affluent areas of society as well (Benson, 2007). This means that as the thousands of asset-builders trained by the Search Institute continue to spread the message of the importance of the assets to child and adolescent well-being, the more areas of society and people of influence in settings of power, the message is going to reach. We can conclude that if those with power and influence receive the message that their children are also at-risk that steps will be taken to bring about change. In addition, let us not lose sight of the fact that this movement will only be strengthened if those who are powerless and voiceless are empowered and valued in the process of change (Garbarino, 1992). Having said this, if we are going to open the dialogue and affect social consensus, one of the most important steps we can take now as advocates is to combine the discussion of the importance of the developmental assets with research, empowered citizens, and its link to the Convention.

In 1986, approximately eight years before it signed and ratified the Convention (January 31, 1992; childjustice.org, 2005), the Chinese government passed the *Law for Compulsory Education Act* (Zhang & Minxia, 2006). Based upon national and international social consensus, the law had two goals: to improve the lives of its rural poor and to stimulate the country's economy by reducing rural poverty through primary education and literacy training.

While China is hostile to many fundamental rights, its commitment to eradicating poverty and illiteracy serves as a good example of how structural change brought about by social consensus can bring about change for the better. This is an important lesson for the United States—itself no paragon of respect for basic human rights when it comes to the current economic situation of millions of impoverished children and families, past policies regarding enslavement, and extermination of the families on the land we now call the US, let alone the use of torture and the occupation of two sovereign Middle Eastern countries in pursuit of the War on Terror.

China took a top-down approach to improving education rates. The burden of educating children was placed on each section of the ecosystem including the Communist government, provinces, communities, schools and families (Zhang & Minxia, 2006). Of course, the involvement of children in this process was for them to attend school. One final note, supplemental financing came from international organizations like UNESCO, the World Bank and UNICEF who shared in China's vision (a clear indication that this was not only the social consensus of the Communist Party but also that of the International community as well).

The results of this shared vision were dramatic. From 1991 to 2002 the number of rural Chinese living in poverty decreased from 200 to 28 million (Zhang & Minxia, 2006). Additionally, the number of people living in rural areas having access to nine-year compulsory education rose from 40% in 1990, to 90% by 2002; educational attainment rose from five years of schooling to nine. From 1985 to 2002 the enrollment rate for primary school-aged children increased from 96 to 98.58%. Finally, between 1990 and 2001, China nearly doubled its gross domestic product increasing significantly from approximately US$58 billion to US$1.16 trillion.

We can conclude that the influence of dramatically reducing the poverty rate by mandating primary education was profound (China, 2004). Through cooperation, communication, goal orientation and trust, China created a snowball effect which positively affected the educational and developmental outcomes of millions of Chinese children.

4.2 Exosystem

Once a social movement for change begins the next course of action is to implement legislated policies and programs. The goal would be to re-center the focus to a national agenda which prioritizes supports for children and families. At the present time the US does not have a nationalized family agenda (Kamerman & Kahn, 2001).

Several articles from the Convention require countries to implement a system of protective supports and resources to help empower parents to successfully raise their children. For example, Article 18 section 2 states: "... States Parties shall render appropriate assistance to parents and legal guardians in the performance of their child-rearing responsibilities and shall ensure the development of institutions, facilities and services for the care of children." In discussing child maltreatment, Article 19 adds, "... the establishment of social programmes to provide necessary support for the child and for those who have the care of the child, as well as for other forms of prevention and for identification, reporting, referral, investigation, treatment." Articles 20 and 21 stipulate that state parties shall implement a system of care for children who are in foster and those awaiting adoptive care. Finally, Article 24 declares children should enjoy the, "...highest attainable standard of health and to facilities for the treatment of illness and rehabilitation of health. States Parties shall strive to ensure that no child is deprived of his or her right of access to such health care services." Again, we must remind ourselves that this is a reciprocal process and no matter how many supports and services are available, it is vital that parents reach out to accept this help (Bronfenbrenner, 1979).

With the passage of federal legislation aligned with the Convention, states, local governments, private organizations, and the legal system would be required to implement policies which place the best interest of children and families at the core of decision making (we acknowledge that many of the tenets are already currently addressed by many local, state and federal laws). Therefore, decision makers at all levels would be required to consider the influence of policy decisions and the corresponding effects on opportunity, status, distribution of fiscal and social resources, participation, familial stability, and time for parenting on children (Limber & Flekkoy, 1995).

From an ecological perspective, a key component of integrating the human rights of children into decision making is the strength of the supportive links which exist between two or more institutions (e.g., state and federal government, local and state school boards, etc.) or two system structures (exo- and meso-, or exo- and macro-systems; Bronfenbrenner, 1979). For policies to have their desired effects, systems would have to acknowledge and communicate with each other, share common goals, establish professional trust, and have an orientation which emphasizes the best interest of children and families (Bronfenbrenner, 2005).

European countries which have ratified the Convention, like Great Britain, Sweden, Finland, Norway, Italy, Germany, and the Netherlands, are committed to interconnected policies which mandate the reduction of risk and the increase in opportunity for children. For example, while not uniform in application, each of these countries has committed themselves to supporting parents through legislated policies which emphasize supports that empower parents to adequately raise their children. These include a comprehensive family leave (Article 18), early childhood education (Articles 28 and 29), cash entitlements (Articles 26 and 27), and housing plans (Kamerman et al., 2003 Melton, 2005; Article 27). Subsequently, at the core of these decisions is the commitment to reduce the leading threat to child well-being: poverty.

4.3 Mesosystem

The same principles which are influential in the exosystem apply to the success of mesosystem structures as well (Bronfenbrenner, 1979). For supports to be effective a bi-directional relationship must be established between a support service like the Home Health Visiting programs, and children and families. Unidirectional systems of supports and the corresponding lack of Home Health Visiting programs in the US place children at risk for unidentified developmental delays, child abuse and neglect, and illness. On the other hand, the efficacy of bi-directional supports empowers parents with the necessary skills to raise healthy children (Kamerman & Kahn, 1993).

What makes European countries like Denmark distinct from the US is that they have an infrastructure supportive of their social policies (Kamerman & Kahn, 1993). In combination with governments who have legally, morally and financially committed to national and international law, child welfare personnel are trained and competent (much like their counterparts in the US), committed to the common goal of improving the well-being of children and families, oriented toward a specific population (mothers with children under the age of three), and establish direct and/or indirect relationships with other programs (Wendt, 1999).

In 1937, as a response to a high infant mortality rate, Denmark began its campaign to improve the well-being of children and families (Kamerman & Kahn, 1993). This movement lead to a social consensus which cascaded into what is perhaps the most comprehensive and universal medical and social supports for children and families in any industrialized country (incidentally, Denmark signed and ratified the Convention, July 19, 1991; UN, 2008). Of course, Home Health Visiting is just one of many interconnected branches of support (Wendt, 1999), but the system here provides a good example of how a mesosystem structure whose primary goal is to promote a child's human right to survival and development (Article 6), health care (Article 24) and social support (Articles 18 and 19) relies upon goal consensus, trust, and orientation to carry out its duty to assure the well-being of children and families.

Under Danish law the birth of a child must be reported to the local municipal health authority (Kamerman & Kahn, 1993; Wendt, 1999). All parents, regardless of income or status, are informed of their right to receive assistance with the care of their child by home health nurses. Upon acceptance, a visiting nurse is assigned and during the first six months of an infant's life a nurse will visit monthly to monitor the development and health of the child. The visiting nurse will focus on identifying possible child abuse, neglect and developmental delays and will offer assistance if needed. Additionally, over the course of the next several years a nurse will continue to visit and provide free advice and assist with health examinations to make sure the child continues developing properly (Wendt, 1999).

Home Health nurses also serve as important links to social services, income maintenance and housing programs, which have been identified as vital resources to strengthening families and assuring child well-being (Bronfenbrenner, 2005; Garbarino, 1991; Kamerman & Kahn, 2001). Of course, parents also have responsibilities in this process including attending regular pediatric appointments, and free educational events. Consequently, one of the most significant indicators of the Home Health Visiting programs effectiveness has been the dramatic reduction in Denmark's infant mortality rate (14.2/1000 in 1970, 5.2/1000 in 1995, 4.5/2007; UNICEF, 2007; Wendt, 1999).

In conclusion, these requirements for child well-being can only be met if the necessary supports and policies are in place to assist parents in meeting the needs of their children. The United Nations Convention on the Rights of the Child supports this thesis, and has therefore laid the groundwork for supporting and nurturing the human rights of children and enhancing child development. The key now is to begin the discourse of what is most important in society-the rhetoric which espouses the well-being of American children and families, or action and progress based on social consensus which permanently supports the creation of environments which nurture the dignity and integrity of children and their families.

References

Adoption.com (2008). Foster care 1999. http://statistics.adoption.com. Accessed 30 June 2008.

Ainsworth, M. D. S., Blehar, M. C., Waters, E., & Wall, S. (1978). *Patterns of attachment: A psychological study of the strange situation.* Hillsdale, NJ: Erlbaum.

Barlett, D. L., & Steele, J. B. (1992). *America: What went wrong?* Kansas City, MI: Andrews McMeel.

Bedard, C. (2007). *Children's rights are human rights.* Chicago: Loyola University Press.

Benson, P. L. (2007). *All kids are our kids: What communities must do to raise caring and responsible children and adolescents* (2nd ed.). New York: Jossey Bass.

Beyer, C. (2008). *Training of trainers: Building developmental assets in school communities.* Seminar attended July 24, 2008, Search Institute.

Bowlby, J. (1969). *Attachment and loss: Vol. 1. Attachment.* New York: Basic Books.

Bronfenbrenner, U. (1974). Development research, public policy, and the ecology of childhood [Electronic version]. *Child Development, 45,* 1–5.

Bronfenbrenner, U. (1979). *The ecology of human development: Experiments by nature and design.* Cambridge, MA: Harvard.

Bronfenbrenner, U. (2005). *Making human beings human: Bioecological perspectives on human development.* Thousand Oaks, CA: Sage.

Brooks-Gunn, J., & Duncan, G. (1997). The effects of poverty on children and youth [Electronic version]. *The Future of Children, 7,* 55–71.

Brown, J., Cohen, P., Johnson, J. G., & Salzinger, S. (1998). A longitudinal analysis of risk factors for child maltreatment: Findings of a 17-year prospective study of officially recorded and self-reported child abuse and neglect [Electronic version]. *Child Abuse and Neglect, 22,* 1065–1078.

Califano, J. A. (1999, October). *What was really great about the great society: The truth behind the conservative myths.* The Washington Monthly.

DeNavas-Walt, C., Proctor, B. D., & Smith, J. (2007). *Income, poverty, and health insurance coverage in the United States: 2006.* US Census Bureau. http://www.census.gov/prod/2007pubs/p60-233.pdf. Accessed 07 August 2008.

Donoghue, J. Child Slavery and the Global Economy: Historical Perspectives on a Contemporary Problem. Paper Presented at the Symposium A Child's Right to a Healthy Environment. Chicago, IL. April 16-18, 2008.

Fagan, P.F. (2001). How U.N. conventions on women's and children's rights undermine family, religion, and sovereignty. The Heritage Foundation Backgrounder Executive summary (No. 1407). Retrieved on June 01, 2008 from, http://www.heritage.org/Research/International/Organizations/upload/95496_1.pdf

Family Medical Leave Act of 1993, Pub. Law. 103-3, 107 Stat. 6.

Frank, M., & Zigler, E. F. (1996). Family leave: A developmental perspective. In E. F. Zigler, S. L. Kagan, & N. W. Hall (Eds.), *Children, families & government* (pp. 117–131). New York: Cambridge University Press.

Garbarino, J. (1976). A preliminary study of some ecological correlates of child abuse: The impact of socioeconomic stress on mothers [Electronic version]. *Child Development, 47*, 178–185.

Garbarino, J. (1992). *Children and families in the social environment* (2nd ed.). New York: Aldine de Gruyter.

Garbarino, J., & Bedard, C. (2001). *Parents under siege: Why you are the solution, not the problem, in your child's life*. New York: Touchstone.

Goldhagen, J. (2003). Children's rights and the United Nations Convention on the Rights of the Child [Electronic version]. *Pediatrics, 112*, 742–745.

Kamerman, S. B., & Kahn, A. J. (1993). Home health visiting in Europe [Electronic version]. *The Future of Children, 3*, 39–52.

Kamerman, S. B., & Kahn, A. J. (2001). Child and family policies in the United States at the opening of the twenty-first century [Electronic version]. *Social Policy & Administration, 35*, 69–84.

Kamerman, S.B. et al. (2003). Social policies, family types and child Outcomes in Selected OECD countries. Paris, France: OECD working paper. Retrieved on June 01, 2008, from, http://www.childpolicyintl.org/publications/SOCIAL%20POLICIES,%20FAMILY%20TYPES, %20AND%20CHILD%20OUTCOMES%20IN%20SELECTED%20OECD%20COUNTRIES. pdf

Limber, S. P., & Flekkoy, M. G. (1995). The U.N. Convention on the Rights of the Child: Its relevance for social scientists [Electronic version]. *Social Policy Report, 9*, 1–15.

Main, M., & Solomon, J. (1990). Procedures for identifying infants as disorganized/disoriented during the Ainsworth Strange Situation. In M. T. Greenberg, D. Cicchetti, & E. M. Cummings (Eds.), *Attachment in the preschool years* (pp. 121–160). Chicago: University of Chicago Press.

McCarthy, J., Marshall, A., Collins, J., Arganza, G., Deserly, K., & Milon, J. (2003). *A families guide to the child welfare system*. Child Welfare League of America. http://www.cwla.org/ childwelfare/. Accesssed 8 May, 2008.

Melton, G. (2005). Treating children like people: A framework for research and advocacy [Electronic version]. *Journal of Clinical Child and Adolescent Psychology, 34*, 646–657.

New York Times. (1992, May 6). *The war against the poor*. Retrieved on July 2, 2008, from www.nytimes.com

O'Connor, J. (1998). US social welfare policy: The Reagan record and legacy [Electronic version]. *Journal of Social Policy, 27*, 37–61.

People's Republic of China. (2004). Permanent mission of the People's Republic of China to the United Nations office at Geneva and other international organizations in Switzerland: Facts and figures show rising prosperity. http://www.fmprc.gov.cn/ce/cegv/eng/qtzz/wtojjzk/t85664.htm. Accessed 37 November 2007.

Prevent Child Abuse of America. (2008). *2006 national child maltreatment statistics*. National Center on Child Abuse Prevention Research. Retrieved on June 15, 2008, from www.preventchildabuse.org

Rutkow, L., & Lozman, J. T. (2006). Suffer the children?: A call for the United States ratification of the United Nations Convention on the Rights of the Child [Electronic version]. *Harvard Human Rights Journal, 19*, 161–190.

Scales, P. C., & Leffert, N. (2004). *Developmental assets: A synthesis of the scientific research on adolescent development*. Minneapolis, MN: Search Institute.

Shaffer, D. B. (2002). *Developmental psychology* (7th ed.). Belmont, CA: Wadsworth.

Sroufe, L. A., Egeland, B., Carlson, E. A., & Collins, W. A. (2005). *The development of the person: The Minnesota study of risk and adaptation from birth to adulthood*. New York: Guilford Press.

Tax Reform Act of 1986. Pub. L. 99-514, 100 Stat. 2085 (1986).

UNICEF. (2007). Child poverty perspective: An overview of child well-being in rich countries. http://www.unicef-irc.org/publications/pdf/rc7_eng.pdf. Accessed 01 August 2008.

United Nations Convention on the Rights of the Child. (1989). United Nations General Assembly Document A/RES/44/25. http://www.cirp.org Accessed 24 October 2005.

United Nations, *Treaty Series*, Vol. 1577, p. 3; depositary notifications C.N.147.1993.TREATIES-5 of 15 May 1993 [amendments to article 43 (2)] 1; and C.N.322.1995.TREATIES-7 of 7 November 1995 [amendment to article 43 (2)]. http://www2.ohchr.org/english/bodies/ratification/11.htm

United States Congress of Catholic Bishops. (2008). How the Census Bureau measures poverty: The poverty threshold. http://www.usccb.org/cchd/povertyusa/povfact13.shtml. Accessed 31 May 2008.

Watson, J. E., Kirby, R. S., Kelleher, K. J., & Bradley, R. H. (1996). Effects of poverty on home environment: An analysis of three-year outcome data for low birth weight premature infants [Electronic version]. *Journal of Pediatric Psychiatry, 21*, 419–431.

Wendt, C. (1999). *Health services for children in Denmark, Germany, Austria and Great Britain.* Working paper available at www.mzes.uni-mannheim.de/publications/wp/wp-4.pdf

Zhang, T., & Minxia, Z. (2006). Universalizing nine-year compulsory education for poverty reduction in rural China [Electronic version]. *Review of Education, 52*, 261–286.

Social Problem Construction and Its Impact on Program and Policy Responses

Karen M. Staller

1 Introduction: From Private Woe to Public Concern

In the small city where I live, I often walk my dogs along a busy four-lane thorough-fare at about the same time that a public school bus deposits its grade school-aged charges in front of a housing project. Routinely I watch the large yellow bus roll to a stop; the lights lining its frame turn from yellow to red, and a huge octagonal stop sign unfolds from the driver's side of the vehicle. Recently—on three separate occasions in less than so many months—I witnessed a car sail by the docked school bus at the posted cruising speed of 45 miles per hour without so much as slowing down, let alone stopping in accordance with the law. Each of these three offending drivers was talking on a cell phone.

While some jurisdictions have begun to enact legislation barring the use of cell phones while driving, many, like mine, have not. To the best of my knowledge, no child in my hometown has been injured under these particular circumstances. However, should it happen (and arguably it is only a matter of time), the local news-paper will face a choice of how to cover the story. It might portray the event as a *private* tragedy and a random accident. Alternatively, the journalist might charac-terize the accident as an illustration of the *public* menace of distracted cell phone drivers, highlighting a broader social issue.

In contrast to the general lack of organized attention around "cell phone drivers," there is a significantly different level of public awareness about the problem of drunk drivers. Scholars who have traced the history of the movement point to the advocacy work of Candy Lightner, who founded Mothers Against Drunk Driving (MADD) in the 1980s after a hit-and-run driver killed her 13-year-old daughter. The driver was intoxicated at the time and on probation for similar offenses (Reinarman, 1988). Reinarman (1988) argues that the public was stirred into action not by a precipitous increase in the actual number of drinking-related accidents, but rather by outrage at the fact that drunk driving had "never been treated seriously by legislatures

K.M. Staller (✉)
School of Social Work, University of Michigan, Ann Arbor, MI 48109, USA
e-mail: kstaller@umich.edu

S.B. Kamerman et al. (eds.), *From Child Welfare to Child Well-Being*, Children's
Well-Being: Indicators and Research 1, DOI 10.1007/978-90-481-3377-2_10,
© Springer Science+Business Media B.V. 2010

and courts" (p. 91) and because advocates zealously brought the issue to public attention.

In the process of building a case about drinking and driving, advocates were able to single out one particular type of car accident—from a variety of possible types—for special treatment. This has given rise to a number of specialized responses. In the United States, we aggressively prosecute drunk drivers and keep statistics on drinking-related accidents. We all know that "friends don't let friends drive drunk" and promote the practice of appointing a "designated driver." Even producers of alcoholic beverages admonish customers to "drink responsibly."

Citizens concerned about cell phone drivers might take note of the history of MADD. They might begin to argue that accidents associated with cell phones are indicative of a particular kind of public nuisance. Alternatively, advocates might build on the existing work of MADD. Hypothetically, MADD could relatively easily become MADDD, Mothers Against Drunk and Distracted Drivers. In this way advocates could join their concerns with the already well-established movement.

As silly as all this might sound, note the significance of the underlying points. First, there is a large and diverse pool of private grievances that *could* be converted into public problems. An unorganized community of people shares these private woes. Second, it is possible to transform these private grievances into public concerns. However, advocates must take up the cause, organize the conversation, and bring it to public attention. Third, once the cause is established in the public mind, policies and practices—both formal and informal—naturally flow. This includes creating statistical categories for measuring the prevalence and incidence of "the problem," researching its causes or consequences, and finding ways to "fix" it. In short, there is a complicated interplay between these activities.

Social scientists often consider these various features in relative isolation and seek empirical answers to questions *within* the domains (e.g., How big is the problem? How effective is the policy? What are the best practices for service delivery? How effective is the intervention?). For example, Joel Best (1995) has argued that *sociologists* have tended to be primarily concerned with how social problems are constructed, while *political scientists* are concerned with how claims shape policy choices. I ask the question, What can *social workers* add to this conversation? Arguably, by professional inclination social workers think environmentally and are concerned with working across levels of intervention. In short, social work naturally covers the expanse from private woes to public problems. Perhaps there is no profession better situated for asking questions that move across these private and public domains. This chapter seeks to challenge social work advocates to consider the entire interconnected nature of social problems and how we "construct" them relative to service delivery (programming) and social policy. I start by looking at the theoretical literature and then move to a comparative case example (of runaway youth and missing children). Next I turn to implications for practitioners and finally, to a brief afterword as to why I hope Dr. Kahn would have seen his intellectual influence in this entire project.

2 Theoretical Perspectives: Social Problem Construction

2.1 Claims-Making Activities and Empirical Research

During the 1970s, Malcolm Spector and John I. Kitsuse inspired a fundamental and significant shift in thinking about the sociology of social problems (Spector & Kitsuse, 1973, 1977). They argued that the day's leading scholars and theorists on social conditions had failed to recognize the political processes associated with formulating and forwarding social claims (Danziger & Staller, 2008). More specifically, they posited that social problems were created, or constructed, as part of ongoing and interactive processes. Their ideas inspired others and gave birth to an entire genre of empirical research on the construction of social problems.

Spector & Kitsuse (2001) used the term "claims-making" to refer to the activity of promoting certain kinds of social concerns as social problems and thus defined social problems not as objective conditions but rather as "the activities of individuals or groups making assertions of grievances and claims with respect to some putative conditions" (p. 75). In doing so, they emphasized the activities of these claims-makers while minimizing the focus on the putative conditions upon which their activities were built.

This had major consequences for empirical researchers. Rather than devoting time to studying the causes and consequences of a variety of social conditions, researchers turned their interests to empirical questions regarding how concerns came to be brought to public attention. Thus there was a fundamental shift from focusing on the social condition as the object of inquiry and onto the activities that promoted certain kinds of claims. From a constructionist perspective, empirical research on social problems "draws attention to the role of interest groups and social movements that contend for ownership of a problem and the power to define and give public prominence to it" (Reinarman, 1988, p. 91). Thus social constructionists are interested in the claims-making activities that make problems visible and viable in public discourse, such as those evident in studies of MADD.

Claims-makers are faced with several distinct tasks, including highlighting an otherwise unnoticed social condition and then promoting it. Of key significance in these claims-making processes are the ideas of *defining*, *typifying*, and *domain expansion* (Best, 1990). First, claims-makers must define the problem by labeling it and specifying its parameters. Once defined, a problem can be *typified*. Individual cases or narratives become useful tools in portraying the "typical" representation of a particular problem. In doing so, claims-makers emphasize some features while minimizing or ignoring others. This selective framing of the social condition is critical in gaining public sympathy and traction. Given competition for public attention, claims-makers often rely on initial claims that evoke widespread sympathy. They provide compelling examples that serve as shorthand for the problem's major characteristics. Children in general, and child-victims in particular, often serve this purpose in public discourse. So in the example above, the death of child by a cell phone talking driver could provide the raw material for typifying the problem of distracted drivers.

Estimating the size of these "typical" problems is yet another claims-making activity, and numbers can serve as claims. As Best (1990) notes, in general, large numbers are more persuasive than small numbers, and official numbers more persuasive than unofficial ones. Not surprisingly, large official numbers are the best of all for convincing the public of the seriousness of a problem. How those numbers come into being and what is counted are often the subject of investigation.

Finally once claims-makers have established a social problem, it is usually easier to *expand* the problem's *domain* than to start a new claims-making activity from scratch. Therefore, an established public problem can serve as "a resource, a foundation upon which other claims can be built" (Best, 1990, pp. 65–66). For example, child abuse was first framed using a medical orientation and labeled the "battered child syndrome." (Nelson, 1984; Pfohl, 1977). Since then, the domain has expanded dramatically to include abuse (physical, sexual, emotional, etc.) as well as neglect (both active and passive forms). Hence in the example employed at the outset, adding cell phone drivers onto the already well-established drunk-driving movement would be an example of expanding the problem domain of a previously established claim.

Players in the process include both "inside" and "outside" claims-makers (Best, 1990). Insiders include lobbying groups, professionals, official agencies, and other pressure groups who have the standing to put pressure directly on policy makers. So MADD could play an insiders role in the cell phone example. Outsiders, on the other hand, are more apt to use the media to bring issues to public attention; influencing the public can secondarily lead to putting pressure on policy makers. Thus, bringing cell phone drivers to public attention as an independently created problem would undoubtedly require media coverage. Reinarman (1988) has argued that the viability of a claim depends, in part, on "the credibility of the claims-makers and the historical context in which such claims become utterable and resonate with the dominant discourse" (p. 91). An internet Google search of the phrase "cell phone accidents" generates a long list of hits, including law firms that specialize in car accidents involving cell phones, and thus provides some evidence, that an organized movement against cell phone driving might well resonate with dominate discourse in this historical moment.

2.2 Linking Social Problems to Policies and Programs

Sociologist Joel Best (1995) has posited that the reason Americans tend to speak about social problems rather than social issues or social conditions is that *social condition* implies a kind of permanence which is impervious to change, while *social problem* conveys a message that "the matter can be solved" (p. 259). It is this implied response, embedded in the way the problem is itself framed, that gives rise to policies, programs, and services. By logical extension, if claims-makers shape our sense of what constitutes a problem, they necessarily influence our understanding of how that problem should be solved or addressed. These solutions flow from the underlying assumptions embedded in the problem framing itself. "Typically, an orientation locates the problem's cause and recommends a solution" (Best, 1995, p. 8).

2.3 Natural History of Social Problems

All these features—that social problems are constructed, typified, and expanded, used as resources—reflect the dynamic nature of social problems. According to Reinarman (1988), "Social problems have careers that ebb and flow independent of the 'objective' incidence of the behaviors thought to constitute them" (p. 91). A number of empirical studies examine the dynamics at play *within* a specific problem domain. Best (1995) notes that "research on the construction of social problems consists largely of case studies, in which sociologists examine how and why particular claims emerged about particular issues. Cases studies draw their data from—and draw attention to—the special features of the substantive case at hand" (p. 189). However, less attention has been paid to the interrelated nature of multiple social problem claims. Therefore, a natural extension to the study of the history of a *specific* social problem is to wonder about the relationship between various *different* but *related* problems. By way of example, this chapter seeks to do just that by engaging in a comparative case study of two independently constructed social problems—that of runaway youth and that of missing children.

3 Comparative Case Study: Runaway Youth and Missing Children

This comparative case example looks at social problem construction, service delivery, and policy responses of two different but interconnected social problems: first that of "runaway youth," which emerged in the late 1960s and 1970s, and second that of "missing children," a phenomena that dominated the advocacy, policy, and program scenes in the 1980s (See Table 1).

My objectives are fourfold: (1) to identify an underlying condition of children who are "absent from home" without the consent of their legal custodians (a social condition in its un-problematized form); (2) to examine how claim-makers in the 1960–70s framed this condition as the "runaway youth" problem and how the same social condition was converted into a problem of "missing children" in the 1980s; (3) to see the relationship of the two problems to the implied "solutions," which include federal policy responses as well as programs and services, by examining the values undergirding the two problems as framed; and (4) to critically consider the implications of framing these two social problems the way we do.

Table 1 Comparing runaway and missing youth movements

Activity	Runaway youth	Missing children
Period of construction	1960–70s	1980
Typified problem	Murdered child prostitutes	Stranger abduction
Breadth of population	Runaways, throwaways, homeless, street youth	Parental abductions, stranger abductions, runaways
Claims-makers	Youth advocates, alternative providers	Parents, police
Media cases	Corll murders, Veronica Brunson	Joanna (Yerkovich), Etan Patz, Adam Walsh
Federal policy	Runaway Youth Act 1974, Runaway and Homeless Youth Act (1978)	Missing Children Act (1982), Missing Children's Assistance Act of 1983
Primary features of construction	Youth independence, confidentiality/privacy, alternative services, outside law enforcement	Concerned parents, police involvement, active public surveillance and networking
Domain expansion	Homeless, street youth	Cyber predators, child pornography
Excluded voices	Parents, police	Youth
National hotline & web address	National Runaway Switchboard, 1-800-RUNAWAY, www.1800runaway.org	NCMEC Hotline, 1-800-THE LOST, www.missingkids.com
Programs/services	Basic centers (crisis shelters), transitional living, street outreach	Milk carton photographs, Amber alerts, missing children reports, cyber tip line

3.1 Runaway Youth Movement

On September 20, 1958, the cover of the *Saturday Evening Post* featured artwork by the much-beloved illustrator Norman Rockwell. It was entitled "The Runaway." The scene depicted an American diner with a little boy perched on a counter stool, his feet dangling in the air, one shoe untied, and his red hobo's stick abandoned behind him. Two adults lean paternalistically toward the boy, one a large police officer and the other a smiling fountain server. The image is iconic.

The Norman Rockwell version of the "runaway" contains many features of the typical 1950s runaway. First, concerned adults (particularly police officers) intervened. Second, their intervention was safe and timely (no harm done). Third, the boy's behavior was characterized as adventurous rather than delinquent (hence the reward of a diner treat rather than handcuffs). Fourth, the child was easily spotted and identified as a runaway (after all, he was carrying his belongings in a manner typical of tramps). Fifth, the depiction is of a boy, not a girl (gender mattered). Not immediately apparent in the illustration are some embedded assumptions that accompany this portrait. The first is that the child does not have sufficient resources or wherewithal to survive away from home for long. Second, he doesn't stray too far. Third, he can and will be returned home safely. Fourth, the child has a safe family home to which he can return. In short, there was no real danger associated with this version of the runaway child. It warranted little, if any, public attention. Every aspect of this quaint runaway narrative would come to be challenged during the 1960s.

3.1.1 Social Condition to Social Problem

I have argued elsewhere that a confluence of factors converged in the mid-1960s and 1970s to produce a new "typical" runaway (Staller, 2003, 2006). I briefly summarize some of these key factors below.

First, demographic pressures during the 1960s produced ideal conditions to promote a new version of the American runaway. The front edge of the baby boomer generation entered their teenage years in 1959. By 1967, baby boomers filled all age groups between 13 and the then-age of majority 21. In 1971 we lowered the federal voting age from 21 to 18 through Constitutional amendment, effectively creating a new, lower national age of majority. This downward shift occurred as baby boomers continued to enter their teenage years and cross the newly declared legal boundary to adulthood. All told, the demographic and social conditions produced an environment ripe for public discussions about growing up, leaving home, and declaring independence from parents. In this context, conversations about the normative experience of leaving home commingled with conversations involving leaving home prematurely (running away).

Second, the cultural and social conditions—particularly those created by the 1960s counterculture—produced an environment that was antithetical to the Norman Rockwell runaway. Counterculture meccas like Haight-Ashbury in San Francisco and the East Village in New York City emerged. Youth spokespersons (claims-makers) and meta-messages (claims) included ideas about peace, love, freedom, brotherhood, doing your own thing, communal living, and dropping out, etc. These claims served as a huge draw for youth in general but had particular appeal for a younger, more troubled population of runaway youth. These conditions essentially undercut every aspect of the Norman Rockwell runaway. Runaways could find resources (such as crash pads and free food) to survive. They found receptive young adults who were unwilling to cooperate with police or with parents in sending them home. They were no longer easily identified at a glance; instead, they blended into the "hippie" scene.

Perhaps worst of all, however, these runaways were exposed to a number of real dangers, including being victimized and exploited. Media claims-makers began to convert the private experience of individual runaway children into a generalized public problem. Aiding them in their efforts were several high-profile and tragic cases. These included the discovery in August 1973 of the bodies of over two dozen boys—most of them runaways, many of whom had been reported missing by their parents—in Texas. The boys had been sexually assaulted, then murdered, by serial killer Dean Corll. In addition, runway girls began to be highlighted and linked to prostitution in the media. For example, in 1977 12-year-old Veronica Brunson, who had lived on the street for so long that she was essentially homeless and had been arrested at least a dozen times in the previous year on prostitution-related charges, died after falling from the 10th floor window of a hotel frequented by prostitutes. The *New York Times*, in its front-page story, noted that her case was illustrative of the "problems and dangers confronting thousands of runaway girls and boys who turn to prostitution to survive alone on the streets of New York" (Rabb, 1977).

By the early 1970s, Norman Rockwell's runway was replaced with a new "typified" version that focused on murdered children who had lived on the street and were driven to "survival sex" because of lack of resources (Staller, 2003, 2006). In short, the social condition of "leaving home without parental permission" was converting into a widely recognized social problem with a particular set of narrative features.

3.1.2 Alternative Services and New Claims-Makers

In gathering places like Haight-Ashbury and the East Village, concerned young adults began experimenting with a new, and decidedly different, kind of service for runaway youth. From these experiments emerged the runaway shelter movement. The runaway crisis shelter was a model borrowed from the crash pads of the counterculture. The early shelters operated completely outside the pre-existing public systems of care for children, such as child welfare and juvenile justice. These alternative agencies shared a set of core values that guided their services. First and foremost, the youth triggered the request for help (it did not come from parents, police, judges, or other adult authorities). Second, it was free. Third, it was confidential (creating some tension between the providers and both parents and police). Fourth, youth autonomy was central to the mission. Thus a primary goal of shelter staff was to aid youth in making their own informed decisions—but not necessarily with the aid of their parents or legal guardians. Fifth, parents were contacted if and only if the youth agreed. Minors who refused to allow parental contact were counseled about their options but not coerced into making a call, nor were they reported to authorities.

In the earliest years, between 1967 and 1974, these alternative agencies walked a fine line between the mainstream culture and the counterculture. They often operated on the fringe of legality, and staff faced the very real possibility of criminal charges for custodial interference or for contributing to the delinquency of a minor by harboring underage youth without parental consent. However, this network of advocates began to emerge as a relatively organized public voice for this alternative approach to services. They argued that shelters provided a safe option to life on the street, a chance to take a break from troubled families, a place to have basic needs met without resorting to illegal activities such as theft or prostitution, and a way to provide youth the opportunity to make wise life decisions.

3.1.3 Policy: Runaway Legislation

When the Federal Runaway Youth Act (RYA) was enacted in 1974, it sought to respond to the newly minted "runaway" problem. Specifically, the RYA legitimized the runaway shelter by accepting claims made by alternative service providers at

Congressional hearings, while rejecting those made by others. This is clearly evident both in the language that was included in the final version of the law as well as in the language that was deleted from it.

First, Congress accepted the typical runaway as one that was on the street, without resources, and endangered. The RYA found that "the number of juveniles who leave and remain away from home has increased to alarming proportions . . . significantly endangering the young people who are without resources on the street." In short, it embraced the newly constructed social problem assumptions that runaway youth would not return home immediately, would live on the street, and were without resources, forcing them to make bad survival choices. The runaway shelter solved that problem by providing basic resources and an alternative to street life.

Second, arguments made that the police did not offer constructive solutions to the runaway problem were fully endorsed. Legislative findings included that runaways were "creating a substantial law enforcement problem," that "the problem of locating, detaining, and returning runaway children should not be the responsibility of already overburdened police departments and juvenile justice authorities," and, furthermore, that it was important "to develop an effective system of temporary care outside the law enforcement structure." This was consistent with youth advocates' claims. Note several related features: first, law enforcement should not be burdened with missing person cases involving runaways; second, they should not be responsible for their return; and, finally, an alternative system of care should be developed. In framing the policy this way, Congress ignored the warnings of at least several police officers who testified at Congressional hearings. These officers argued that police were, in fact, in the best position to spot and intervene with street-based runaways; they believed that the communication systems between local law enforcement units should be strengthened; and they expressed some unhappiness with the unwillingness of shelter providers to cooperate with authorities. In support of this final argument, officers noted the difficulty they faced when being placed between uncooperative shelter staff protecting adolescents' confidentiality, on the one hand, and worried parents, on the other.

Third, the role of parents was essentially ignored. The original RYA bill proposed in 1971 included the following justification: "that the anxieties and fears of parents whose children have run away from home can best be alleviated by effective interstate reporting services and the earliest possible contact with their children." This language was deleted in the final version of the law. In doing so, three things happened. First, the parental perspective—and their "anxieties and fears"—were virtually eliminated from the "runaway" problem and solution. Second, interstate reporting, which would provide a way of locating runaway children, was rejected. Third, the presumption that early parental contact was important was diminished.

3.1.4 Services Associated with Runaway Policy

As noted above, once a social problem is constructed and has a firmly established place in policy and practice, it is often easy to use it as a resource to expand its domain. The RYA of 1974 was no exception. The act was quickly amended to include "runaway and homeless" youth, and later street youth. In response to the population domain expansion, new services were added (Staller, 2004). Ultimately, the act embraced five types of services: (1) basic centers or short-term runaway crisis shelters, (2) a runaway "hotline" or crisis telephone line that was based on the same core values as the shelter (free, confidential, and readily available 24 hours a day), (3) street outreach programs for youth who were at-risk of sexual exploitation, (4) transitional living programs for homeless youth, and (5) aftercare counseling for youth who had utilized services and return home.

3.1.5 Absent Players: Parents and Police

I argue here that the Runaway Youth Act, and its expansion, has largely excluded the voices of two major constituencies—parents and police. It is logical, even predictable, that these parties would find a way back into the public conversation through claims-making efforts of their own. The scholarship on the social construction of "missing children" lends support to this theory and is directly linked to that of "runaway" youth. I take this movement up next.

3.2 Missing Children Movement

3.2.1 Private Concerns to Public Problems

On December 20, 1974, Gloria Yerkovich's 5-year-old daughter Joanna disappeared from her home in upstate New York. Ms. Yerkovich would not see her daughter again until 1984, when the teenager was produced in an Ulster County Courthouse by her biological father (Child Find Official Regains Daughter, 1984). On May 25, 1979, 6-year-old Etan Patz disappeared in New York City on his way to school. He was never found, in spite of massive search efforts and national media attention. Just two years later, on July 27, 1981, another 6-year-old boy, Adam Walsh, disappeared from a shopping center in Hollywood, Florida. Adam's decapitated head was found two weeks later about 120 miles away from the spot he had gone missing. His case was not officially closed until 2008, 27 years later (Almanzar, 2008).

In each of these three cases, it seemed unlikely from the outset that the relatively young children had run away from home. Instead, suspicions were that children had been abducted. Nonetheless, they illustrated two different kinds of suspected abductions. Yerkovich believed that her daughter had been taken by the girl's natural father. But when she turned to the police for help, she found them unresponsive. At the time, there were no parental abduction laws, and while custodial parents might have a clear *legal* right to their children because of a court order, there were few options for tracking down or regaining control of a child taken by a non-custodial parent.

In contrast, both little boys, Etan and Adam, were believed to have been snatched by an unrelated stranger. To the worried parents, law enforcement agencies did not seem to act fast enough. For example, although the FBI had the discretion to get involved in cases where kidnapping was suspected, it declined to do so in Walsh's case because there was "no ransom note, nor any evidence of kidnapping or travel of the child across state lines" (Elliott & Pendleton, 1986, p. 681, fn. 67). When closing the case nearly three decades later, the Hollywood Chief of Police acknowledged "flaws in his department's investigation" (Almanzar, 2008).

This trio of cases and the advocacy efforts launched in their aftermath gave rise to the construction of a new social problem—that of the "missing" child. Although the nature of the abductions was of two different types (non-custodial parent and stranger), what the cases seemed to share was an inability of concerned parents to effectively work with law enforcement agents to obtain a timely and successful outcome on behalf of their "missing" children. Advocates highlighted a number of complaints: the lack of law enforcement attention and resources; the built-in delay required before police would accept missing persons reports; the lack of coordination between local, state, and federal law enforcement agencies; and the lack of policy of any sort dealing with missing children.

Yerkovich and the Walshs soon found themselves spearheading major advocacy efforts on behalf of other aggrieved parents facing similar situations. In 1981 Yerkovich founded Child Find, Inc., a national not-for-profit agency devoted to locating missing children, particularly those who are the subject of custody disputes. This agency grew to one with national standing and still exists today (http://www.childfindofamerica.org).

The Walshs' advocacy is legendary in the United States. John Walsh appeared on local and national news stations. The family established the Adam Walsh Outreach Center for Missing Children (later renamed the Adam Walsh Child Resource Center), from which they launched local and national advocacy efforts (Elliott & Pendleton, 1986, p. 673, fn. 15). John Walsh lobbied for legislation in his home state of Florida. He testified, along with several prominent law enforcement agents, for a law providing that "a police agency would act immediately on any missing child report filed with the agency" (Elliott & Pendleton, 1986, p. 673). Furthermore, Walsh testified at state legislative hearings on similar bills in New York, Illinois, Indiana, Kentucky, Georgia, California, and Louisiana, among others (Elliott & Pendleton, 1986, p. 673, fn. 15). He eventually lobbied for federal legislation as well. Walsh hosts the popular television show America's Most Wanted, a program devoted to solving notorious cases. In short, these parents used the circumstances of their children's individual cases as a basis to galvanize a movement.

3.2.2 Numbers Claims

A number of notable scholars have tackled various aspects of the construction of the missing child problem (Best, 1990; Elliott & Pendleton, 1986; Fritz & Altheide, 1987; Gentry, 1988). But perhaps there is no element of the problem that has been more studied by scholars and journalists than the use, or arguably misuse, of numbers in making claims about missing children.

Early advocates in the missing children movement supported their concerns by relying on the purported fact that "that 1.5 million children *vanish, disappear* or are *abducted* each year" from their homes (Fritz & Altheide, 1987, p. 477). This number was repeated in news accounts, docudramas such as "Adam," which was aired in 1983 and featured the Adam Walsh case, as well as in the social science literature. Advocates argued that of the one and a half million missing children, about 100,000 per year involved child snatchings while another 50,000 were the result of stranger abductions (Best, 1990). The remainder were runaway youth.

In spite of the substantial number of runaways included in this claim, advocates did their best to focus public attention on the stranger abduction cases to highlight their cause. At the outset, advocacy organizations such as Child Find stood by the figure that 50,000 stranger abductions occurred each year. Even more alarming, Child Find estimated that "only 10% of abducted children returned to their parents, another 10% were found dead, and the remaining forty thousand cases per year remained missing" (Best, 1990, p. 46). In addition, according to Best (1990), the "American Bar Association's president stated that Americans buried five thousand unidentified children each year" (p. 46). In short, claims-makers began building a dramatic case for large numbers of seriously endangered missing children.

There was virtually no empirical evidence to support these numbers. In fact, the huge number of purported stranger kidnappings claimed by advocates flew in the face of the few official statistics that existed. For example, the FBI's National Crime Information Center (NCIC) reported that there were 35 cases of child-abduction in 1981, 49 cases in 1982, and 67 in 1983 (Elliott & Pendleton, 1986; Fritz & Altheide, 1987). Initially undaunted, advocates countered with arguments that the FBI's NCIC data were inadequate and misleading (Fritz & Altheide, 1987). They attacked the tracking systems, suggesting that the actual number of missing children was far greater than the existing data indicated. Elliott & Pendleton (1986) wrote, "Walsh and others maintain that the FBI's figure is low because they believe the vast amount of missing children cases are not entered into the National Crime Information Center (NCIC) computer" (pp. 688–689).

Not surprisingly, this number discrepancy was taken up by investigative journalists and scholars. In particular, in 1985 *Denver Post* journalists and Pulitzer Prize winners Griego and Kilzer quickly exposed a serious numbers gap (Gentry, 1988). They concluded, "The bottom line is clear. There are not tens of thousands of children snatched away each year to be beaten, tortured, or murdered, the common perception of many parents" (cited in Fritz & Altheide, 1987, p. 480). The journalists went on to note, "These numbers reflect the confusion and complexity of missing children numbers that often fail to differentiate between three types of cases: runaways, parental abductions, and stranger abductions" (cited in Finkelhor, Hotaling & Sedlak, 1990).

Joel Best (1990) has systematically worked through the numbers claims made by missing children advocates, utilizing a variety of existing official public data and effectively demonstrating that the extent of the problem—particularly kidnapping and homicide numbers—had been greatly exaggerated. In the end, he concludes that the "combination of big numbers, broad definitions, and horrible examples made these claims compelling" (p. 60). In fact, there is some beauty and skill in the way advocates forwarded the missing child claims. First, advocates typified the "missing" child by relying on stranger abductions. These cases were particularly compelling and awful, although ultimately few in number. Second, they included within the "missing child" label not only stranger abductions but also non-custodial parent abductions and runaway youth. The distinctions between these populations mostly eluded the public. Third, by combining these populations, advocates could make large number claims about missing youth.

Advocates eventually retreated from these large number claims but not before federal legislation was enacted based on the wildly inaccurate figures and perceptions. As Fritz & Altheide (1987) noted, "Notwithstanding the lack of systematic research on the topic, decision makers proposed sweeping policy changes.... How the nature of the problem could be clearly understood without an awareness of the range and extent of cases was apparently never an issue" (p. 477).

3.2.3 Policy: Missing Children Legislation

President Ronald Reagan first signed the Missing Children Act (MCA) into law on October 12, 1982. He did so in the presence of John and Reve Walsh who, as the president noted, "came to the cause of all exploited children because of their own family tragedy" and who had "rallied thousands of others to this noble cause." Also present was Sergeant Richard Ruffino, a member of Bergen County, New Jersey's sheriff's office and recognized as "an expert in missing persons" who had "contributed countless hours of his own time in the effort to assist searching parents" (Reagan, 1982). In short, both parents and police officers were present at the signing ceremony.

Reagan promised that "the Missing Children Act will reassure parents that every effort is being made to find, or in more tragic circumstances, to identify their children" and noted that "finding missing children" had "become a national problem. Because of overlapping jurisdictions and the lack of centralized information, parents of missing children have faced frustration and anger in their attempts to locate their children" (Reagan, 1982). The law, he went on to say, "attempts to lessen these problems by mandating a system to allow parents access to a central computer file designed to help trace missing children. The act also will aid in identifying deceased children . . . and at least ease the parents' pain of not knowing" (Reagan, 1982).

Indeed, this act sought to strengthen reporting systems by creating a national clearinghouse for missing person investigations. The FBI has been responsible for operating the NCIC since 1967 and had added the category of "missing persons" to its database in 1975. However, information on missing persons was not recorded by age or by circumstances of disappearance. Therefore, there was no way to tell how many of the "missing person" cases involved minors. MCA authorized the "division of missing persons file into four categories: disability, endangered, involuntary, and juvenile" at the NCIC (Elliott & Pendleton, 1986, p. 675, fn. 27). Theoretically this meant that, for the first time, the federal government could begin tracking the number of children who were missing "involuntarily" (abducted) as well as those who were "endangered" no matter what the circumstances causing their absence from home.

Although the Missing Children's Act was a significant first step in keeping statistical records on missing youth, it was the Missing Children's Assistance Act (MCAA) of 1983 (and its subsequent amendments) that really created a service structure for dealing with the problem. First, MCAA defined a "missing child" as "any individual less than 18 years of age whose whereabouts are unknown to such individual's legal custodian if (a) the circumstances surrounding the individual's disappearance indicate that such individual may possibly have been removed by another from the control of such individual's legal custodian without such custodian's consent; or (b) if the circumstances of the case strongly indicate that such individual is likely to be abused or sexually exploited" (42 U.S.C. §5772 (1)). In doing so, the act explicitly identified abducted youth in the definition, but it also implicitly implicated runaway youth who were at-risk of abuse or exploitation. Second, it noted the importance of aiding both parents and law enforcement officers, stating, "In many cases, parents and local law enforcement officials have neither the resources nor the expertise to mount expanded search efforts" (42 U.S.C. §5772 (3)). Third, it noted that abducted children are frequently moved from one locality to another, requiring the cooperation and coordination of local, state, and federal law enforcement efforts (42 U.S.C. §5771 (4)).

In short, MCAA highlighted the dangers facing "missing children" and advocated for aid, better coordination between parents and police, and better cooperation between and among all law enforcement agencies.

3.2.4 Services Associated with Missing Children Policy

MCAA authorized the creation of and ultimately funded the National Center for Missing and Exploited Children (NCMEC). Among other things it mandated the operation of a 24-hour toll-free telephone line "by which individuals may report information regarding the location of any missing child, or other child 13 years of age or younger whose whereabouts are unknown to such child's legal custodian, and request information pertaining to procedures necessary to reunite such child with such child's legal custodians." In addition, NCMEC serves as a national resource center and clearinghouse; is responsible for coordinating public and private programs that locate, recover, or reunite missing children with families; provides technical assistance and training to law enforcement agencies; provides assistance to families and law enforcement agencies in locating and recovering missing children; and operates a cyber tip line to receive reports on Internet-related child sexual exploitation (42 U.S.C. §5773(b) (1)). NCMEC is required to work in partnership with the Department of Justice, FBI, and Department of Treasury to help find missing children and prevent their victimization.

3.3 Comparing the Movements

Sociologist David Finkelhor and his colleagues have spent almost two decades trying to make sense of "missing children" data using several iterations of the National Incidence Studies of Missing, Abducted, Runaway, and Thrownaway Children (NISMART) (Finkelhor et al., 1990; Hammer, Finkelhor & Sedlak, 2002). The difficulties in defining and counting these various overlapping categories of "missing" children are numerous, although several evidence-based facts appear to have emerged with some consistency over time that are relevant to the discussion at hand.

First, the vast majority of "missing" children are runaways. According to Hammer (2002), "Runaways/thrownaways constitute the largest component of children reported missing to authorities. They make up almost half (45%) of all children reported missing and greatly dwarf the numbers who are reported missing because of family or non-family abductions or who are lost or injured" (p. 9). Second, the vast majority of runaways are gone for a short period of time, do not travel far from home, often "run" to the homes of friends or family, and return home safely. For example, Hammer, Finkelhor & Sedlak (2002) report that 77% of all runaways/thrownaways are gone for less than one week. In the end, the numeric portrait of "runaway" youth may be better supported by the Norman Rockwell version of the runaway narrative than what was typified in the 1970s.

However, "runaway" youth are important for this chapter because they serve as the bedrock upon which both the "runaway youth" and the "missing children" movements were built. Claims-makers associated with these two movements used "runaways" as a starting point to frame their problems in two very different directions. In doing so, two diametrically opposed sets of solutions emerged.

The runaway youth movement was framed from the youth's perspective and took a rights-based approach. Therefore core values associated with services included youth autonomy, confidentiality, and privacy, which extended to all runaway services including shelters, hotlines, and outreach efforts. Advocates assumed the right of youth to make decisions independent from their families. Service providers sought to offer alternative systems of care outside existing public sector systems, including law enforcement, juvenile justice, and child protective services.

Conversely, the missing children movement took a parent-rights perspective. Worried parents sought help locating children. Core services include a hotline, website, and clearinghouse where the public can see photographs of missing children, report sightings, and get other assistance in locating children. In addition, policies and practices sought to strengthen law enforcement networking and promote faster action and better communication among policing agencies and with the public. Taken together, these responses sought to promote broader, more aggressive systems of surveillance in order to locate missing youth.

The two movements took shape through the acts of claims-makers shaping very different images of typified social problems. Arguably, both movements focused public attention on particularly endangered child-victims but at different ends of a spectrum of missing youth—with homeless street youth on one side and stranger-abducted children on the other. What links the two extremes is a middle ground population of relatively safe "runaway" children. Nonetheless, the net result of building social problems in two different directions was two diametrically opposed sets of programs, services, and policy responses. In many ways, these two responses appear to work at cross-purposes. One promotes the independence of youth and shields their movements via confidential services and privacy rights; the other seeks to track them down through shared information and public surveillance.

Examining the intersection of these two independently constructed social problems invites questions about at least two foundational assumptions. First, arguably whenever a minor is "missing" from his or her legal residence (for whatever reason), both the legal custodians *and* the child are implicated. Therefore, both sides of this dyad are critical to assessing the problem at hand. Framing policies and services exclusively from one perspective or the other may unduly complicate response to the problem. Second, the two framings may fail to appreciate the multi-faceted societal role of police officers. Certainly they investigate crimes (including kidnappings and abductions) but they also perform community-policing roles as well. For better or worse, police officers often find themselves mediating all sorts of family issues. Furthermore, they are often in position to first spot runaway youth. It might be more effective to recognize their role as first responders on all sides of the missing children/runaway youth problem.

My major objective in this comparative case study, however, is not to criticize the outcome of these two movements. Perhaps they offer the best range of services for both youth and parents that we could hope for. Instead, my goal has been to unpack the relationship between problem, service, and policy in both movements and then to consider the interconnected nature of the two.

Although I have used a topic of particular interest to me in this comparative case study, it is meant only as an example. Readers are invited and challenged to substitute any social issue of interest to them, place it in a domestic or global context, and engage in a similar intellectual exercise of examining how the problem has been shaped and responded to.

4 Implications for Practitioners

Subscribing to the notion that social problems are the product of various claims-making groups' activities and that the way the problem is shaped has implications for the corresponding services, programs, and policies that attempt to solve that problem, offers a wide range of opportunities for social reformers. First, it puts advocates in a position to think about the entire conceptual framework linking problem to service to policy. Second, this integrated conceptual framework can provide advocates with a logical and comprehensive strategy for intervening, consistently and forcefully, at all systems levels. Third, if advocates are trained to think flexibly about alternative framings of problems and solutions, rather than taking pre-existing formulations as given, they are better prepared with the analytic skills to re-frame problems, programs, and policies in ways that best serve their agendas.

All this bodes well for social workers. Social workers stand in a very unique relationship to social conditions and claims-making activities. First, as front-line practitioners working with some of the most vulnerable and marginalized clients, social workers are likely to see recurring but un-problematized social conditions in their daily practice long before other social actors take notice. As such, they have a special responsibility to think about framing those conditions as problems to advance clients' interests. Second, because social workers deal with individual cases, they are likely to have the raw material to provide compelling case examples that engage the public when building claims. Third, because social workers are trained in community organizing, they are in a good position to move social problem agendas forward in public discourse. They have the skill set to organize and promote claims in community settings. Fourth, because social workers are in a position both to implement policy and to observe its impact on individuals, they can claim a unique expertise in making claims. Fifth, because social workers are interested in micro, mezzo, and macro practice, they stand in a strong public position to communicate and organize across these levels of practice while framing and forwarding a social problem of interest. Sixth, because social workers are employed in very diverse institutional settings, they are in a unique position to observe, organize, and act on social problems that cut across service domains. For all these reasons, it seems particularly appropriate that social workers be trained in thinking about social problem constructions and encouraged to develop the analytical skills to take this theoretical knowledge and put it into action.

5 An Afterword on Alfred Kahn's Influence

News of Dr. Kahn's death reached me as I was revising this chapter. I appreciated the eventual inevitability of such news, but I was stunned and deeply saddened nonetheless. In my life, he was a larger than life figure, an inspiration because of his enormous intellectual energy and personal generosity; a mentor and a role model. Like so many generations of CUSSW doctoral students, I took his history and philosophy of social welfare course as well as Dr. Kamerman's social welfare policy course early in my doctoral studies.

As good fortune would have it, I was invited to continue to work with them. In particular, they engaged me in two different projects—one examining the impact of welfare reform on children and the other a comparative case study of services for families and children in big cities—both projects entailed bringing together a star studded list of prominent scholars, practitioners, and policy-makers to discuss, debate, and share their insights and concerns (Kamerman & Kahn, 1996a, 1996b, 1996c, 1996d; Kahn & Kamerman, 1998). Under Dr. Kahn and Kamerman's tutelage, these experiences shaped my intellectual future.

So what is the point of bringing this up now? As different as my scholarship may appear, at its core are the trace elements of the intellectual gene pool from which it springs. Perhaps drawing out the generic lessons—which are evident in the work I have presented in this chapter—might be of use to others.

First, among them is the importance of the "case" and of case-based studies. It is in the particular and applied details that much practical and useful information may be gleaned. Second, and related, is the importance of thinking comparatively. It is the act of comparing and contrasting that permits exploring the range of what is available to us and provides the opportunity to notice what might be missing. Third, is the importance of listening—with both respect and curiosity—to the voices of others, including those with very diverse political and cultural views. It is in the breadth of these vantage points that the widest range of options and ideas can emerge. Fourth, is the importance of capitalizing on the moment while still appreciating its historical place in an ever-continuous evolution of ideas and practices. Fifth, is thinking broadly across boundaries be they systems, institutions, or policies and not to be constrained by narrowly constructed domains. Finally, is to think conceptually and embrace big ideas. In this outset of this book, Dr. Kahn's own chapter demonstrates many of these very elements: thinking historically and contextually, looking backwards as a springboard for looking forward; asking big questions, at the same time pondering how advocates should organize services and policies to best serve children.

After re-reading much of Dr. Kahn's earlier work—and it does not really matter which of six decades of his work you pick up and look at—for me, one final significant attribute of his scholarship emerged. It is his eternal optimism, his sense of wonderment and unbridled excitement in seeing what the future would bring. So it is very fitting that in his final first chapter he prods us ever-forward by demanding we consider: what next in the service of children? It is a question I will keep in the fore as I move forward in my own work.

References

Almanzar, Y. (2008, December 17). 27 years later, case is closed in slaying of abducted child. *The New York Times*, A14.

Best, J. (1990). *Threatened children: Rhetoric and concerns about child-victims*. Chicago: University of Chicago Press.

Best, J. (1995). *Images of issues: Typifying contemporary social problems* (2nd ed.). New York: Aldine de Gruyter.

Child Find Official Regains Daughter. (1984, August 28). *The New York Times*.

Danziger, S. K., & Staller, K. M. (2008). Social problems: Overview. In T. Mizrahi & L. Davis (Eds.), *Encyclopedia of social work* (20th ed.). Washington, DC: NASW and Oxford.

Elliott, S. N., & Pendleton, D. L. (1986). S. 321: The Missing Children Act—Legislation by hysteria. *University of Dayton Law Review, 11*, 671–708.

Finkelhor, D., Hotaling, G., & Sedlak, A. (1990). *Missing, abducted, runaway and thrownaway children in America. First report: Numbers and characteristics national incidence studies*. Washington, DC: Office of Juvenile Justice and Delinquency Prevention and Westat.

Fritz, N. J., & Altheide, D. L. (1987). The mass media and the social construction of the missing children problem. *Sociological Quarterly, 28*, 473–492.

Gentry, C. (1988). The social construction of abducted children as a social problem. *Sociological Inquiry, 58*, 413–425.

Hammer, H., Finkelhor, D., & Sedlak, A. J. (2002, October). Runaway/thrownaway children: National estimates and characteristics. National incidence studies on missing, abducted, runaway and thrownaway children (NISMART). Washington, DC: Office of Juvenile Justice and Delinquency Prevention.

Kahn, A. J., & Kamerman, S. B. (1998). *Big cities in the welfare transition*. New York: Cross National Studies Research Program. Columbia University School of Social Work.

Kamerman, S. B., & Kahn, A. J. (1996a). *Confronting the new politics of child and family policy in the United States*. Report 1: *Whither American social policy?* New York: Cross-National Studies Research Program. Columbia University School of Social Work.

Kamerman, S. B., & Kahn, A. J. (1996b). *Confronting the new politics of child and family policy in the United States*. Report 2: *Planning a state welfare strategy under waivers or block grants*. New York: Cross-National Studies Research Program. Columbia University School of Social Work.

Kamerman, S. B., & Kahn, A. J. (1996c). *Confronting the new politics of child and family policy in the United States*. Report 3: *Child health, medicaid, and welfare "reform"*. New York: Cross-National Studies Research Program. Columbia University School of Social Work.

Kamerman, S. B., & Kahn, A. J. (1996d). *Confronting the new politics of child and family policy in the United States*. Report 4: *Child welfare in the context of welfare "reform"*. New York: Cross-National Studies Research Program. Columbia University School of Social Work.

Nelson, B. J. (1984). *Making an issue of child abuse: Political agenda setting for social problems*. Chicago: University of Chicago Press.

Pfohl, S. J. (1977). The discovery of child abuse. *Social Problems, 24*, 310–323.

Rabb, S. (1977, October 3). Veronica's short, sad life—Prostitution at 11, death at 12. *New York Times, 1*, 36.

Reagan, R. (1982, October 12). Remarks on signing the Missing Children Act and the Victim and Witness Protection Act of 1982. http://www.reagan.utexas.edu/archives/speeches/1982/101282c.htm. Accessed 8 January 2009.

Reinarman, C. (1988). The social construction of an alcohol problem: The case of Mothers Against Drunk Drivers and social control in the 1980s. *Theory and Society, 17*, 91–120.

Spector, M., & Kitsuse, J. I. (1973). Social problems. *Social Problems, 21*, 145–159.

Spector, M., & Kitsuse, J. I. (1977). *Constructing social problems*. Menlo Park, CA: Cummings.

Spector, M., & Kitsuse, J. I. (2001). *Constructing social problems*. New Brunswick, NJ: Transaction Publishers.

Staller, K. M. (2003). Constructing the runaway youth problem: Boy adventurers to girl prostitutes, 1960–1978. *Journal of Communications, 53*, 330–346.

Staller, K. M. (2004). Runaway youth system dynamics: A theoretical framework for analyzing runaway and homeless youth policy. *Families in Society, 85*, 379–491.

Staller, K. M. (2006). *Runaways: How the sixties counterculture shaped today's practices and policies*. New York: Columbia University Press.

The Development of International Comparative Child and Family Policies

Shirley Gatenio Gabel

In the 1970s, Sheila B. Kamerman and Alfred J. Kahn pioneered a new field of study: comparative child and family policy. At the time they wrote,

> Interest in family policy and its potential development as a field or as offering a criterion to guide public action also is clearly growing. Whether or not the two are directly related, and whether or not there is a natural progression from concern with the family to interest in family policy, is not yet clear. Nor is there consensus on exactly what is happening to the family in the industrialized world, how family change should be regarded, or what is meant by family policy (Kamerman & Kahn, 1978, p. 1).

In the decades following Kamerman and Kahn's observations, the field of comparative child and family policy blossomed in both the industrialized and developing world. Today, child and family policies are an essential component of most countries social welfare schemes, though the scope, types of benefits and the allocation of resources vary widely. There is growing attention paid to evidence-based child-centered comparative research in both the industrialized and developing parts of the world and on the transferability of policies from one country to another. Interest in the portability of policies is not only among like-developed countries, but also from developed to developing countries and the visa-versa.

This chapter reviews the international developments in policies affecting children and their families. It begins with definition of child and family policies and then a brief summary of the growth in family policy in industrialized countries and its attention to increasing family size and well-being. This is compared to the development of child and family policies in the developing world. Among developing countries, child and family policies are often framed from a child rights perspective. The impetus for a child rights approach is considered and a summary of the major international documents promoting this perspective are presented. The chapter concludes with a discussion of how changing in perspectives on child and family needs has affected the evolution of policies in both developing and developed countries.

S.G. Gabel (✉)
School of Social Services, Fordham University, New York, USA

S.B. Kamerman et al. (eds.), *From Child Welfare to Child Well-Being*, Children's
Well-Being: Indicators and Research 1, DOI 10.1007/978-90-481-3377-2_11,
© Springer Science+Business Media B.V. 2010

1 Defining Child and Family Policy

Characteristic of child and family policies today globally is, a concern for *all* children and their families, not just poor families, atypical families or families with problems, although these and other family types may receive special attention. Child and family policies may be explicit (policies and programs deliberately designed to achieve specific objectives directly targeted at improving the well-being of children or regarding individuals in their family roles or the family unit as a whole) or implicit (actions taken in other policy domains, for non-family related reasons, which have important consequences for children and their families as well). Child and family policy assumes a diversity and multiplicity of policies rather than a single, monolithic, comprehensive legislative act affecting child and family well-being (Kamerman, forthcoming).

Today child and family policies may include: income transfers and housing allowances directly and indirectly benefitting children; policies assuring time for parenting, including paid and job protected leaves from employment following childbirth or adoption, and during children's illnesses or school transitions; child protection and prevention from abuse and neglect; early childhood care and education; laws of inheritance, adoption, guardianship, marriage, separation, divorce, custody, and child support; family planning and services; family support programs; and health services.

2 Child and Family Policies in Industrialized Countries

The initial focus of family policy in industrialized countries centered on actions the state could take to increase the falling birthrates of mothers. Fertility declined steadily in most European countries during the late 19th century and went into a steep descent by the early 1920s. The fertility rates varied by country yet on average more than half of Europe had fertility rates below replacement rates (Bavel, 2008). In Sweden, Alva and Gunnar Myrdal's' book, *Kris I befolkningsfrågan (Crisis in the Population Question)*, was one of the earliest efforts to apply modern social science research to develop family policy responses. The Myrdals debated what an ideal family structure should be and in response considered policies and programs that would promote married couples having more children (Carlson, 1990).

In contrast to the explicit family policies debated in Sweden and elsewhere in Europe at the time, other countries such as the United States developed implicit social policies affecting children and their families (Kamerman & Kahn, 1978). Less concerned with fertility rates because of the influx of immigration, the focus of U.S. efforts in the early part of the 20th century was on "child saving" and family preservation among poor children and their families (Katz, 1986).

After World War II, family policy was part of social policy discussions about what governments might implicitly and explicitly provide for families with children, in particular those laws, regulations, benefits, and programs that affect the situation of families with children (Kamerman & Kahn, 1999; Gauthier, 1996). In the building of post-war welfare states, debates centered on the role of women in the family and with regard to employment, social solidarity across income groups and classes; ideal family size; and equalizing the social costs of child rearing.

After brief rise in fertility rates following World War II, Europe was once again experiencing lowered fertility rates and a simultaneous increase in its elderly population. Across Europe, this was accompanied by changes in family composition, structure and roles; changing labor market needs that affected women's participation in the labor market; and evolving notions of optimal child rearing and child development (Kamerman & Kahn, 1978). All countries witnessed a decline in the prevalence of married couple, one breadwinner families. Family policy had the potential to modify the vulnerability of the growing numbers of single parent and economically vulnerable families and as Kamerman and Kahn have noted it also had "the potential of conservation or regressive application and use to support what some people define as the traditional family exclusively and to acknowledge only traditional family roles." (Kamerman & Kahn, 1978, p. 8).

Troubled economies, reorientation of policies and policy goals, and new sociodemographic trends affecting children and families contributed to a growing interest in comparative child and family policies by the late 1970s. Child and family policies were at once contracting and expanding. A move away from universal provision of child and family policies occurred although family allowances remained the key cash benefit transfer, its value increasingly varied across countries and it was often supplemented by other child and family benefits such as means-tested cash benefits targeted at low-income or single-parent families (Gauthier, 1996). The increased labor force attachment of mothers heightened interest in the expansion of maternal and later parental leaves and benefits, child rearing benefits and child care options.

Early childhood education and care experienced a surge of policy attention during these years. As mothers of young children were joining the labor market in increasing numbers, the need for early childhood education and care grew. Access to quality early childhood care and education could both support the social needs of families and strengthen the foundations of lifelong learning for all children.

No longer limited to fertility issues, the attention to public policies and families turned to: increasing female employment to support, at least in part, the rise in single parent families, sustaining economic growth and pension systems; promoting gender equity; enhancing and promoting child development; addressing fertility concerns; and tackling child poverty. OECD referred to these policies as "family-friendly"[1] policies.

Since the 1980s, another approach to understanding the needs of and responsibilities to children grew more popular. This framework, known as children's rights, grew from concerns for children's well-being worldwide but particularly in developing countries. The Convention on the Rights of the Child (CRC) sparked a new

---

[1] A term used earlier by Sheila B. Kamerman in *Parenting in an unresponsive society: Managing work and family life*. New York: Free Press (1980).

lens on childhood, family and societal needs and responsibilities. There was concern about how industrialized countries would incorporate this perspective that for
at least some countries seemed to be in conflict with family-centered policies and
benefits. Expressing the opinion of the European Observatory on National Family
Policies, Ditch, Barnes and Bradshaw noted, "Whilst family policies and the impact
of emerging trends on families are issues which remain at the heart of policy
debate, it is also the case that there is a degree of tension between the discourse
of supporting families and a tendency to individualisation of citizenship rights; as
workers, women, children, and increasingly, fathers" (Ditch, Barnes, & Bradshaw,
1996, p. 3).

Political and economic pressures created a climate to curtail social spending in
the 1990s while the proportion of children in the population of many industrialized countries declined. Despite this, public investment in children and families
increased in most countries in the 1990s and into the turn of the century (Gatenio
Gabel, & Kamerman, 2006). Although cash transfers continue to be the dominant
policy instrument, increased spending on parental leave benefits and services; specialized cash family benefits and early childhood education and care benefits, reflect
changing child and family policy goals. The current goals of family policies have
expanded to include reconciling work and family responsibilities; providing incentives to work; enhancing and strengthening the development of young children;
targeting help to families considered most vulnerable due to age or disability of
children, family size, or family structure; and preparing young children for formal schooling (Gatenio Gabel, & Kamerman, 2006). The increased proportion of
social expenditures spent on in-kind benefits and services reflects the interest in
going beyond alleviating income poverty and the general economic situation of
children and families to support other aspects of well-being. Recent policies also
acknowledge the importance of the early years in a child's life as an opportunity for
modifying social and economic inequities (Heckman & Masterov, 2007).

The focus also shifted from reducing child poverty, which in many industrialized countries was now low, to increasing child well-being. Policies were not only
to care for children who were materially vulnerable, but increasingly policies are
called upon to enhance the potential of children by promoting their economic, social,
developmental, and emotional situations.

3 Beyond the Industrialized Countries

In contrast to the development of child and family policies in industrialized countries that began with an interest in family welfare and population growth, the initial
focus in developing countries was child-centered. Cross-national study of child policies in the developing world is grounded in children's rights and less evolved as a
field of study though increasingly used to guide policy development in developing
countries. Child and family policy in the developing countries is also more likely
to be influenced and shaped by international NGOs. In both the developing and

developed world, government and non-government agencies play important roles in shaping child and family policies, yet the role of NGOs in many developing countries today is often critical in the enactment and implementation of child policies (Oberdörster, 2008).

3.1 The Framework for Children's Rights and Early International Documents

The original documents acknowledging the special rights of children were first conceived of and drafted by advanced industrialized countries. Two international documents provided early piecemeal protection against international economic and sexual abuse of children: the International Labor Conference adopted the Minimum Age (Industry) Convention in 1919, and; the League of Nation adopted the Convention for the Suppression of Traffic in Women and Children in 1921 (Bueren, 1998). Two years later, Eglantyne Jebb, co-founder of Save the Children who worked with Balkan refugee children, drafted the first international declaration of children's rights. The League of Nations adopted the Declaration of the Rights of the Child in Geneva in 1924 (Ensalco, 2005). In five principles, the Declaration covered the needs of children such as food, health care, shelter, and emergency relief; rallied against the exploitation of children with regard to work, delinquency, and service; and linked these to the developmental needs of children. The Declaration viewed children's rights mainly with regard to socio-economic and psychological needs and made children the objects not subjects of these rights—a perspective that continues to dominate even today (Bueren, 1998).

Attention to the rights and needs of children was suspended as the world's attention turned to the rise of fascism in the ensuing decade and then to World War II.

3.2 The Creation of UNICEF

The formation of the United Nations (UN) in 1945 rekindled interest in the needs of children. According to Maggie Black, the postwar emergency in Europe and the Far East was protracted and millions lacking adequate shelter, fuel, clothing and nutrition struggled to survive the bitter winter of 1946–47 (Black, 1986). The situation was particularly harsh on children, many of who orphaned because of the war and had no means of support. In certain regions, famine spread and half of all babies born alive died before their first birthday.

In 1944, the allied powers established the UN Relief and Rehabilitation Administration (UNRRA) to help those in Eastern and Western Europe but by the end of 1946 replaced this with the Marshall Plan for Western Europe only. Many of the postwar relief functions were progressively transferred to newly created, specialized UN agencies, such as the Food and Agricultural Organization (FAO), the World Health Organization (WHO), the United Nations Educational, Scientific, and Cultural Organization (UNESCO), and the International Refugee Organization (which became the UN High Commission for Refugees in 1951).

At the last meeting of UNRRA, several individuals raised concern that the fate of children should be of special concern regardless of what part of Europe they lived (Jackson, 1986) and proposed that UNRRA's residual resources be used to fund a UN International Children's Emergency Fund (ICEF). The newly formed UN passed a resolution in December 1946 creating ICEF (later to become known as UNICEF). The creation of ICEF established the principle that the needs of children were above any international conflict and refocused attention on children's needs (Black, 1996).

ICEF's earliest programs were located in Poland, Yugoslavia, and Romania but by the late 1940s, Unicef was assisting children on both sides of the civil wars in China and Greece, as well as in the Middle East. The intention of ICEF was to provide temporary aid to children in the postwar emergency yet ICEF soon took on projects that extended beyond helping children to survive the aftermath of war to providing relief to children living in poverty. ICEF became increasingly active in addressing children's public heath concerns in developing countries and its popularity grew. It became a permanent UN agency to safeguard children in 1953. "International" and "emergency" dropped from its title and its new name was the United Nations Children's Fund, commonly referred to as Unicef (Black, 1996).

Unicef's primary focus in the 1950s was to help control or eradicate epidemic disease in Asia, Africa and Latin America and in doing so; it broadened its scope both regionally and thematically (Black, 1996). By the early 1960s attention shifted to child well-being more generally and eradicating child poverty. There was strong interest in aiding children in the newly independent African nations who were overwhelmed by poverty and potential disease. Unicef worked with other UN agencies such as the WHO, FAO, UNESCO, the Bureau of Social Needs, and the International Labour Office (ILO) to develop strategies for development on both on national and broader regions. Unicef took the position that children's needs should be considered in entirety and addressed in national development plans along with the needs of their parents and caretakers. It objected to the compartmentalization of children's needs (United Nations Children's Fund, 2006).

3.3 1959 Declaration of the Rights of the Child

The UN's General Assembly adopted a Declaration of the Rights of the Child in 1959. The 1959 Declaration incorporated the fundamental concerns expressed for the material and spiritual development of children in the 1924 document. It went beyond this by promoting education for all children including those with disabilities, and by calling for the protection of children against all forms of exploitation, neglect and cruelty including trafficking and in work (Ensalco, 2005). It also prohibited discrimination and gave children the right to a name and a nationality (Black, 1996).

Like its predecessor, the 1959 Declaration lacked enforcement mechanisms and continued to treat children as the subjects of rights not holders and participants.

3.4 International Momemtum for Children's Well-Being and Rights—1970s

An international momemtum for children's welfare and rights formed in the 1970s fueled by the efforts of NGOs to promote the rights of children and by the growing numbers of NGOs formed to provide relief to children in developing countries. Unicef was reluctant to advocate for children's rights during these early years because it feared antagonizing government partners who were not commited to recognizing the human rights of children and Unicef did not want to become entangled in controversy around women's reproductive rights (Black, 1986; Black, 1996; Gerschutz & Karns, 2005).

NGOs serving children lobbied the UN to declare 1979 as the "International Year of the Child" (IYC). According to Black, the NGO community also resusciated a child-centered focus within Unicef (who became the lead agency for IYC) because in striving to be part of national development plans, Unicef's emphasis on the needs of children had diminished (Black, 1986). The idea for a special year for children was first presented by Canon Joseph Moerman, Secretary General of the International Catholic Guild Welfare Bureau, who felt, "there was a fatigue among people regarding the situation of children. The attitude seemed to be: in our countries (i.e. the West), it's not so bad, and in the Third World, it's hopeless." (National Commision International Year of the Child, 1980).

Some 170 developed and developing countries and territories representing 1.5 billion children participated in the International Year of the Child by assessing, developing and implementing programs, and reporting on children's needs at international, national and local levels. The International Year of the Child also ushered the use of children's rights as a framework for children's needs around the world (Black, 1996).

Unicef's new Executive Director, James P. Grant seized the momentum coming from the International Year of the Child to mobilize Unicef to lead the international community advocating for child and famiy well-being. Unicef's top priority in the 1980s became child survival and development. Within his first couple of years at Unicef he published the first *State of the World's Children 1980–81* (Grant, 1982). This *State of the World's Children* summarized the living conditions and challenges confronting children around the world using available statistics and research. Over the years, it has become a benchmark of childhood inidcators and the main vehicle for Unicef to publicize the policy directions it was advocating. The success of policy initiatives would become measured against the the family and childhood indicators that became staples of the State of the World's Children reports. The availability of this information, expanded Unicef's role to increasingly include measuring and publicizing the impact of macroeconomic policies in the developing world on the well being of children in the 1980s (Black, 1996).

3.5 1989 the Convention of the Rights of the Child

The economic recessions around the world, increasing urbanization and industrialization, restructuring of production and growth away from agriculture, and changing demographics resulted in the increased vulnerability of children in the 1980s. Economic dependence on children as laborers increased and new social issues such as street children developed. Children's rights activists publicized these situations and other exploitative situations of children to promote the need to declare and restate the rights of children, this time with enforcement mechanisms (Gerschutz & Karns, 2005). Activists and NGOs worked with Unicef over the course of the 1980s to draft a document specifying the rights of children. The prompt and widespread ratification of the the children's rights convention is attributed to the influence of international NGOs and their ability to develop grassroots support (Oberdörster, 2008).

In 1989 the Convention of the Rights of the Child (CRC) was adopted by the General Assembly of the UN. The CRC was the first international document with legally binding force to detail children's rights and methods for their implementation. The CRC has been noted for its breadth and sensitivity to diversity of children's lives, situations, communities, and needs (Melton, 2008). In contrast to the 1924 Declaration of Children's Rights, the CRC is comprised of 54 articles encompassing a wide range of situations. The document recognizes the societal responsibility to provide children with the socioeconomic, physcial and psychological supports needed to become individuals with dignity, tolerance, freedoms and the abilities to sustain themselves. It states that this is best accomplished when children are raised in family environments, the family being the fundamental unit of society. At the same time, the CRC reflects the involvement of government and others in the raising of children in today's societies. The CRC extends to all "actions concerning children, whether undertaken by public or private social welfare institutions, courts of law, administrative authorities or legislative bodies" (United Nations General Assembly, Art. 3).

The participation of children in decisions affecting their welfare is promoted. Any child "who is capable of forming his or her own views" has a right to be heard (Art. 12; see also Arts. 13–15 and 17). The rights and needs of children are also to be understood from the perspective of children (Arts. 6(2), 18(2), 27(2), 5, 9, 10, 18 and 22).

A key aspect of the CRC is to facilitate the enactment of domestic laws and policies that improve the welfare of children. All but two nations, the United States and Somalia, have signed the CRC.

Two optional protocols, one eliminating the sale of children, child prostitution and pornography, and the other dealing with the involvement of children in armed conflicts, were added in 2002.

Periodic reports on the status of the Convention's implementation are required and to be reviewed by the UN Committee on the Rights of the Child but inadequate resources hamper the Committee's ability to enforce timeliness and to sanction governments has compromised the effectivesness of the CRC (Gerschutz & Karns, 2005).

Concern regarding how the information generated by the reports would be handled and used prompted the formation of the Children's Rights Information Network (Children's Right Information Network (CRIN). Representatives from Unicef Geneva and New York, Save the Children Sweden and the Defence for Children International (DCI) began meeting in 1991 to tackle this issue. DCI and Save the Children Sweden spearheaded this effort. In 1992 a Facilitating Group was created to establish CRIN that included global representation from human rights and child focused NGOs.[2] Today, CRIN has over 2,000 members and is a key vehicle in helping countries and activists to implement the UN Convention on the Rights of the Child. CRIN educates and leads advocacy efforts to support the implementation of the CRC by hosting petitions, publishing status reports on issues and by country, and providing a platform for joint campaigns.

3.6 Renewed Advocacy for Children in the 1990s

In 1990, a World Summit for Children (WSC) was held at the United Nations. It was an impressive gathering of world leaders to promote the well-being of children chaired by Brian Mulroney of Canada and Mussa Traoré of Mali. There were 159 countires represented, with 71 heads of state in attendance, as well as 45 NGOs participating.

At the summit, a World Declaration on the Survival, Protection and Development of Children and a Plan of Action comprising a detailed set of child-related human development goals for the year 2000, was signed by many of the governments represented at the WSC. These included targeted reductions in infant and maternal mortality, child malnutrition and illiteracy, as well as targeted increases in access to basic services for health and family planning, education, safe water and sanitation. Many of these goals were further developed and incorporated in the Millenium Development Goals (MDGs). The WSC generated a high level of commitment on behalf of children around the world, and helped to create new partnerships between governments, NGOs, donors, the media, civil society and international organizations in pursuit of a child well-being.

WSC participants adopted a set of goals to promote the welfare of children recognizing that many countries lacked the capacity to accurately measure progress

---

[2] Included were representatives from: DCI, International Centre for Childhood and the Family, International Save the Children Alliance, NGO Group for the Convention on the Rights of the Child, Office of the High Commissioner for Human Rights, Save the Children Sweden, Save the Children UK, UNICEF Innocenti Centre, Unicef, African Network for the Prevention and Protection Against Child Abuse and Neglect, Arab Resource Collective, Butterflies, Concerned for Working Children, and the Instituto Interamericano del Ninos. CRIN was founded in 1995 and is housed in Save the Children UK in London.

toward these goals. Unicef developed a household survey known as the Multiple Indicator Cluster Survey (MICS) to assist countries in monitoring the situation of children and women through statistically sound, internationally comparable estimates of socioeconomic and health indicators. MICS surveys are conducted every 5 years. Each round of surveys builds upon the last and offers new indicators to monitor current priorities in addition to monitoring trends. Since the initiation of the MICS, nearly 200 surveys have been implemented in approximately 100 countries. The latest round of surveys (MICS3) is generating data representative of close to one in four children living in developing countries.

As more parties became interested in meeting the needs of children and policies developed in response, the need for policies to integrate the developmental needs of children was interpreted as critical to the promotion of children's rights. Unicef formed the International Child Development Centre (ICDC) in Florence, Italy in 1988 to integrate the concepts of human development and human rights into policies affecting children (Black, 1996). ICDC conceptualized children's rights as the criteria around which social policies were to be measured (UNICEF Innocenti Research Centre, 2008).

ICDC's work in Central and Eastern Europe, commonly known as the MONEE project, is illustrative of this approach. Following the fall of the Soviet Union in 1989, ICDC took the lead in analyzing the effects of the newly independent countries transition to open markets and new political systems. Using economists, sociologists, demographers, and policy specialists, ICDC helped train specialists in the transitioning countries on tools to be used for social policy analysis as new policies were being formulated. ICDC is now known as UNICEF's Innocenti Research Centre (IRC).

3.7 Acknowledging the Changing Needs of Families

The changing needs of families, while evident in policy developments in industrialized countries, were less formed globally and particularly in developing countries. In 1989, the UN General Assembly proclaimed that 1994 was the International Year of the Family (IYF). Recognizing the family as the basic unit of society, the UN sought to promote the the realization of family human rights through policies and local, national and international actions to strengthen family viability. The UN Commission for Social Development was designated the preparatory body and the Economic and Social Council as the coordinating body for the Year. The IYF raised awareness of family needs and prompted greater attention to family issues at all levels in developed and developing countries. Families, unlike children, did not have a UN agency devoted to their welfare and definitions of families were controversial. Controversies continue around definitions of a family and whether and if family planning should be promoted. All this increases the challenges of implementing family related policies within countries.

To maintain the interest in family related policies, the UN celebrated the Tenth Anniversary of the International Year of the Family in 2004. Coinciding with this, the Programme of the Family, which is under the Division for Social Policy and Development within the Department of Economic and Social Affairs of the United Nations, identified five trends that explicitly affect family life around the globe and called upon nations to address these needs: (1) changes in family structure, which includes shift from extended to nuclear families as well as rise of one-person households, falling fertility rates, increases in single parent families; (2) demographic aging, specifically lower fertility rates and higher life expectancy affecting intergenerational solidarity, housing, social security systems, care giving and health costs; (3) increased migration due to violence, discrimination, natural disasters and the hope for better economic opportunities and the resultant increases in female-headed households around the world, trafficking and sexual exploitation of women and children; (4) the HIV/AIDS pandemic increasing adolescent and grandparent headed households in some regions of Africa; and (5) the impact of globalization. Most countries vowed to enact policies to ameliorate the negative effects of these trends and have used other UN and NGO resources to implement responses. Lack of funding has prevented the systematic monitoring of the responses.

3.8 Recent Developments

Most developing countries today pay particular attention to the needs of chilren and have in place public policies to respond to these needs. Scarce resources have fueled interest in using evidence-based research from developed and other developing countries regarding the effectiveness of child-centered policies. Severe income poverty continues to be a dominant social issue in developing countries (Gatenio Gabel & Kamerman, 2009). Of all age groups, children are the most likely to be omitted or offered the least social protection even though children are often the largest population group developing countries (Gatenio Gabel & Kamerman, 2009).

The range of child-centered policies is very wide among developing countries and can be controversial. The low-income countries, especially those in sub-Saharan Africa and South East Asia, have achieved the least, largely through targeted, categorical, and means-tested benefits and often in partnership with and at the initiation of non-governmental organizations (Gatenio Gabel & Kamerman, 2009). Unlike the past when in-kind benefits (such as food and clothing) were favored as a means of meeting the needs of poor children in developing countries, today means-tested cash benefits have become the major strategy for addressing poverty. New policy responses linking means-tested cash benefits to human capital investments of health and education for children are popular but far from a panacea. The importance of early care and education has been assimilated by most countries though the availability of programs may be limited due to scarce resources.

While attention to child policies has grown appreciably in the developing world, the lack of a comparative database on child policies constricts further cross-national research and policy development. Recently, Unicef has taken on a more active role in advocacting for child-conditioned policies around the world (Fajth, 2008). In September 2007, Unicef launched a global study on child poverty and disparities.

The Global Study aims to find context-specific evidence to assess policy responsiveness to outcomes related to child poverty and disparities. Child poverty experts in over 45 countries have analyzed the living conditions of poor children by country. The findings are being summarized in country specific reports and will be used to advocate for stronger child policies within the nations and to measure the overall implications of international policy frameworks on the rights and lives of poor children. At the same time, Unicef is reviewing the effectiveness of child-conditioned social protection strategies worldwide on child well-being and together with NGOs and scholars pursuing an evidence-based approach to child policy development.

Today, there are thousands of domestic and international NGOs contributing to the development of child and family policies. These NGOs range from being: international to grassroots organizations, issue specific to all encompassing, and population specific to covering issues affecting all children and their families. Some NGOs work cooperatively with governments, others are critical agitators of government policies. Never has the influence and scope of NGOs on the development of child and family policies been greater yet further research on their role and influence is needed.

4 Summary and Discussion

Today, almost all countries give consideration to the effects of policies on children and families, though the type of attention, scope and methodology for measuring the effects varies considerably across countries. In both industrialized and developing countries, the scope of policies affecting children and families has grown and are increasingly scrutinized for their effectiveness in achieving stated goals. This movement toward accountability-based public policy requires accurate measures of the conditions children face and the outcomes of programs designed to address those conditions. The growing demands for accountability reflects greater awareness of economic constraints as well as the emergence of new normative and conceptual theories about childhood and children's needs. The normative concept of children's rights, the sociological conceptualization of childhood as an independent stage, and ecological theories of child development, have contributed to the increased attention to children, their needs, child indicator measures, and the development of the child social indicator movement (Ben-Arieh, 2008).

The study of child and family policy in industrialized countries began with a specific concern regarding policies that would foster increased fertility and soon after regarding equalizing the social costs of raising children. As family life became more complex, new policy goals for children and families were established and research on how these goals would best be achieved followed. A range of policy tools evolved. The needs of young children, especially those whose mothers were employed, demanded greater attention both in terms of the type of care that was best for children's development and with regard to how working parents were expected to manage their time as both earners and nurturers. As the situation for most children improved in industrialized countries, newer policies differentiated and responded to the needs of children who were left vulnerable due to family composition, disability or other circumstances. Learning from the experiences of other countries became instrumental to the development of child and family policy.

The introduction of human rights, more specifically children's rights, in the latter part of the twentieth century raised public awareness of the needs of children in both developing and developed countries. For the first time in modern history, children were no longer seen as appendices of their families, the state or charitable institutions. The CRC is a powerful tool for challenging existing power relationships and enforces the view that policies enhancing chidren's development are, or should be, entitlements. Although difficult to monitor its implementation, the CRC has been a critical force in the development of explicit and implicit child and family policies among developing countries. The monitoring of the CRC has made policymakers more aware of the interdependence of nations. Domestic and international NGOs play a critical role in policy formulation around the world, especially in developing countries. Unicef has been a driving force in influencing the development of child-conditioned policies and responses to children's needs around the world but future analyses should examine the contributions and influence of NGOs in policy development affecting children.

The variety of child and families policies is enormous. Some countries have been more interventionist in relation to the family, while others have adopted a "hands off" approach to what are considered private matters, and most lie somewhere in between the two. As interest in comparative research grew, so did the availability of data on child and family policies, particularly for industrialized countries. Increasingly, policymakers at every level, demand evidence regarding the effects of various policies on outcomes for children. This is likely to encourage the development of comparative child and family databases globally and regionally. Today, efforts are underway to extend this type of information to child and family policies in the developing world and from a child rights perspective.

References

Bavel, J. V. (2008). *Subreplacement fertility in the West before the Baby Boom current and contemporary perspectives*. Interface Demography Working Paper 2008-1. Belgium: Vrije Univesiteit Brussel.

Ben-Arieh, A. (2008). The child indicators movement: Past, present, and future. *Childhood Indicators Research, 1,* 3–16.

Black, M. (1986). *The children and the Nations: The story of Unicef.* Sydney, Australia: UNICEF.

Black, M. (1996). *Children first: The story of UNICEF, past and present.* Oxford: Oxford University Press.

Carlson, A. (1990). *The Swedish experiment in family folitics: The myrdals and the interwar population crisis.* New Brunswick and London: Transaction Publishers.

Ditch, J., Barnes, H., & Bradshaw, J. (1996). *A synthesis of national family policies 1995.* York: European Observatory on National Family Policies, University of York.

Ensalco, M. (2005). Children's human rights: Progress and challenges for children worldwide. In M. Ensalco, L. C. Majka, M. Ensalco, & L. C. Majka (Eds.), *Children's human rights: Progress and challenges for children worldwide* (pp. 9–30). Maryland: Rowman & Littlefield Publishers.

Fajth, G. (2008). UNICEF's global study on child poverty and disparities. *Rethinking poverty: Making policies that work for children*. New York: The New School.

Gatenio Gabel, S., & Kamerman, S. B. (2006). Investing in children: Public commitment to children in twenty-one industrialized countries. *Social Service Review, 80*(3), 239–266.

Gatenio Gabel, S., & Kamerman, S. B. (2009). A global review of new social risks and responses for children and their families. *Asian Social Work and Policy Review, 3*, 1–21.

Gauthier, A. H. (1996). *The state and the family*. New York: Oxford University Press.

Gerschutz, J. M., & Karns, M. P. (2005). Transforming visions into reality: The convention on the rights of the child. In M. Ensalaco, L. K. Majka, M. Ensalaco, & L. K. Majka (Eds.), *Children's human rights*. Lanham, MD: Rowman and Littlefield Publishers.

Grant, J. P. (1982). *The state of the world's children 1980–81*. New York: UNICEF.

Heckman, J., & Masterov, D. V. (2007). Productivity argument for investing in young children. *Review of Agricultural Economics, 29*(3), 446–493.

Jackson, R. (1986). In M. Black, *The children and the nations* (Foreword). New York: UNICEF.

Kamerman, S. B. (forthcoming). Families and family policies: Developing a holistic family policy agenda. *Hong Kong Journal of Pediatrics*.

Kamerman, S. B., & Kahn, A. J. (1997). *Family change and family policies in Great Britain, Canada, New Zealand, and the United States*. Oxford: Oxford University Press.

Kamerman, S. B., & Kahn, A. J. (Eds.). (1978). *Family policy: Government and families in 14 countries*. New York: Columbia University Press.

Katz, M. (1986). *In the shadow of the poorhouse: A social history of welfare in America*. New York: Basic Books.

Myrdal, A., & Myrdal, G. (1941). *Nation and family: The Swedish experiment in democratic family and population policy*. New York: Harper and Brothers.

National Commision International Year of the Child. (1980). *Report to the president: United States National Commision on the International Year of the Child*. Washington, DC: U.S. Government Printing Office.

Oberdörster, U. (2008). Why ratify? *Vanderbilt Law Review, 61*(2), 681–712.

Organization of Economic Cooperation and Development (OECD). (2007). *Babies and bosses – reconciling work and family life a synthesis of findings for OECD Countries*. Paris, France: OECD.

Unicef Innocenti Research Centre. (2008, December 2). *Unicef innocenti research centre – About us*. Unicef Innocenti Research Centre: http://www.unicef-irc.org/aboutIRC/. Accessed 2 December 2008.

United Nations Children's Fund. (2006). *1946–2006 sixty years for children*. United Nations Children's Fund. New York: United Nations Children's Fund.

United Nations General Assembly, Convention of the Rights of the Child. (1989).

Using Child Indicators to Influence Policy: A Comparative Case Study

Lawrence Aber, Juliette Berg, Erin Godfrey, and Catalina Torrente

1 Introduction

Economic indicators have guided economic policymaking for almost a century. A wide range of social indicators have become increasingly important to policy debates over the last half century. But child indicators are only recently having impact on the policy process. This is likely due to the relative recency of children's issues as a formal focus of policy making and to the relative conceptual and methodological immaturity of child indicator data systems. But, as evidenced by new journals, books, data series and practices, the child indicator movement and its relevance to policymaking is undergoing rapid transformation and change. Increasingly, governments and non-governmental organizations throughout the world recognize that children are their nation's (and the world's) future. And indicators of children's welfare and well-being, if designed and used in particular ways (Aber & Jones, 1997; Ben-Arieh, 2008; Moore & Brown, 2006), are increasingly influential in the policy formulation, implementation and evaluation processes. Over the last decade, by deliberate design and directed effort, this "child indicators for policy change" movement has become increasingly international in scope and character.

This chapter hopes to make a contribution to this emerging movement. Two overarching goals motivate this chapter: (1) to begin to understand those critical features of child indicator systems and their use to influence policy which may be common across nations and those which may be unique to specific nations; and (2) to generate a modest number of recommendations about how to improve the use of child indicators for use in policymaking that may prove relevant to a broad number of countries.

The chapter is decidedly not a systematic comparison across a large and representative sample of nations. Rather, it represents something of a comparative case study. We focus on three nations, Colombia, France and South Africa, which

L. Aber (✉)
Insititute for Human Development and Social Change, New York University, New York, NY, USA

Each author made nearly equal contributions to this chapter. Authors are listed in alphabetical order.

S.B. Kamerman et al. (eds.), *From Child Welfare to Child Well-Being*, Children's Well-Being: Indicators and Research 1, DOI 10.1007/978-90-481-3377-2_12, © Springer Science+Business Media B.V. 2010

are quite different regionally, politically, demographically and developmentally. We have chosen these countries because one or two authors work intensively in each of them and therefore have both the motivation and knowledge to delve deeply into the child indicator systems of that country and their use (detailed descriptions of each country's recent economical, political and historical context are available from https://www.cia.gov/library/publications/the-world-factbook/).

After an in-depth scan of the child indicators systems of each country, we made the decision to focus on one domain of indicators and policy: the domain of education. We focus on the education domain for three reasons. First, a comparative analysis of multiple domains across all three countries is well beyond the scope of a single chapter. Second, we wished to focus on a domain considered fundamental to children's well-being everywhere in the world. This led us to a consideration of the three dimensions in common among major international data systems (e.g. UNDP's Human Development Index; Unicef's State of the World's Children reports; UN's Millennium Development Goals project). Among these three common dimensions—of health, education and livelihoods—we selected education because it is relatively the most child-specific. Also, as Ben-Arieh (2008) and Bottani (1996) have noted, education is an area in which indicators have grown rapidly in recent years and is a primary example of the impact of the global-indicator and child-centered movements on the development and collection of increasingly nuanced and comprehensive data. Third, by selecting a single domain—education—we were able to bring much greater specificity to our task of comparative analysis. Finally, we focused our analysis on the primary period of indicator growth in this area, from 1990 to the present. If this comparative case study exercise is at all helpful to others in the field, perhaps it will stimulate comparative case analyses focusing on other countries and other domains of children's welfare and well-being. A small series of such case studies could be a valuable prelude to a more systematic analysis of the use of child indicators in policymaking across a number of domains and in a larger representative sample of countries.

A web-based approach was used to explore the role of educational indicators in the policy process in Colombia, France and South Africa. Our first step was to conduct a brief scan of national media sources and child advocacy websites to gain a better understanding of the educational system in each country as well as the primary issues and concerns in this area. With this as background, we then consulted a number of sources to look for evidence of the use of indicators throughout the policy process. We reviewed documents and reports acquired from the websites of education departments, parliamentary and legislative institutions, child advocacy groups and other national and international agencies and initiatives collecting, managing and analyzing indicators. These documents included annual reports, departmental documents, strategic plans, indicator summaries and evaluation reports, as well as legislative bills, acts, amendments, thought-pieces and transcripts of recent activity. This review was conducted with the aim of characterizing and comparing the philosophical perspectives, goals and priorities of educational policy, the extent to which indicators are used at various stages of the policy process and the quality of indicator systems across the three countries. We wish to acknowledge at the outset that reliance on web searches and documents and report reviews constitutes an important limitation of our research method. We would have preferred to complement this method with interviews and field observations that could help confirm and challenge government's perspectives and to better understand how socio-political factors influence the use of indicators in the policy process.

The chapter is organized to help us meet our two overarching goals. In the second section, we describe the philosophical perspectives on policy goals and priorities for children of each country. As will become clear, we do not believe one can evaluate the quality of child indicator systems and their utility in the policymaking process except in the context of national values, goals and priorities for child policy.

In section three, we turn to the child indicator systems themselves in the education domain in each of the three focal countries. We describe both common and unique features of their content, timing, sources and disaggregation.

Next, in section four, we explore the relevance of these indicators for policymaking. Because we could not do in-depth interviews or surveys of policymakers or actually participate extensively in the policy process, we rely in this section on an analysis of policy documents and reports designed for the public and evaluate the quality of indicators.

Based on our analyses in sections two to four, we present a small number of recommendations about how to improve child indicator systems and their use to have improved impact on the policy process. To anticipate our major conclusions, we recommend that national child indicator systems privilege: methodological rigor over comprehensiveness; within-domain comprehensiveness over across-domain comprehensiveness; and the use of policy to influence the design and quality of child indicator systems (as well as the use of child indicator systems to improve the design and positive impact of policy on children's welfare and well-being).

Throughout Al Kahn's career, he encouraged colleagues and students alike to speak truth to power. He championed the use of reliable, valid indicators of children's welfare (truth) in persuading policymakers and politicians (power) to do the right thing by children. He also championed comparative analysis of child and family policy as a tool for identifying better ways of meeting the needs of children and families throughout the world. We derive our inspiration for this chapter from these two features of Al Kahn's illustrious career.

2 Philosophical Perspectives, Goals and Priorities

We begin our analysis with a discussion of the philosophical perspectives, goals and priorities of child policy in general, and education policy in particular, across the three countries. As representations of a country's prevailing values, norms and objectives, these conceptual frameworks have important implications for indicator systems. At least in theory, indicators should be developed, collected and used to assess whether the country is adhering to its basic philosophical principles and succeeding in reaching its policy goals and priorities.

2.1 Philosophical Perspectives on Policy

Despite considerable historical, economic and political differences across the three countries comprising this analysis, all tend to emphasize the *rights of children* as citizens. This is true across child development policy in general and is particularly noticeable in the area of education. Each country has ratified the 1989 United Nations International Convention on the Rights of the Child (CRC), and incorporates rights-based language into their policy and legislative documents.

For example, France's educational reform documents use rights based language both in stating the goals of the education system and in justifying the need for reforms: the legislative code of education states that the right of all children and adults to an education is guaranteed (Reiss, 2005). In principle, this right is directed towards personality development, an increase in the level of ongoing development (formation), integration into social and professional life, and active citizenship, no matter social origin, culture, and geography. In recent years, France has also introduced a *capabilities based approach* (Alkire, 2002) by laying out a set of goals involving the acquisition of a number of diverse competencies thought to be important to children's development. Rather than focus exclusively on the rights of all citizens to a basic education, this reform initiative implies that all children should have the opportunity to develop a more well-rounded and more advanced set of competencies through the education system.

In Colombia, the CRC, approved and elevated to constitutional principle by the Colombian Congress in 1991, introduced the notion of children as social subjects and citizens with rights, and assigned to the state and to society as a whole the role to protect and guarantee the rights of children (ICBF, 2006). Moreover, the new Constitution gave children a special protected status, which prioritizes their rights above those of other members of society. Thus, even though some aspects of Colombian policy were based on a rights perspective prior to 1991, the integration of the CRC into the Constitution, and the subsequent subscription to several international treaties supported by the Convention, marked a fundamental shift in the focus of public policy from a framework of *children's survival* to one of children's rights (ICBF, 2006). All policy documents reviewed as part of this study reflect this shift, as they incorporate rights based language and make explicit references to children's rights to justify the need for policy (e.g. Código de la Infancia y la Adolecencia de, 2006).

Ratified in 1996, the South African constitution is one of the most progressive in the world, specifically guaranteeing a wide array of human rights to its citizens. From a historical perspective, the rights-based philosophy espoused in the constitution is seen as crucial to redressing the injustices of the apartheid era, and ensuring the continued protection of all South Africans. Almost all subsequent national legislation and policy has reflected this approach, directly referencing the constitutional mandate to protect human dignity and rights. In addition, South Africa has endorsed and incorporated into national law numerous international treaties designed to support basic human rights, including the CRC, the MDG, and the International Covenant on Economic, Social and Cultural Rights (1996), among others.

Child rights figure prominently in South Africa's policy perspective. South Africa not only ratified the CRC but incorporated its language directly into the constitution. Moreover, as in Colombia, children enjoy a special protected status in the constitution. This rights-based perspective has dominated policy-making in the area of education as well, as evidenced in both the South African Constitution (Section 29 (1) (a) and (b) and the DoE 1995) guiding policy framework, the White Paper on Education and Training. In these documents, basic education is defined not simply as basic literacy and numeracy skills, but as the skills that underlie human rights and the principles of the Constitution, including civic engagement, arts education, mutual respect, the values underlying the democratic process, and independent and critical thinking. In addition, policy-makers see education as a primary vehicle through which the nation can be reconstructed and reconnected.

2.2 Goals and Priorities of Education Policy

Although all three countries share a similar philosophical perspective, the particular goals and priorities of education policy vary in accordance with the characteristics of the country, such as its level of economic development and sociopolitical reality.

In France, the main goals have for a long time been citizenship formation, equality of access and opportunity, and the transmission of knowledge and general culture to children of all social classes. Schools are also supposed to serve as a complement to the family system by fostering tolerance and respect, hard work and effort, and motivation (Reiss, 2005). A national education system was formed during the French Revolution around the objective of supporting the new democracy through the transmission of the values of the Republic and the formation of cultured citizens. Since then, the education system has undergone a number of reforms that parallel the goals of a strong, democratic government, from the institutionalization of free, secular, and compulsory education at the end of the 19th century to the goal of creating a more equal society in the 20th century by reducing the strong correlation between social background and educational attainment. Today, the government continues to balance socialist goals with liberal ideals, while facing pressure to maintain a competitive place in the global economy and new struggles with social inequalities related to the influx of immigration As such, the particular focus of the two major education reforms in the last 20 years (1989, 2005) has been to; reduce inequalities; provide an indispensable base of knowledge, competencies, and rules for behavior; to enable all students to successfully enter the workforce; and to improve school functioning.

These goals of instruction, advancement, and integration are admittedly not being fully met and new ways of addressing them have been proposed (CNDP, 2004). For example, the latest major education reform in 2005 calls for the establishment of a common base of knowledge defined by a set of competencies made up of a combination of knowledge, aptitudes, and attitudes (e.g., in language skills, this refers to knowledge such as vocabulary and the capacity to use this knowledge in concrete situations) (Haut Conseil de L'Education, 2005). These competencies (e.g., the mastery of the French language, acquisition of a foreign language, civic competencies, autonomy and initiative) are intended to address shortcomings in the acquisition of basic qualifications, greater school failure among children of disadvantaged backgrounds, greater insertion in the workforce, and school violence. The main implication of these reform efforts is that the advanced set of measurable competencies identified above, that go beyond basic academic skills, are necessary for the country to instill its values in its citizens and for these citizens to become fully functioning and integrated members of society.

In Colombia, education is seen as the basis for human, cultural, economic and social development. Therefore, the overall goals of the education system are to form whole human beings who will be able to contribute to the construction of a peaceful and more equitable society and who will use scientific knowledge to further the country's and its citizens' development (Ministerio Nacional de Educación, 1996). These overarching goals do not come as a surprise, given the country's struggle with a long-standing internal conflict rooted in conditions of extreme poverty and a history of unequal access to resources.

Colombia's current education policy is called Revolución Educativa (Educational Revolution), and its concrete goals and commitments are outlined in a document called Revolución Educativa: Plan Sectorial 2006–2010 (Ministerio Nacional de Educación, 2008). According to this document, four dimensions comprise the main focus of current policy, namely *coverage, quality, relevance and efficiency.* Briefly, coverage refers to facilitating access to high quality and equitable education for all children, regardless of social, economic and cultural background. Quality means providing education that enhances children's academic performance and nurtures their civic, socio-emotional and academic competencies. Relevance means that education should contribute to the country's increased productivity and competitiveness in the global economy. Finally, efficiency refers to the modernization of the education system, which involves the movement towards decentralization and increased autonomy of educative institutions; the provision of educational, physical and technical resources for institutions to provide high quality services; and the improvement of information networks that will strengthen policy design, monitoring and evaluation.

In South Africa, education has undergone a major change since the first democratic elections in 1994. The first priority of education policy was to transform the fragmented and racially divided education system under apartheid into a single unified system based on the principles of equity and redress. Since that time, the government has focused considerable attention on establishing a new legal and policy framework for education and training based in the principles of the constitution and the overarching Reconstruction and Development Programme.

The early period of democracy in South Africa was characterized by an emphasis on improving access to education. Inclusivity was one of the basic principles of the South African education system, and was considered necessary to meet the requirements of the Constitution by eliminating discrimination, providing universal access to basic education and progressively extending access to further education (DoE, 1995, 2008c). Early education policies also incorporated the goal of equity in schooling, aiming to bring into the mainstream of educational opportunities various vulnerable groups in danger of marginalization and exclusion. In addition to racial groups disadvantaged by Apartheid, these include orphans and vulnerable children, those infected or affected by HIV/AIDS and other serious diseases, those living in poverty, those in deprived rural and urban areas, and schoolgirls who become pregnant. Access and equity continue to be the primary goals and priorities of the South African Department of Education. However, in recent years, the quality of education, especially in math, sciences and technology, has become an increasingly important policy priority (DoE, 2005a, 2008c). As laid out in its strategic plan for 2007–2011 (DoE, 2007b), the department's current goals include improving access to quality education for families in poverty, improving quality through a newly implemented curriculum and improved infrastructure and broadening the health and wellness of educators and learners.

3 Indicator Systems

In this section, we discuss the recent state of educational indicator collection in Colombia, France and South Africa. We focus on three dimensions of indicator systems: content, timing and aggregation, which often reflect the goals and philosophical perspectives of education policy in each country and facilitate (or hinder) the use of indicators in policy development. Rather than offer an exhaustive inventory, the aim of this section is to present the educational indicators most commonly found in national educational reports and policy documents and highlight important similarities and differences across countries.

3.1 Content of Indicators

Our cross-country analysis revealed a number of educational indicators that are commonly collected across the three countries. We group this set into three broad categories corresponding roughly to the stages of policy implementation. The first category, *input indicators*, refers to the investments governments make in the educational system. France, Colombia and South Africa all collect indicators measuring their fiscal investment in education. These include expenditures on education at national and regional levels as well as the percentage of gross domestic product (GDP) spent on education. The second category, *process indicators*, refers to measures of intermediate educational activities and conditions. An important characteristic of these indicators is that they are expected both to be influenced by government investments in education and to have an influence on child outcomes. All three countries collect a number of process indicators, including: the total number of schools, students and educators; enrollment ratios; gender parity;

student-to-educator ratio; student and educator characteristics and attitudes; classroom practices; physical infrastructure; and school policies and programs. The third category, *outcome indicators*, refers to the final outputs of the educational system such as students' academic achievement, skill acquisition, and social and educational attainment. Commonly collected indicators in this category include measures of academic achievement, attainment of educational qualifications, graduation rates and enrollment in secondary and tertiary education.

In addition to these commonalities, our analysis revealed interesting cross-country differences in the specific indicators routinely collected. For example, of the three countries, France was the only one to regularly collect data on school attendance, which is differentiated from enrollment in that it measures children's presence in school on a regular basis. France was also the only country to regularly collect indicators on the number of violent acts occurring in schools. In addition, Colombia was the only country routinely collecting indicator data on access to education for children displaced by internal conflict and South Africa was the only country collecting data on school fees, social grants, and educator, learner and parental illness and death.

We also found interesting cross-country differences in the depth and emphasis placed on indicator collection within common domains. For example, while all three countries gather process indicator data about the physical infrastructure of schools, South Africa places considerably more emphasis on collecting indicators in this domain. In addition to measures of building integrity and access to technical resources, South Africa collects a wide array of indicators of more basic infrastructure conditions in schools such as access to clean water and basic sanitation, number of toilets, desks and chairs, road quality, and number of classrooms. In addition, whereas South Africa and Colombia focus on more basic outcome indicators such as graduation rates and enrollment in higher education, France gathers a more comprehensive set of indicators to document the usefulness of the education system for integrating youth into social and economic life. These include measures of achievement in higher education, as well as employment and career outcomes of students leaving secondary and higher education. Finally, although all three countries collect indicators of student skills and knowledge, in South Africa these are most often limited to academic areas such as literacy, math, and science. Both Colombia and France collect achievement indicators in a wider array of skill areas, including civic competencies.

These differences in content and emphasis appear to us to reflect not only each country's primary policy goals but also their current needs, and historical and economic circumstances such as recent patterns of immigration in France and the pursuit of post-Apartheid social equality and the toll of the HIV/AIDS pandemic in South Africa. In Colombia, indicators about displaced children reflect the country's political struggles with its ongoing internal conflict. Finally, in South Africa, the post-Apartheid goal of redressing the injustices of the past and increasing access to education is manifested in the collection of data on social grants and school fees. Likewise, indicator data on illness and death among learners, families and educators is a response to the toll of the HIV/AIDS pandemic.

3.2 Timing and Source of Indicator Collection

Regarding timing of indicator collection, we found that across all three countries indicators gathered from departmental administrative data are generally collected on a yearly basis. Examples include: total number of schools, educators and students in the educational system, gross enrollment and gender parity statistics, attainment of qualifications, graduation rates, physical infrastructure and some student and teacher characteristics.

In France, a number of different indicator systems operate simultaneously. Many of the output indicator systems are managed by DEPP, a government body created in 1987 to quantitatively evaluate the education system and particular education initiatives. Thirty-one summary indicators that include the activity, operation, and results of the education system have been collected yearly since 1991 (Santos, Gibert, & Yacoub, 2007). These indicators report on access to education, the acquisition of basic skills and knowledge, school functioning, inequalities in the system and the usefulness of the education system in integrating young people. Another government body (IGAENR), created in 1965 within the ministry of education, collects input and process indicators on the functioning of the school system that are summarized in an annual report to the government (http://www.education.gouv.fr). A number of indicators are also collected yearly that conform to EU standards and are monitored by Eurostat, the Statistical Office of the European Communities that oversees the European statistical system (ESS) aimed at collecting comparable data across the EU (http://epp.eurostat.ec.europa.eu/). While these data are collected by each individual country, the Statistical Programme Committee (SPC) oversees the quality and content of indicator systems by creating a common and regionally and internationally comparable dataset. Educational indicators monitored by Eurostat include financial ones such as the annual expenditure on public and private education per pupil, and non-financial ones such as student enrollment by level, student-teacher ratios, and foreign language learning. Most of these data have been collected every year since 1998.

In Colombia, the National Ministry of Education recently is making efforts to generate more reliable and timely indicators covering other areas of education. Such efforts include the creation of a set of systems in charge of collecting information about education. SINEB (National Information System about Basic and Middle Education[1]) and SINIES (National Information System for Higher Education), for example, gather information assessing the coverage, quality, equity and efficiency of education services from elementary to higher education. Indicators collected on a yearly basis include the number of school-aged children, the number, type and location of educative institutions as well as the population they serve, the academic status of students at the end of the academic year, school personnel and

---

[1] In the Colombian education system, Basic elementary and secondary education includes grades 1st–9th, and "Middle" education refers to grades 10th and 11th. Unlike in the U.S, there are only 11 grades as opposed to 12.

their qualifications, and schools' expenses and resources (Decreto 1526 de Julio 24 de 2002). SINCE (National Information System of Educational Contracts) is another noteworthy example, for it intends to provide timely information to monitor the progress and efficiency of initiatives to improve education coverage for vulnerable populations such as displaced and indigenous children (Ministerio de Educación Website).

In South Africa, the national and provincial DOEs house a system-wide monitoring system, the Educational Management Information System (EMIS) that collects annual school survey data from principals on a variety of school characteristics including enrollment, promotion, transfers, educator, learner and family characteristics, basic instructional practices and school governance and policy. Data on graduation rates and certificate and matriculation pass rates is also captured via EMIS. The department has also recently established the National Education Infrastructure Management System (NEIMS) which will collect yearly data on the physical infrastructure needs of schools.

We also found that in all three countries a set of indicators are collected at longer intervals of 2–5 years. These take the form of systematic studies which generally yield a more comprehensive set of indicators and/or more detailed indicators in an area of particular interest. In addition to collecting national statistics for selected age cohorts (e.g., for 5th and 9th graders), these more comprehensive efforts often focus on a subset of children, such as in a sample of schools. While the sampling and data collection procedures inherent in these studies limit the generalizability and utility of the indicators they generate, they still have the potential to provide valuable information for policy makers, practitioners and students.

In France, an in-depth assessment of skills in particular academic areas has been carried out since 2003 among children at the end of primary school and at the end of *college* (equivalent to middle school in the United States, 8th grade) (DEPP, 2007). The study has covered a variety of areas, from written and oral comprehension in 2003 to foreign languages, history and geography and civic education in 2006. Of particular note is the study that was conducted in 2005 (and previously in 1995 and among secondary school students in 1998) on students' attitudes towards life and society (*"Les attitudes a l'egard de la vie en societe des eleves en fin d'ecole primaire et en fin de college"*) among a representative sample of students at the end of primary school and at the end of 9th grade (Santos et al., 2007). This study asks students to report on their own perceptions and attitudes towards schooling and their role in society and includes questions related to students' perceptions of efficacy towards their peers, the school ecology, individual rights in society, and school norms. This child-centered approach to indicator data collection is rare.

In Colombia, the most comprehensive indicators come from Pruebas Saber (Knowledge Tests), a set of tests administered at least every 3 years to every 5th and 9th grader in the country, and to a sample of 3rd and 7th graders in some regions. These tests measure children's competencies in math, social and natural sciences, language, and civic competencies, and place Colombia among the first countries in Latin America and the Caribbean conducting censual evaluations of its student population (UNESCO, 2006—OEI document).

In South Africa, systemic evaluation studies are conducted by the DoE at the foundation phase (Grade 3) and intermediate phase (Grade 6) and is planned for the senior phase (Grade 9) (DoE, 2005b). The primary goals of the systemic evaluation are to measure the extent to which the education system achieves specific social, economic, and transformational goals by assessing student achievement at selected grades while taking into account the context of teaching and learning. Informed by a four-part conceptual model, indicators are collected in 4 domains: the context of teaching and learning; the human and material inputs and resources available; the quality of teaching (and learning) processes and practices; and the quality of outputs (outcomes) of the education system, specifically language, mathematics and natural sciences. So far, the Grade 3 evaluations have been conducted in randomly sampled schools in 2001 and 2007. The Grade 6 evaluation was conducted in 2004 and the Grade 9 evaluation was planned for 2005/2006.[2]

All three countries also make use of a number of international and regional evaluations that gather comparable information every few years from subsets of students in selected grades by different international organizations. These include the PIRLS (Progress in International Reading Literacy Study) conducted every 5 years among 9–10 year olds, and the Trends in International Mathematics and Science Study (TIMSS). France and Colombia both conduct the International Association for the Evaluation of Educational Achievement (IEA) study, and the PISA study, conducted every 3 years among 15-year olds. Other region-specific studies are conducted, including studies by the OECD, Unesco and Eurydice in France, (Abriac et al., 2007); the Laboratorio Latinoamericano de Evaluación de la Calidad de la Educación (LLECE) and the Civic Education Study of the International Association for the Evaluation of Educational Achievement (IEA) in Colombia; and the Monitoring Learning Achievement (MLA) project and the Southern and Eastern Africa Consortium for Monitoring Educational Quality (SACMEQ) in South Africa.

Finally, each of the three countries has additional unique methods of educational indicator collection. For example, South Africa relies on indicators collected as part of commissioned reports on particular aspects of the educational system, such as learner retention and school safety (e.g. Ministerial Committee on Learner Retention in the South African Schooling System, (MCLRSASS, 2008; DoE, 2008b). These studies are often initiated through special legislative committees and tend to produce indicators with relatively limited use. Many of these reports apply sophisticated statistical techniques to existing data to create higher-quality indicators. Others collect primary data but only do so once, typically from small subsamples that are not easily generalizable to the nation as a whole. In France, longitudinal panel data that monitor performance and progress of students across time have also been in place since 1989 (1989 and 1995 panels). This panel data is particularly useful for following gender and social background inequalities across schooling. In Colombia, the government is now conducting "Evaluaciones Estratégicas" (strategic evaluations, in English) in which data is exhaustively collected and systematically analyzed

---

[2] Further detail and results of the Grade 9 systemic evaluation have yet to be released.

with the aim of better informing decisions about resource allocation and design and implementation of policy reforms and programs. These evaluations examine the impact, relevance, efficiency, sustainability and costs of specific policy initiatives and have the potential to constitute a very useful tool for policy makers (http://www.dnp.gov.co).

3.3 Indicator (Dis)aggregation

Another dimension of educational indicators is the way in which they are aggregated and disaggregated. As was the case with the content of indicators, this is to some extent a reflection of the goals and priorities of education policy and the structure of the educational system. All three countries examined here disaggregate indicator data by significant categories such as gender, education sector, grade level, geographic region, institution type, and special needs populations. Gender is the most consistent and prominent way to break down indicator data in all three countries. This is likely influenced by international agreements stressing the importance of gender parity in education (e.g. CRC, MDG). However, they vary in the extent to which particular categories are most commonly used to present the data. For example, indicators are consistently presented by province in South Africa and by department and municipality in Colombia, whereas in France regional breakdowns are less common. This may reflect differences in the structure of the educational system: South Africa's and Colombia's educational systems are run at both the national and regional level, whereas the system in France is nationalized. Finally, Colombia and France consistently break down indicators based on socioeconomic background, which is relatively rare in South Africa. This difference may stem in part from national rhetoric about whether the underlying cause of educational disparities is socioeconomic or racial in nature.

4 Relevance of Indicators for the Policy Process

Scholars have identified a number of roles for the use of indicators in the policy process. Brown & Corbett (2003) describe five purposes of indicators for policy-makers to: (1) provide background information on the lives of children to set the stage for policy planning; (2) monitor needs and establish trends; (3) set specific concrete goals; (4) create standards of accountability; and (5) systematically evaluate, monitor and refine policies and programs.

In this section, we evaluate the extent to which each of our three countries use indicator systems for the five purposes described above. Specifically, we focus on three areas essential to this process where our analysis revealed potentially important cross-country differences: the prominence of indicators in policy documents; the use of international indicators; and the extent to which the quality of indicators limits and facilitates their use in the policy process.

4.1 Indicators in Policy Documents

Our approach was to evaluate publicly available educational policy documents for their reference to indicators. As the end product of a complex and lengthy process, policy documents are a public record of the policy process and a representation of what policy makers and government officials deem most relevant for public consideration. Although limited in some ways, our method of assessment is useful for evaluating the importance countries place on using indicators in policy formation and implementation, and provides an objective metric to make cross-country comparisons. We examined a number of types of policy documents, including departmental documents such as annual reports and strategic plans and legislative documents such as policy white papers and reports and acts, bills and amendments.

4.1.1 Departmental Documents

In France, newly proposed programs are introduced with a report by the Ministry of Education that usually includes a section that calls for an improved indicator system or a set of indicator benchmarks to measure the success of a program. For example, a 2008 priority in the domain of education in the *banlieues* (French suburbs) is to deal with the problem of school drop out rates through the reduction of absenteeism among secondary school students, thought to be the most direct cause of drop out rates (Ministere de l'Education, 2008). The report calls for the elaboration and diffusion of an indicator system that measures levels of school disengagement in the presence of the newly proposed initiative. The report also proposes a set of quantitatively measured benchmarks in order to assess the success of the program (e.g., 10% yearly reduction in drop outs from priority zones in each region). The systematic inclusion of a call for the use of existing, improved, or newly created indicators to evaluate program effectiveness is indicative of France's commitment to developing indicator systems and using them to inform policy.

In Colombia, indicators are very frequently found across all types of policy documents, and are commonly used to describe the current situation, to justify the need for improvements and to decide what areas to prioritize. "El Plan Nacional de Desarrollo" (National Development Plan), a document published every 4 years at the beginning of each presidential period, is a good example as it frequently uses indicators to delineate and justify the government's economic and social policy. The "Plan Sectorial de Educación" (Educational Sector Plan), also published every 4 years, is another good example of the presence of indicators in policy documents, as it outlines concrete policy goals and commitments regarding education which are partly based on the examination of current indicators. Moreover, these two documents usually make reference to the importance of using indicators to monitor the progress of policy initiatives and to evaluate the impact of policy implementation. Emphasis on the importance of developing evaluation and monitoring mechanisms is also clearly reflected in other documents, such as a mayoral guide for policy design created by the Ministry of Education in concert with other governmental institutions. In this guide, mayors are encouraged to use indicators in every stage of policy design. There is information about the specific indicators to be collected, as well as the institutions responsible for data collection and analysis.

In South Africa, indicators are most explicitly detailed in DoE documents such as annual reports and strategic plans (e.g. DoE, 2003, 2007a, 2007b, 2008), which are reviewed and approved by ministerial committees in Parliament. The indicators referenced in these documents are most often performance measures that track departmental progress on specific policy goals and lay out targets over time. These performance indicators consist largely of relatively subjective indicators such as "most schools are implementing curriculum" that are most appropriate for internal departmental use. Although more rare, departmental documents also specify a select number of more objective performance indicators such as "X% of age-eligible children enrolled in Grade R (Kindergarten)" that can be more widely utilized.

4.1.2 Legislative Documents

In France, indicators are also often cited in legislative documents prepared by the Senate and the National Assembly (e.g., Reiss, 2005). These indicators point out shortcomings in the system and are used to justify the need for improvements. In these documents, a set of benchmarks are frequently proposed that set clear goals and can be used to assess the success of a program. For example, in October of 2004 a report was presented to the prime minister by the *Commission du debat national sur l'avenir de l'ecole* led by Claude Thelot, to organize and summarize the national debate on the future of schooling (Thelot, 2004). The report lays out a set of policy initiatives based on a combination of sources, including consensus from a public debate that involved more than a million people and data from qualitative and quantitative surveys whose results were publicly accessible on the Commission's website (www.debatnational.education.fr). In 2005, the National Assembly issued a policy report regarding the future of schooling (Report Number, 2085) and in April, 2005, an education reform law (*Loi Fillon*) followed. In this National Assembly policy document, specific indicators are presented throughout the introduction to make the case for the need for reforms. An annex of indicators, including bachelor degree attainment by disadvantaged families, number of students pursuing a scientific graduate degree, number of girls in the scientific and technology track, and computer and internet competencies, that are attached to concrete objectives is included in the report that is intended to mobilize and measure progress (Reiss, 2005). These indicators include international comparisons of academic achievement based on the 2003 PISA study, the historical evolution of educational attainment and job access based on national data, regional breakdowns of degree completions, the evolution of education expenditures, and educational attainment by socio-economic background. In addition to explicitly making use of indicators to justify the need for reforms, the National Assembly also calls for the need to track and evaluate successfully implemented initiatives, less successful reforms, and those that were never applied in order to better understand feasibility. Again, France's commitment to using indicators to inform policy is suggested by their inclusion and use across a variety of legislative documents.

In Colombia, the presence of indicators in legislative documents is relatively uncommon. Nonetheless, Colombia's acknowledgment of the importance of indicators is reflected in a set of legislative documents that mandate and regulate the creation of evaluation mechanisms to monitor the education system. The most basic document regulating education policy is the Political Constitution of 1991, which stipulates that it is a duty of the State to inspect the education system, with the aim of monitoring its quality and the fulfillment of its goals, as well as providing the necessary conditions to guarantee the access to, and permanence in the system for all children (Article 67th). Similarly, "La Ley General de Educación" (General Law of Education), the most important law regulating the education sector, restates the mandate of the Constitution and orders the creation of the National Information System. In Articles 75 and 80, this law makes explicit the connection between indicators and policy, by asserting that the National Information System will provide the community with information about the quality, quantity and characteristics of educative institutions, and will serve as a guide for the administration and planning of public educational policy at the national and regional level. In addition to these documents, there are Acts that regulate in more detail the characteristics and functioning of the Information System (e.g. 1526 Act of July 24th, 2002, and the 2707 Resolution of June 26th, 1996). Additionally, since the Constitution of 1991 there is a set of documents called "Exposición de Motivos" (Explanatory Preambles), in which the rationale underlying the creation of particular laws is carefully presented. In these documents, indicators are frequently used to develop and support the argument. In general, legislative documents reflect Colombia's appreciation of the importance and usefulness of evaluation systems and the indicators they produce for the improvement of the education system.

In South Africa, the primary legislative acts in the area of education, such as the South African Schools Act (1996) and the Education Laws Amendment Bill (2007), make little reference to indicators either in justifying the need for policy or in monitoring policy implementation and evaluating success. Instead of referencing indicators, legislative acts, bills and amendments tend to justify policy in terms of upholding constitutional and international human rights and redressing the inequities of Apartheid.

Moreover, the only policy document to reference indicators in the use of monitoring or evaluating of policy is the 1996 National Education Policy Act, which ties the need to protect fundamental human rights to the enhancement of quality education and educational innovation through systematic research and development, monitoring, and evaluation of provision and performance. Although this act recognizes the need for indicators of the educational system, its only proviso is to grant authority to the minister of education to establish indicator systems. By failing to specify the content, timing or source of data collection the act implicitly divorces indicators from the legislative process. This divide is represented in subsequent legislation, which fails to make any reference to indicators for monitoring or evaluation purposes.

Other policy documents, such as white papers that establish the guiding principles of the policy area, also largely reflect South Africa's limited reliance on indicators to justify and monitor policy. For example, the seminal white paper on education and training (1995) makes little mention of indicators, echoing instead national rhetoric about upholding citizen's rights and redressing past injustices. However, the language of more recent white papers suggests that indicators may be playing an increasingly important role in the policy process. For example, White Paper 5 on Early Childhood Education (2001) presents indicators gathered from a nationwide audit of early childhood development (ECD) provisioning to describe the state of early education and justify policy to improve service delivery (William & Samuels, 2001). In addition, the white paper lays out specific policy goals to be achieved in the form of indicators. However, the paper still relies heavily on the need to uphold the fundamental rights of young children and does not include any discussion of long-term indicators of the policy's success or detail important input or process indicators.

4.2 Indicators in International Comparisons

All three countries use internationally relevant indicators to compare the state of their educational system within an international and regional framework, evaluate the effectiveness of policies implemented in other countries and justify implementing within-country reforms. This is a reflection of a common view across the three countries that access to and quality of education is a measure of the country's economic progress and future competitiveness.

Most commonly, international indicators are used to establish the country's position compared to other economically or regionally similar nations. For example, France often cites the PISA study as a way to compare the country's performance on educational achievement to other countries' performance. As mentioned before, Colombia has recently participated in several international studies that allow for comparisons with countries inside and outside the region. Results from these studies are often referenced to describe how critical the national situation is and to justify the need for policy-initiated reforms. In South Africa, the SACMEQ is widely reported and often used to point out the relatively poor achievement outcomes of South African learners, despite the relatively high percentage of GDP spent on education. One result of this situation is that the improvement of educational quality in schools—especially schools serving the poor—has become one of the most important drives of the DoE (DoE, 2008c). International comparative studies are also used as method of gathering indicator data for internal use, although this practice is more prevalent in South Africa than in France or Colombia.

In France and Colombia, international indicators are also used to make more nuanced and in-depth analyses of particular educational policies. For example, in their 2004 report, the French National Assembly used an international comparative approach to address the achievement gap problem. Specifically, the influence of system-wide policies on differences in classroom heterogeneity were compared across three sets of European secondary school level models to understand how these policies may contribute to more or less opportunities for social integration. At one extreme are central European countries such as Germany and Belgium where classes tend to be most homogenous because of tracking and same-sex classrooms. At the other extreme are the Scandinavian countries and Portugal, where no transition exists between primary and secondary school and where policies such as tracking and grade retention are either illegal or rarely used. Based on achievement data from the PISA study, the report concluded that systems that involve greater performance heterogeneity within classes benefit the lowest performing students without affecting the highest performing students. Conclusions from this comparative analysis were used to provide an example for how the French system might be improved.

Although it is not a common practice, Colombia has also taken the international comparative approach a step further by analyzing the diverse conditions under which polices can be effective. The purpose of such analysis is to evaluate the applicability and likelihood of success of particular policies in the Colombian context. The "Balance del Plan Decenal de Educación" (Ministerio Nacional de Educación Nacional, 2006), an evaluation of the impact of educational policy from 1996 to 2005, presents comparisons with four countries (Finland, Korea, Chile and Mexico) that have shown outstanding outcomes in the area of education. The study describes and contrasts the education systems and policies that are believed to explain the educational achievements of these four countries and draws conclusions about the suitability of current Colombian policy for achieving its intended goals.

4.3 Quality of Indicators

Lastly, the quality of indicators plays an important role in the ability of policy-makers to successfully use them in the policy process (Ben-Arieh, 2008). In recent years, scholars have proposed several guidelines to enhance the relevance of indicators in policy formation and implementation. Based on recommendations by Ben-Arieh (2008) and Moore & Brown (2006), we evaluate the quality of the educational indicators collected in Colombia, France and South Africa according to the following criteria: (1) comprehensiveness of coverage and relatedness to significant consequences for children's well-being; (2) impartiality and soundness of scientific methods; (3) regularity and timeliness of data collection; (4) clarity and accessibility; (5) adequacy of disaggregation and (6) alignment with policy objectives and initiatives.

France. The collection of indicators on the education system in France is overall comprehensive. These indicators are collected across a range of domains, are fairly comprehensive within domains, and involve data that assesses both children's well-being as well as their well-becoming (e.g., current achievement and attitudes towards school and society, as well as the connection between academic qualifications and future employment). The indicators collected on a yearly basis since at least 1989 tend to be more basic, but even these are collected across a range of domains and include a number of input, process, and outcome indicators. The more recent indicators that are being collected less frequently are increasingly focusing on positive outcomes and children's experiences. In terms of comprehensiveness, therefore, France's indicator system is relatively advanced and continues to make improvements. In addition, it seems like statistical institutions generally use methodologically sound and impartial methods and disseminate their findings within 2 years both in France, regionally, and internationally. Nonetheless, as with all data collection and dissemination efforts, we recognize that methodological rigor may be compromised by both field conditions and political and institutional interests.

Most of the findings are easily accessible via the internet, either through Eurostat or through the Ministry of Education website where a number of indicator reports are available for free that provide a diversity of colorful tables and graphs. These reports include the comprehensive report entitled *Reperes et references statistiques* (RERS) published every year since 1984 that includes all statistical information available on the processes and outcomes of the education system (Ancel et al., 2008); and the *State of Education* report published every year since 1991 that presents 30 summary indicators with the goal of describing the evolution over time of the education system and geographical comparisons (Abriac et al., 2007). These reports are readable and provide definitions of the constructs that make up the indicators, describe the sample and where the data comes from, when and by whom the data was collected, and precisely how the data was analyzed.

Despite the high quality of the indicators being collected and disseminated, as with all indicator systems, there are also a number of shortcomings. These shortcomings exist less in the quality of data collection and public accessibility as in the extent to which the indicators that are currently being collected reflect the specific goals of the system. There are two major domains in which the French indicator system is lacking in this way. First, disaggregated data is limited to only a few subgroup breakdowns. One omission that has gotten substantial media attention recently is the absence of disaggregation by race/ethnicity or religion. The government has recently explicitly outlawed the collection of this demographic information, specifically in the census. On the one hand, the government argues that inequalities can be measured in other ways and that the collection of this information risks putting members of minority groups in danger of discrimination. On the other hand, researchers argue that given the presence of discrimination and such great inequalities based on these characteristics, this data should be collected and used to address these inequalities ("La Statistique", 2007). The recent emphasis on reducing inequalities through education (Thelot, 2004) suggests that this is a problem that needs to be carefully understood and addressed. The disproportionate number of religious and ethnic minority groups living in disadvantaged neighborhoods (known as "priority zones") suggests that disaggregation of process and outcome data by these groups would be useful in identifying the ways in which inequalities can be reduced.

The second shortcoming lies in the absence of indicators aimed at measuring specific policy objectives. First, although the development of competencies across multiple learning domains have been recently emphasized, only a select number of these domains (e.g., civic education) appear to be tied to specific indicators. Outcome data on other targeted domains (e.g., autonomy and initiative, humanistic culture) are not yet being systematically collected, particularly within individuals across time. These competencies are related to personality development, a commonly stated goal of the education system. Second, while France does have some child-centered indicators (i.e. attitudes about education), this data is not being systematically collected either, particularly across age groups and across time. Third, timely data that tracks individual students longitudinally has been identified in policy documents as useful for educators and students to improve student outcomes (e.g., EduSCOL, 2008, Ministere de l'education, 2006). While some longitudinal data is currently being collected, this type of systematic and accessible data collection initiative, while under development, has not yet been implemented. Finally, achievement indicators are only available starting in the primary school years. The collection of indicators that provide information on children before they enter primary school would be useful in assessing the development of and the factors that contribute to inequalities in school success.

Overall, France has two decades of particularly high quality educational indicators, based on the criteria identified above. Furthermore, the increasing presence of indicators in reform and policy documents indicates a growing national discussion on the importance and usefulness of indicators to inform policy and suggests that the country is headed in the direction of using indicator data to inform future initiatives and evaluate current and past reforms. The ministry of education appears to be making clear efforts to improve the indicator system with this goal in mind. However, a level of resistance and skepticism impedes the collection of some potentially important information (i.e., religious and ethnic disaggregation). Furthermore, indicators that are longitudinal and utilized by educators and students to track within-person progress are still under development.

Colombia. In general, indicators in Colombia are fairly comprehensive and relevant to children's well-being, and include both positive and negative aspects of child development (e.g. number of new slots for children from vulnerable populations; children attitudes towards democracy). However, compared to input and process indicators, there seem to exist relatively few outcome indicators. For example, there are no indicators monitoring children's academic performance throughout school. While Pruebas Saber are a good starting point, they only assess children in a few selected grades, do not track individuals' progress over time, and are not administered on a yearly basis.

The existence of documentation describing the development of instruments like Pruebas Saber suggests that indicators collected by responsible agencies are based on rigorous procedures. However, we are aware that realities in the field may differ significantly from the accounts presented in official documents, and acknowledge the possibility that data collection efforts may be hindered by corruption and inefficiency, among many other factors.

Regarding the timeliness of educational indicators in Colombia, basic information about schools and students (e.g. enrollment, graduation rates) as well as results from state exams are collected and released annually and lend themselves to time trend analyses. In some cases the release of data is delayed for a few months and this can potentially limit policy makers' ability to use updated information (e.g. www.dane.gov.co—Ficha técnica de la información de recolección del año 2007 de la investigación de educación formal del Dane). Nonetheless, timeliness of indicator collection and dissemination may improve in coming years, as a result of recently created norms that, if successfully implemented, will result in a more efficient information system (e.g. "Resolución 166"). Another important limitation is that, as we mentioned before, fundamental indicators about student performance over time is lacking and we did not find any evidence of efforts heading in that direction. This is problematic because without this kind of information it is difficult to capture change and to fully understand what factors facilitate or hinder the achievement of educational goals.

In reference to clarity and accessibility, education indicators found in official documents that are widely disseminated are often presented in appealing tables and charts and accompanied by information about the source and agency responsible for data collection, and by a concise definition or explanation that guides interpretation. The situation is the same for most indicators found in the websites of the Ministry of Education, ICFES, DANE and DNP. In the best of cases, indicators are also linked to a record card that includes the periodicity of data collection, the indicator's unit of measurement, the variables and equations used to create it, the way in which the data is grouped, guidelines to interpret graphs and figures, and samples of the instruments used to collect the data (e.g. Forms C600A and C600B, used by DANE to collect general information about schools, students and teachers). However, this rich descriptive information about indicators goes back only a few years, when systems of information were subject to significant transformations. Information about the sampling universe and number of units from which data was actually collected is still rarely provided (www.dane.gov.co) and data collection procedures are not as accessible as basic descriptions of indicators are. For example, a description of procedures to ensure the veracity and accuracy of the data is rarely available, making it impossible to determine whether the information may be biased due to data collection errors and/or reporters' personal, institutional or political interests. Overall, given the information publicly available, it is difficult to make a precise assessment of the accuracy, reliability and validity of the information.

Finally, at least from what we can observe in official documents, it appears that education indicators in Colombia are increasingly becoming more aligned with public policy. One reason for this increased alignment may be the fact that most policy documents make explicit reference to specific indicators required to inform and evaluate policy. Categories used to disaggregate data are a good example of such alignment. In most situations, data are broken down in a way that allows for the assessment of the situation of vulnerable populations, which are the target of current governmental reforms.

South Africa. Our review of South Africa's educational indicator system suggests that there is considerable room for improvement, particularly in the areas theorized to enhance the relevance of indicators in policy formation and implementation. Ours

in not an isolated finding; there is growing recognition among South African academics, analysts and policymakers that educational indicator systems, especially those
implemented and supported by the provincial and national DoE, need further development (e.g. Chrisholm, 2004; Dawes, Bray, & Van der Merwe, 2007; DoE, 2008c; MCLRSASS, 2008).

Perhaps the most striking limitations in the quality of educational indicators collected by the DoE regard the methodological rigor and timeliness of data collection. While relatively comprehensive, EMIS, the primary yearly data collection system supported by the DoE, is beset with reporting and formatting difficulties that limit the accuracy, impartiality and availability of the indicators it produces. Because data are reported in aggregate from school principals, they are subject to reporting bias, errors of estimation and between-school differences in data tabulation. In addition, poor coordination between provincial and national departments of education creates a considerable time lag between data collection and data accessibility. Finally, although data are collected every year, they are not designed to account for changes in key indicators between the current and previous years. These features of EMIS severely limited the ability to create an accurate assessment of learner retention, a basic and important indicator of the performance of the educational system (MCLRSASS, 2008).

In contrast to the system-wide indicator collection in South Africa, smaller data collection initiatives launched by the DoE as well as other governmental departments and international organizations tend to produce educational indicators that are more methodologically and scientifically sound, impartial, accessible and clearly aligned with policy objectives and initiatives. For example, the DoE's Grade 3 and 6 systemic evaluations are guided by a comprehensive four-part model of indicator collection that documents multiple phases of the policy process, including inputs, processes and outcomes. Schools are sampled representatively and data are aggregated from individual response to create overall statistics. Indicators are methodologically rigorous, easily interpretable and grouped into substantive areas that are clearly aligned with stated education policy goals. Unfortunately, the indicators produced by these initiatives are also limited in key ways that constrain their utility in the policy process. First and foremost, these initiatives often collect data from only a subset of the population in certain grades and do so at only a few points in time. Thus, there are limits to the generalizability and timeliness of the indicators they generate, as well as their ability to capture change. Second, the indicators produced through special data collection initiatives such as ministerial committees tend not to be incorporated into on-going indicator systems.

As previously discussed, South African educational policy tends not to rely heavily on indicators to justify or monitor initiatives. In this way, the limitations of the educational indicator systems in South Africa could be considered a reflection of the country's rights-based approach to policy. However, it is notable that limitations in the comprehensiveness and disaggregation of educational indicators in South Africa constrain their alignment with the policy foci of redressing the injustices of apartheid and ensuring equal access to quality education for all. For example, indicators of access to education are surprisingly few. Although basic enrollment data is collected, the ability to use this data to track change over time and calculate key indicators of grade promotion and learner retention is severely limited. Even more surprising, data regarding day-to-day attendance at school is virtually non-existent. And, while a set of important access indicators such as school transportation and exemptions from school fees are being collected via EMIS; the quality of that data collection system hinders the extent to which they are publicized and utilized in the policy process. In addition, the categories that are most commonly used to disaggregate indicators do not always speak to the goals of educational policy. Indicators are most often presented by province and gender, and only rarely (if at all) presented by other vulnerable populations of interest or by racial/population group. The latter is particularly striking given South Africa's interest in tracking whether the educational system is indeed redressing the injustices of the past.

We end by noting that in recent years South African department officials and policymakers focused efforts on making sustained improvements to facilitate the use of indicators in the policy process. For example, in the past few years the DoE implemented the National Education Infrastructure Management System (NEIMS), which improved the methodology and timeliness of indicator collection on the physical infrastructure of schools. In addition, the DoE Strategic Plan 2007–2011 indicates that the department has recently created an internal system planning and monitoring division. The specific goals of this division include strengthening EMIS to enhance planning and monitoring and developing a monitoring and evaluation framework. Finally, the DoE is planning to implement a system-wide individual learner tracking system to collect more accurate data about learner mobility, promotion, retention and achievement and enable outcome indicators to be linked to individual and school characteristics.

Overall, while educational indicators across the three countries seem to cover a wide array of dimensions relevant to children's well-being, we can also identify a number of shortcomings that are common across at least two if not all three countries examined here. First, in Colombia and South Africa basic indicators, such as attendance, are missing or are not being regularly collected. Second, in all three countries, some outcome indicators that are relevant for evaluating specific policy goals are absent or unsatisfactory. Third, longitudinal indicator data, which assess the same child across multiple points in time, is either absent from indicator systems or not systematically collected. Finally, in France and South Africa, the demographic breakdowns that are typically used to disaggregate educational indicators do not fully reflect the country's social realities and are therefore not aligned with policy goals.

Some of the shortcomings described above are a reflection of the inherent challenges associated with collecting high quality and timely indicator data, especially in countries with limited resources. Despite these challenges, it is noteworthy that each country is currently planning and/or implementing modifications to their indicators systems. If successfully applied, these modifications are likely to produce higher quality indicators and increase the probability that indicators are effectively used at different stages of the policy process. However, we also recognize that the development, reporting and use of a country's indicator system is embedded within its political process. Even with the most high quality indicators available, political interests and economic circumstances may prevent decision-making based on this data.

5 Recommendations and Conclusions

Through the comparative analysis conducted here, we identified important commonalities and differences in the scope and quality of indicator systems and their relationship to public policy across three politically, regionally and developmentally diverse countries. This analysis has allowed us to assemble a set of recommendations for enhancing the use of indicators in the policy process. Although they have been drawn from the particular experiences of the education sector in Colombia, France, and South Africa, our aim is for these recommendations to be applicable to child indicators in general and informative for a broader array of countries.

As discussed above, scholars have identified a number of distinct characteristics which contribute to the strength and effectiveness of indicator systems and improve the use of indicators in developing and implementing policy. However, our analysis of Colombia, France, and South Africa revealed inherent tensions between these characteristics. This is not unexpected in the context of limited fiscal resources when countries must balance competing interests. Because it is unlikely that countries will be able to meet all of the standards of quality indicators that have been identified, our first set of recommendations incorporate suggestions on how to prioritize standards of quality to create the most successful indicator systems.

First, there is a tension between the comprehensiveness of indicators and their reliability, validity, and timeliness. The effectiveness of the use of indicators in the policy process is limited by a lack of timeliness and weak methodology. These features undermine policymakers' trust in indicators and impede their ability to use them to make well-informed decisions and accurately evaluate policies. When resources are limited, there is the potential that methodology will be compromised in order to collect a wider range of indicators. Therefore, we suggest that countries should prioritize the investment of resources in methodological rigor over comprehensiveness.

Second, in the education sector, indicators can be grouped into a number of content domains, including those measuring access, attainment, achievement, qualifications, resources, and infrastructure, among others. In terms of comprehensiveness, we believe a distinction should be made between collecting indicators across multiple domains versus collecting multiple indicators within a particular domain. Ideally, countries should collect indicators that are comprehensive both across and within domains. However, in the context of limited resources, we argue that priority should be given to comprehensiveness within domains. When resources for indicator collection are spread across multiple domains, there is an inherent risk to indicator quality; indicators are more likely to be basic, less valid and therefore not as informative or influential. In contrast, when more comprehensive indicators are collected within a particular domain, quality is likely to improve; indicators may be more nuanced and methodologically sound and thus of greater utility in the policy process. Because this prioritization limits the number of domains across which indicators are collected, there is a danger that potentially important domains of indicators will be neglected. Therefore, we stress that indicator domains should be judiciously chosen to reflect the areas of greatest policy importance.

One way to ensure indicators are highly relevant to policy goals is to foster a bi-directional relationship between indicator development and policy formation. Indicators can be used to shape and monitor policy, but policy can also be used to influence decisions about which indicators to collect and use. When introducing new policies and programs, government officials should explicitly link them to relevant existing and new indicators and establish quantitative benchmarks. As we have observed in France and Colombia, this practice can facilitate the collection of effective and informative indicators that are aligned with specific policy objectives. The experience of South Africa suggests that misalignment between indicator collection and policy goals could result in inefficient spending of a country's resources and inability to appropriately evaluate the impact of policy decisions. However, as we mentioned before, we recognize that the use of indicators is embedded not only in a policy process, but also in a political process. Because indicators are politically sensitive, statistics produced by office bodies are often selectively analyzed and released. Establishing enduring benchmarks of child well-being is necessary to ensure that indicators are appropriately and accurately capturing children's status across political administrations. In addition, it is critical to foster the collection of indicator data by independent researchers and agencies.

Our second set of recommendations includes suggestions for additional types of indicators that if collected would provide policymakers with richer and more nuanced information about children's well-being. To begin, we underscore the importance of collecting indicators not only about presumed policy outcomes, but also about the *intermediate* processes expected to lead to those outcomes. This is important for three reasons. First, collecting methodologically sound input, process and outcome indicators will allow for increased efficiency and effectiveness in the policy process by ensuring the ability of policymakers to track policy implementation, monitor the achievement of goals, identify the need for adjustments, and evaluate if policy is having the intended consequences. Second, specifying key indicators at each stage of the process will surface implicit assumptions about the mechanisms through which policy is expected to lead to change and lead to greater consensus around goal setting. Third, this approach inherently recognizes that societal change does not occur overnight. Specifying and collecting intermediate outcomes ensures that policies are not prematurely discarded because final outcomes have not yet been achieved. As a key part of this process, we propose that non-governmental organizations involved in the policy process such as the media and advocacy and research groups also focus more attention on input and process indicators. Focusing as much attention to intermediate outcomes as is generally paid to final outcomes will help ensure public accountability at each stage of the policy process.

Next, we propose that indicators should not only involve objective measures of the system such as percent GDP spent on education, but should also reflect the subjective experiences of students and educators such as their perceptions of available resources. Oftentimes, traditional indicators collected via administrative data do not capture this perspective. Subjective perceptions of the schooling experience may differ significantly from conclusions made from more objective indicators. Thus, policy decisions based off of these traditional indicators may not fully address the needs of students and educators. Indicators that measure subjective experiences are important in accurately assessing programs and policies.

Across all three countries, we also found that longitudinal data following the same children over time was either absent or lacking. There are several reasons why longitudinal indicator data is useful for informing policy. First, analytic methods available to analyze longitudinal data can provide more causal assessment of the impact of newly implemented programs on educational outcomes than cross-sectional data. Second, following the same students over time can help inform how student economic and geographical mobility can impact student achievement over time. This data can help policymakers disentangle the effects of economic, school, and neighborhood factors on students' educational outcomes. Third, data that tracks particular students, teachers, and schools over time, can help inform local policy that can make more direct, immediate policy decisions in the face of struggling students and schools. We acknowledge that, while effective, longitudinal data can be costly to collect. However, even something as basic as an individual student identification number would allow education departments to track individual students through the educational system and more accurately calculate indicators of student retention, promotion and mobility.

Our last recommendation concerns the use of internationally comparable indicators. Based on our findings, Colombia, France and South Africa tend to use these kinds of indicators to identify their ranking in an area of interest, such as math or reading achievement. We suggest that international comparisons can be more powerful tools when they are used more analytically and thoughtfully. As evidenced by France, a more nuanced comparative analysis of cross-country educational policy can inform decisions about national policy selection and implementation. These types of comparisons are most effective when they take into account similarities and differences between the countries being compared in their economic, social and political context. We argue that conclusions based on this type of comparative analysis should be directly used to inform policy. In particular, international comparisons can be useful in selecting potentially effective national policies.

Acknowledgments The authors are grateful to several colleagues who read an earlier version of this manuscript and gave us helpful feedback: LaRue Allen, Andrew Dawes, Maria LaRusso and Patricia Camacho.

References

Aber, J. L. & Jones, S. M. (1997). Indicators of positive development in early childhood: Improving concepts and measures. In R. M. Hauser, B. V. Bown, & W. R. Prosser (Eds.), *Indicators of Children's Well-Being* (pp. 395–408). New York: Russel Sage Foundation.

Abriac, D., Braxmeyer, M., Braxmeyer, N., Brun, A., Brutel, C., Caille, J.P., et al. (2007). *The state of education from nursery school to higher education: 30 indicators on the French education system*. Report prepared by the Ministry of National Education and the Ministry of higher Education and Research.

Alkire, S. (2002). Dimensions of human development. *World Development, 30*(2), 181–205.

Ancel, F., Bourny, G., Bouvier, J., Brezillon, G., Brun, A., Brutel, C., et al. (2008). *Reperes et references statistiques sur les enseignements, la formation et la recherché – edition 2008*. Report prepared by RERS.

Ben-Arieh, A. (2008). Indicators and indices of children's well-being: Towards a more policy-oriented perspective. *European Journal of Education, 43*(1), 37–50.

Bottani, N. (1996). OECD International education indicators. *International Journal of Educational Research*. Indicators of Educational Performance, Chapter 8, Vol. 25, No. 3, Oxford: Pergamon Press.

Brown, B., & Corbett, C. (2003). Social indicators as tools of public policy. In R. Weissberg, H. Walberg, M. O'Brien, & C. Kuster (Eds.), *Long-term trends in the well-being of children and youth*. Washington, DC: CWLA Press.

Chrisholm, L. (2004). *The quality of primary education in South Africa*. Paper prepared for the UNESCO EFA Global Monitoring Report.

Dawes, A., Bray, R., & Van der Merwe, A. (2007). Monitoring child well-being. A South African Rights-based approach. Cape Town: HSRC Press. (www.hsrcpress.ac.za).

Decreto 1526 de Julio 24 de 2002. (2002). Ministerio de Educación Nacional. Bogotá, DC.

Departamento Administrativo Nacional de Estadística (DANE- DIRPEN). (2005). Caracterización de la información en el sector educación. DANE, Colombia.

Department of Education (DoE). (1995). *White paper on education and training*. Pretoria, South Africa: Author.

Department of Education (DoE). (2001). *White paper 5 on early childhood education*. Pretoria, South Africa: Author.

Department of Education (DoE). (2003). *Strategic plan for the department of education 2003–2005*. Pretoria, South Africa: Author.

Department of Education (DoE). (2005a). *Education for all – 2005 country status report: South Africa*. Pretoria, South Africa: Author.

Department of Education (DoE). (2005b). *Grade 6 intermediate phase systemic evaluation*. Pretoria, South Africa: Author.

Department of Education (DoE). (2006). *Monitoring and evaluation report on the impact and outcomes of the educational system on South Africa's population: Evidence from household surveys*. Pretoria, South Africa: Author.

Department of Education (DoE). (2007a). *Annual report 2006–2007*. Pretoria, South Africa: Author.

Department of Education (DoE). (2007b). *Strategic plan 2007–2011*. Pretoria, South Africa: Author.

Department of Education (DoE). (2008a). *Annual report 2007–2008*. Pretoria, South Africa: Author.

Department of Education (DoE). (2008b). *Progress report on Ministerial Safe and Caring Schools*. Pretoria, South Africa: Author.

Department of Education (DoE). (2008c). *South Africa: Country report on the development of education*. Pretoria, South Africa: Author.

Haut Conseil de l'Education. (2005). *Recommandations pour le socle commun*. Paris, France: Author.

Instituto Colombiano de Bienestar Familiar (ICBF). (2006). Colombia por la primera infancia: Política pública por los niños y niñas, desde la gestación hasta los 6 años.

La statistique, piege ethnique. (2007, November 10). *Le Monde*. Retrieved from http://www.lemonde.fr

Ministere de l'education nationale, de l'enseignement superieur, et de la recherche. (2006). *Enseignements elementaires et secondaire.* Paris, France: Author.

Ministere de l'education nationale, de l'enseignement superieur, et de la recherche. (2007). *EduSCOL – Socle commun de connaissances et de competences.* Paris, France: Author.

Ministere de l'education nationale, de l'enseignement superieur, et de la recherche. (2008). *Programme d'action triennal du ministere de l'Enseignement superieur et de la Recherche.* Paris, France: Author.

Ministerial Committee on Learner Retention in the South African Schooling System. (2008). *Learner retention in the South Africa schooling system.* Cape Town, South Africa: Author.

Ministerio de Educación Nacional. (2008). *Revolución Educativa: Plan Sectorial 2006–2010.* Documento No. 8.

Ministerio de Educación Nacional. (1996). *Plan Decenal de Educación 1996–2005.*

Ministerio de Educación Nacional. (2006). *Balance del Plan Decenal de Educación 1996–2005: La educación un compromiso de todos.* Colombia.

Moore, K. A., & Brown, B. (2006). Preparing indicators for policymakers and advocates. In A. Ben-Arieh & R. M. Goerge (Eds.), *Indicators of children's well-being: Understanding their role, usage, and policy influence* (pp. 93–104). Dordrecht, Netherlands: Springer.

Reiss, F. (2005). *Le project de loi (n° 2025) d'orientation pour l'avenir de l'ecole.* Report prepared by the Commission des Affaires Culturelles, Familiales et Sociales for the Assemblee Nationale.

Santos, S. D., Gibert, F., & Yacoub, S. (2007). *Les attitudes a l'egard de la vie en societe des eleves en fin d'ecole primaire et en fin de college.* Report prepared by the Direction de l'Evaluation, de la Prospective et de la Performance (DEPP), Ministere de l'Education Nationale.

Thelot, C. (2004). *Pour la reussite des eleves.* Report prepared by the Commission du Debat National sur l'Avenir de l'Ecole.

UNESCO. (2006). Colombia. *World data on education* (6th ed.).

William, T., & Samuels, M. L. (2001). *The nationwide audit on ECD provisioning in South Africa.* Pretoria, South Africa: Department of Education.

Main Websites

Children's Institute: http://www.childrencount.ci.org.za

Eurostat: http://epp.eurostat.ec.europa.eu/

Departamento Nacional de Planeación: http://www.dnp.gov.co

Departamento Administrativo Nacional de Estadística: www.dane.gov.co

Ministerio de Educación Nacional: www.mineducacion.gov.co

Instituto Colombiano para el fomento de la Educación Superior: http://www.icfes.gov.co/

In Children's Voices

Peter Burton and Shelley Phipps

1 Why Do We Need to Listen to Children?

Economics, as a discipline, has paid relatively little attention to children. Several explanations for this inattention are plausible: (1) economics tends to focus on models of individual choice and children are typically given limited agency; (2) economics focuses on analysis of markets while children live in a world largely outside the market as traditionally defined (e.g., home production activities and publicly provided schools and parks are central for children's well-being); (3) households are often taken as the basic unit of account in studies of income or poverty, perhaps since data are seldom available at any other level (Phipps, 1999). Where attention has been paid to children, it has typically been in the context of "investing in children" to secure better outcomes in the future (e.g., Haveman & Wolfe, 1995). Particular attention has been given to the study of children at risk for future negative attainments as a result of growing up poor (e.g., Duncan & Brooks-Gunn, 1997).

While understanding and investing in positive future outcomes for children is without doubt extremely important, this does not mean we should neglect the study of children's well-being now, while they are children. As Jen Qvortrup (1999) argues, children should not be reduced to "human becomings." Too much focus on the future might, for example, mean children are drilled for very long hours in school, leaving no time for socialization and fun in the present. Childhood is, in itself, an important life stage to be lived and enjoyed. It has its own unique characteristics, both biological (e.g., children are small and rapidly growing both mentally and physically) and cultural (e.g., children in Canada must attend school; parents have authority over most aspects of a child's life, from residence to medical treatment; children can't choose their political leaders). Thus, being a child "makes a difference in terms of one's activities, opportunities, experiences and identities"

S. Phipps (✉)
Canadian Institute for Advanced Research, and Department of Economics, Dalhousie University, Halifax, Nova Scotia, Canada
e-mail: Shelley.Phipps@dal.ca

S.B. Kamerman et al. (eds.), *From Child Welfare to Child Well-Being*, Children's Well-Being: Indicators and Research 1, DOI 10.1007/978-90-481-3377-2_13,
© Springer Science+Business Media B.V. 2010

(Alanen, 2001, p. 2).[1] We need a balanced understanding of both what promotes future life chances and what generates present well-being for children (Ben-Arieh, "From Child Welfare to Children Well-being: The Child Indicators Perspective" of this book).

How, then, do we go about understanding the current well-being of children? We can set children tests in math or reading to assess numeracy and literacy, we can measure their height and weight and assess whether or not they are obese, we can ask their teachers about their behavior or their parents about family income. Certainly, these data will all provide valuable indicators of child well-being. But, in this chapter, we argue that we should also ask the children. If we want to know, for example, if children are happy or what makes children happy we should listen to the voices of the children themselves.

2 Are Children Capable of Assessing Their Own Well-Being?

Although there are many individual domains of well-being that individuals could be asked to assess (e.g., health, home life, school life, etc.), to keep things manageable, in this chapter we focus on global assessments of well-being. Specifically, we consider questions such as "Are you satisfied with your life?" or "Are you generally happy?" Some readers might question if anyone, adult or child, can actually make assessments of their own well-being that are meaningful for the purposes of either science or public policy formation. However, it is well-established that answers provided by adults to single questions of this type "have credible claims as primary objects of policy-oriented research" (Helliwell, 2006, p. 36); moreover, such questions have the advantage of being extremely easy to include in national surveys at relatively low cost. Thus, for adults, there is a rapidly growing body of research making use of subjective assessments of personal well-being (see Diener, Lucas, Schimmack, & Helliwell, 2009; Frey & Stutzer, 2002 or Layard, 2005 for overviews of this literature).

The literature on the subjective well-being of children and youth, on the other hand, is still relatively small (see Huebner, 2004 for a review of the child literature). Ben-Arieh (2005) argues that since the near-universal adoption of the United Nations Convention on the Rights of the Child, children's rights have become part of the general discourse on social and human rights; yet, scientific acceptance of children's right to speak for themselves is less wide-spread. There is, nonetheless, a small body of existing research on self-reported quality of life for children and youth that has established a number of important points. First, child/youth self-assessments of their own quality of life are meaningful from about age eight

---

[1] To the extent that "childhood" is socially constructed, it may have different meanings at different times or in different places; children of different gender or race may experience childhood in different ways (Prout, 1997).

(Huebner, 2004). Self-assessed quality of life scales for children/youth are significantly correlated with, yet are distinct from, other measures of mental health or well-being (Huebner et al., 2000b; Huebner, 2004). There is stability across time in how children/youth answer questions about their own well-being (Huebner et al., 2000). Child/youth reports of own quality of life are predictive of important future outcomes (Huebner et al., 2000b). Parent and child assessments of the child's well-being correlate well (Gilman & Huebner, 1997), but yet are far from identical (Curtis, Dooley, & Phipps, 2002), so it is important not only to ask parents to provide assessments of their children's lives, but also to ask the children.

If children are to be asked to participate in research in which they describe their feelings, experiences and perceptions of life, an important ethical issue is that they not be put in any emotional or physical danger. While this is, of course, true for respondents of any age, the power imbalance between an adult researcher/ interviewer and a child respondent is particularly large, making the child potentially particularly vulnerable. Research methods must ensure that the child can meaningfully give informed consent to his or her participation, parents must also give consent, and both the privacy and safety of the child must be guaranteed (see Ben-Arieh, 2005).

3 Do Canadian Children Say They are Satisfied with Life?

As an illustration of how we *can* "ask the children" about their own well-being, we use microdata from a very large cross-sectional survey carried out by Statistics Canada (the Canada Community Health Survey for 2005). The CCHS is representative of the Canadian population aged 12 and over. For children, interviews were only carried out if the privacy of the child's responses could be guaranteed (i.e., parents were not able to see the child's responses).[2] Since we only have data from the CCHS starting at age 12, we focus here on young people from age 12 to 17 (since 18 is the legal age of majority in Canada).

In Fig. 1, we compare answers to the question: "How satisfied are you with your life in general?" for 12–17 year-old children with answers to exactly the same question provided by adults who are over the age of 30 and parents.[3] We use the public access version of the CCHS which provides 8,832 observations for teens and 20,979 observations for adults. Respondents were offered five possible responses to the life

---

[2] When children aged 12–15 were selected as respondents to the CCHS, interviewers were obliged to obtain permission from parents/guardians to carry out the interview.

[3] The parents are not, however, the parents of the teens in the sample since the CCHS selects only one family member for the interview; "parents" can also have younger children but with the age restriction on the adults we hope they approximate parents of children in the age range of our child sample. We choose to compare teens to adults who are parents rather than all adults, since households will be more similar than would be the case if we compared, for example, teens with elders.

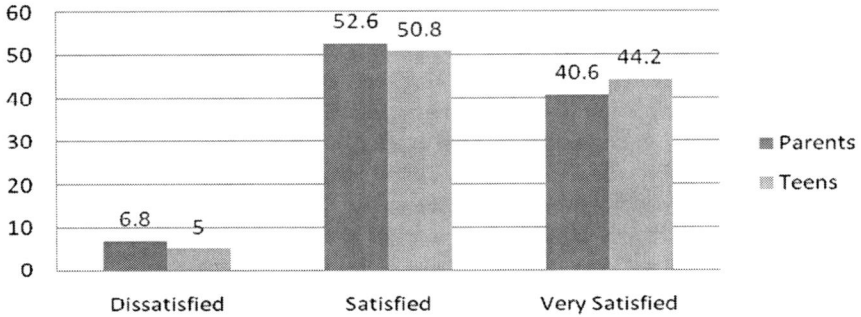

Fig. 1 Life satisfaction for parents compared to teens
Source: Author's calculations using the Canada Community Health Survey 2005.

satisfaction question: (1) very satisfied; (2) satisfied; (3) neither satisfied nor dissatisfied; (4) dissatisfied or (5) very dissatisfied.[4] Since very few respondents (adults or children) report themselves in the bottom three categories, these are aggregated for presentational purposes. Note that both adults and children were very willing to answer this question. Non-response was only 2.3% for teens compared to 1.7% for adults.

As is evident in Fig. 1, the pattern of response is quite similar for Canadian 12–17 year olds and for Canadian parents—the most likely choice in either case is to be "satisfied" (but not "very satisfied") with life. However, it is nonetheless true that Canadian 12–17 year olds are happier than Canadian parents (the difference is statistically significant). For example, 44.2% of teens report themselves "very satisfied" compared to 40.6% of parents; only 5.0% of teens are "dissatisfied" with life compared to 6.8% of parents.

4 What Makes Children Happy? Key Correlates of Child Well-Being

In this section of the chapter, we provide an overview of key themes in existing research on the correlates of self-assessed child well-being. In addition to surveying the literature which has used multivariate analysis, we illustrate key points using simple cross-tabulations based on the CCHS (described above). Throughout this discussion, we compare findings for children with those in the literature on adult well-being. An important point, however, is that since adults and children inhabit worlds that differ in some key dimensions, there are correlates of well-being that make sense for adults but not for children (and vice versa). For example, for many Canadian adults, the world of paid work is central; for most Canadian children, the world of school is more important.

---

[4] Survey weights are used for these calculations.

4.1 Health

A first key point, not surprisingly, is that own health status is one of the most important correlates of teen self-assessed life satisfaction (see Burton & Phipps, 2008a or 2008b). This is also true for adults and the magnitude of estimated associations between life satisfaction and personal health are very similar for teens and adults (see, for example, Helliwell & Putnam, 2004). Figure 2 illustrates much lower reported life satisfaction for Canadian 12–17 year olds who have general activity limitations compared to those who do not (similar patterns are evident if we compare teens with chronic health problems to those without such conditions).

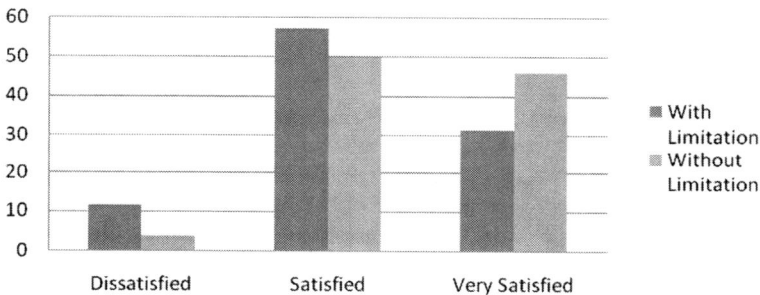

Fig. 2 Life satisfaction for teens with and without activity limitations
Source: Author's calculations using the Canada Community Health Survey 2005.

Notice that this association has the potential problem of "spurious correlation" since the same person (the teen) reports both life satisfaction and whether or not he/she has a general activity limitation. Thus, a teen with a very cheerful disposition may both under-state health problems and over-state life satisfaction, compared to a teen with a more gloomy disposition. However, in earlier research, we have found the same strong association using mother's report of the teen's health and teen's assessment of his/her happiness (Burton & Phipps, 2008a, 2008b).

4.2 Gender

Figure 3 illustrates that 12–17 year-old girls are less satisfied with life than boys of the same age. For example, 6.6% of girls are not satisfied, while only 3.6% of boys are not satisfied. At the other end of the satisfaction spectrum, 46.2% of boys are very satisfied while only 42% of girls are very satisfied (again, differences are statistically significant). The same pattern of girls being less happy than boys is also apparent in a sample of 12–15 year old children in a different Canadian survey (see Burton & Phipps, 2008a, 2008b), in a Spanish survey of 10–16 year olds (Casas et al., 2007),[5] as well as in an international survey which asks children

---

[5] Other earlier research has suggested that demographic variables such as age, gender and race have only weak associations with adolescent subjective well-being (e.g., Huebner et al., 2000a).

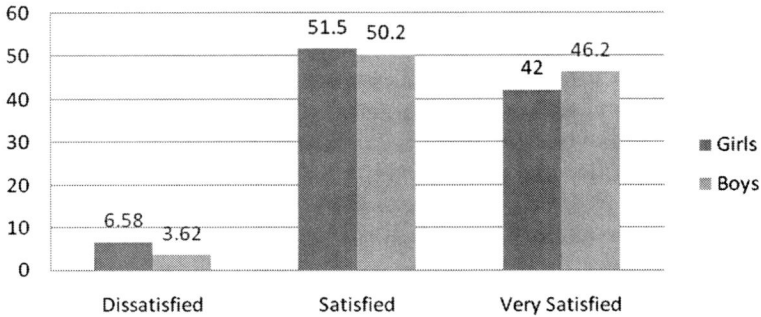

Fig. 3 Life satisfaction for teen girls compared to teen boys
Source: Author's calculations using the Canada Community Health Survey, 2005.

about happiness (Currie et al., 2008). This is in interesting contrast with the adult literature which has consistently found, at least perhaps until recently (Stevenson & Wolfers, 2009) that women are happier than men. It remains an open research question as to why this adult/child difference in patterns of well-being should exist. Is puberty particularly difficult for girls? Are social pressures to "look good" especially hard for girls during the teen years (see Burton & Phipps, 2008a, who find "looking good" to be a strong correlate of young teen happiness). Will this gender difference also "switch" for the current generation of girls and boys as they grow older, or will these girls remain less happy than their male counterparts over their entire life-course?

4.3 Family Income

A third important correlate in the small literature on child self-assessed well-being is family income level. Notice, however, that while we certainly expect family income to be important for children, this is a case where the relationship between family income and child well-being might be different than the relationship between family income and adult well-being. First, family income is less likely to be a "marker of personal success" for young people than for adults. Second, children are often given only limited information about family finances. Third, although we do not know a great deal about how family income is shared within families (see Burton, Phipps, & Woolley, 2007), there is evidence that parents may attempt to shield their children from economic hardship. A British survey of spending within families found poor parents, especially mothers, to be significantly more likely to "do without" basic necessities such as clothing, entertainment or even food than their children. When asked why they had "gone without" these things, overwhelmingly the most common response was "to provide shoes or clothing for my children" (Middleton, Ashworth, & Braithwaite, 1997). But, there is a limit to how far resources can be stretched and the evidence seems clear that low family income is associated with lower life satisfaction for teens. For example, Ash & Huebner (2001) find that adolescents with lower socioeconomic status (proxied as being eligible for a free school lunch

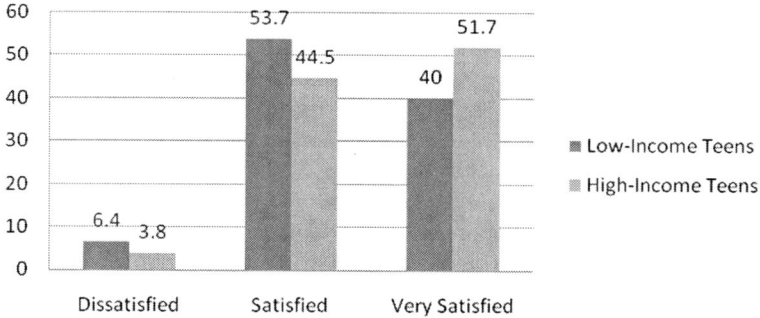

Fig. 4 Life satisfaction for low versus high income: teens
Source: Author's calculations using the Canada Community Health Survey, 2005.

program) have lower levels of subjective well-being. Using longitudinal data and multivariate techniques, Burton & Phipps (2008b) find a strong negative association between self-assessed happiness of young teens (12–15 year olds) and, especially, multi-period average family income.

This pattern is illustrated in Fig. 4 which again uses the CCHS data to compare self-assessed life satisfaction for teens from families with incomes in the top 20% of the Canadian income distribution with teens from families in the bottom 20% of the Canadian income distribution. (Parents/guardians were asked about family income when the child had completed his/her interview.) Over half (51.7%) of high-income teens report themselves to be "very satisfied" with life compared to only 40% of low-income teens.[6] Figure 5 presents the same comparison of reported life satisfaction for parents with family income in the top and bottom of the Canadian income distribution. Consistent with the idea of parents "sheltering" children discussed above, we find a much larger association between family income and parental life

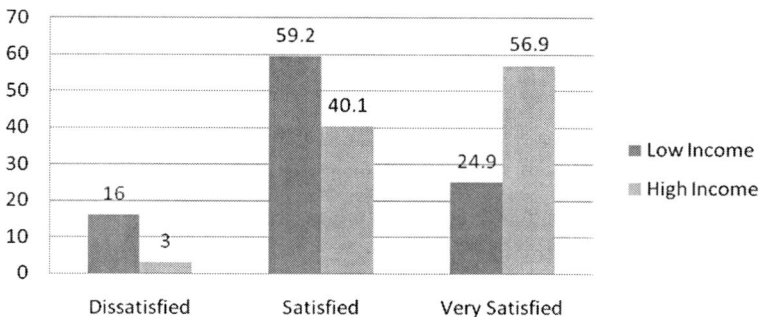

Fig. 5 Life satisfaction for low versus high income: parents
Source: Author's calculations using the Canada Community Health Survey, 2005.

[6] Similar, though smaller, associations are apparent for parental education.

satisfaction than is evident for the teens. For example, only a quarter of parents with family income in the bottom quintile report themselves to be "very satisfied" with life compared to 40% of teens in the same family income category.

A perhaps more surprising finding in the literature for adults is that, holding constant own family income, life satisfaction declines as the incomes of neighbors increase (e.g., Barrington-Leigh & Helliwell, 2008; D'Ambrosio & Frick, 2004, 2007; Ferrer-i-Carbonell, 2005; Luttmer, 2005). And, the size of this relative income effect is roughly as large (and negative) as the positive association with own income. Perhaps not surprisingly, given the susceptibility of teens to both peer pressure and marketing, Burton & Phipps (2008b) also find a large negative association between youth happiness and median income in the teen's neighborhood for Canadian 12–15 year olds, especially boys.

4.4 Social Relationships

Finally, as is also true for adults (e.g., Helliwell & Putnam, 2004), social relationships have the strongest associations with adolescent subjective well-being:

> Their relationships and connections with others are central to how children understand well-being (NSW Commission for Children and Young People, 2009, p. 2).

Figure 6 illustrates, for teen respondents to the 2005 CCHS, that having a "very strong" sense of "belonging to the local community" has very large associations with teen life satisfaction.[7] Indeed, for teens, this is the largest association evident in the CCHS data. (While also large for adults, the teen association is, in this case, the larger.)

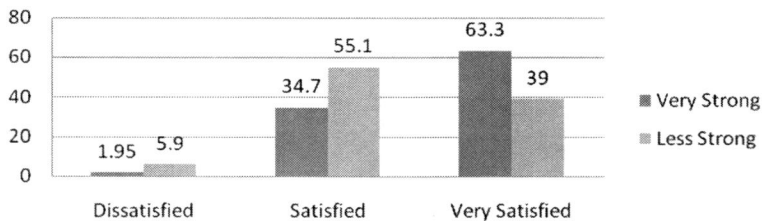

Fig. 6 Life satisfaction for teens with a "very strong" versus less strong sense of belonging to community
Source: Author's calculations using the Canada Community Health Survey, 2005.

Although this is a case where "spurious correlation" is a possibility (i.e., teens with cheerful dispositions may report high life satisfaction and high levels of belonging), the finding remains robust in multivariate analysis that also include an

---

[7] The exact question asked is: "How would you rate your sense of belonging to your local community? Would you say it is very strong, somewhat strong, somewhat weak or very weak?" In our sample of teens, 21% responded that they have a "very strong" sense of belonging.

indicator that the teen reports himself/herself to have "excellent" mental health (the top category on a 5-point scale) as a proxy for "cheerfulness."

Moreover, the basic point about the centrality of different kinds of social relationships to child well-being is evident in other studies using a variety of more sophisticated methods. Good relationships with both parents and peers predict higher life satisfaction, with the parental relationships being the more important (e.g., Nickerson & Nagle, 2004, 2005; Ma & Huebner, 2008). For children in married-couple families, the youth's assessment of how well parents are "getting along" is THE most important correlate of youth self-reported well-being (Burton & Phipps, 2008a). Having a teacher who is perceived to be "unfair" has a large, negative association with young teen self-reported happiness (Burton & Phipps, 2008a), perhaps paralleling findings for adults that having trust in key social institutions is important for well-being (e.g., Helliwell & Huang, 2008). Finding social relationships to be the most important correlate of young teen well-being is very consistent with social psychology's "social identity theory" which argues that group memberships that are important to the individual are in fact central to a young teen's understanding of "who he or she is" (Haslam, 2007).

5 Conclusions

This chapter has focused on child reports of current happiness and life satisfaction for Canadian 12–17 year olds. Our approach has been to review major themes in the adult literature on subjective well-being and to ask if key findings extend to children. We find that personal health status matters equally for adults and children. Gender patterns differ, with adolescent girls less happy than adolescent boys and the reverse true for adults. Higher family income is correlated with higher levels of happiness for both adults and children, but income has much larger associations for adults (perhaps because income is perceived as a marker of personal attainment for adults; perhaps because parents attempt to shelter their children from economic hardship). However, the most important correlate of young teen well-being in these data is having a sense of belonging to the local community. As is also true for adults, social relationships are central to well-being.

Notice, though, that by asking if key findings in the adult literature also hold for children we are still to some extent projecting an adult perspective onto the children. If we really want to understand more of the "child's perspective" about current well-being, we might also ask the children what we need to know (see Ben-Arieh, 2005). An interesting step in this direction has recently taken by the New South Wales Commission for Children and Young People (Fattore, Mason, & Watson, 2009) which has engaged children in a conversation about what, from their perspective, are the questions we should ask.

There has, internationally, been growing interest in the use of indicators of child well-being to guide and monitor policy (e.g., Ben-Arieh & Goerge, 2006). Often, indicators reflect adult concern about future outcomes for children. And, as adults, we may both have more information about what will lead to better outcomes in the future and be less inclined to discount the future as "a long way off." Thus, (in Canada) we tell children to dress warmly, to eat their vegetables and to do their homework. It is clearly vital that we monitor indicators we, as adults, know are important for the future outcomes of children. However, if we take seriously the idea that children's well-being ought to matter in the present as well as the future, then we need to include in our sets of indicators reports from the children themselves about their lives today. It is encouraging that there have already been some steps in this direction. For example, the World Health Organization has started reporting on child life satisfaction across countries using the Health Behavior of School-Aged Children (HBSC) database (Currie et al., 2008). We argue that expanding the use and study of self-reports of child well-being is an important direction for the future.

Acknowledgments We thank Lihui Zhang for her excellent research assistance, Asher Ben-Arieh and John Helliwell for most helpful comments, and the Canadian Institute for Advanced Research for funding.

References

Alanen, L. (2001). Childhood as a generational condition. In L. Alanen & B. Mayall (Eds.), *Conceptualizing child-adult relations* (pp. 26–49). London: Falmer.

Ash, C., & Huebner, E. S. (2001). Environmental events and life satisfaction reports of adolescents: A test of cognitive mediation. *School Psychology International, 22*, 320–336.

Barrington-Leigh, C. P., & Helliwell, J. F. (2008). Empathy and emulation: Life satisfaction and the urban geography of comparison groups. National Bureau of Economic Research, Working Paper 14593.

Ben-Arieh, A. (2005). Where are the children? Children's role in measuring and monitoring their well-being. *Social Indicators Research, 74*, 573–596.

Ben-Arieh, A., & Goerge, R. M. (2006). Indicators of children's well-Being: Understanding their role, usage and policy influence. *Social Indicators Research Series* (Vol. 27). Dordrecht: Springer Press.

Burton, P., & Phipps, S. (2008a). Economic resources, relative socioeconomic position and social relationships: Correlates of the happiness of young Canadian teens. *Child Indicators Research, 1*, 350–371.

Burton, P., & Phipps, S. (2008b, August). *From a young teen's perspective: Income and the happiness of Canadian 12 to 15 year-olds*. Paper presented at the 30th General Conference of the International Association for Research in Income and Wealth, Portoroz, Slovenia.

Burton, P., Phipps, S., & Woolley, F. (2007). Inequality within the household reconsidered. In S. Jenkins & J. Micklewright (Eds.), *Inequality and poverty re-examined* (pp. 103–125). Oxford: Oxford University Press.

Casas, F., Figuer, C., Gonzalez, M., Malo, S., Alsinet, C., & Subarroca, S. (2007). The well being of 12 to 16 year-old adolescents and their parents: Results from 1999 to 2003 samples. *Social Indicators Research, 83*, 87–115.

Currie, C., Gabhainn, S., Godeau, E., Roberts, C., Smith, R., Currie, D., et al. (2008). Inequalities in young people's health. HBSC International Report from the 2005/2006 Survey. World Health Organization.

Curtis, L., Dooley, M., & Phipps, S. (2002). *Does parent or child know best? An assessment of parent/child agreement in the Canadian national longitudinal survey of children and youth*. Statistics Canada. Analytical Studies Branch, Catalogue No. 11F0019MIE – No. 181.

D'Ambrosio, C., & Frick, J. R. (2004). *Subjective well-Being and relative deprivation: An 'empirical link.* IZA Discussion Paper No. 1351.

D'Ambrosio, C., & Frick, J. R. (2007). *Individual well-being in a dynamic perspective.* IZA Discussion Paper Series No. 2618.

Diener, E., Lucas, R., Schimmack, U., & Helliwell, J. (2009). *Well-being for public policy.* Oxford: University Press.

Duncan, G., & Brooks-Gunn, J. (Eds.). (1997). *Consequences of growing up poor.* New York: Russell Sage Foundation.

Fattore, T., Mason, J., & Watson, E. (2009). When children are asked about their well-being: Towards a framework for guiding policy. *Child Indicators Research, 2*(1), 57–78.

Ferrer-i-Carbonell, A. (2005). Income and well-being: An empirical analysis of the comparison income effect. *Journal of Public Economics, 89*, 997–1019.

Frey, B. S., & Stutzer, A. (2002). *Happiness and economics: How the economy and institutions affect human well-being.* Princeton: University Press.

Gilman, R., & Huebner, E. S. (1997). Children's reports of their life satisfaction: Convergence across rates, time and response formats. *School Psychology International, 18*, 229–243.

Haslam, A. (2007). *Psychology in organizations: The social identity approach* (2nd ed.). London: SAGE Publications.

Haveman, R., & Wolfe, B. (1995). The determinants of children's attainments: A review of methods and findings. *Journal of Economic Literature, 23*, 1829–1878.

Helliwell, J. F. (2006). Well-being, social capital and public policy: What's new? *The Economic Journal, 116*(510), C34–C45.

Helliwell, J. F., & Huang, H. (2008). *Well-being and Trust in the workplace.* National Bureau of Economic Research, Working paper 14589 (forthcoming in Industrial and Labor Relations Review).

Helliwell, J. F., & Putnam, R. D. (2004). The social context of well-being. *Philosophical Transactions of the Royal Society of London, 359*(1149), 1435–1446.

Huebner, E. S. (2004). Research on assessment of life satisfaction of children and adolescents. *Social Indicators Research, 66*, 3–33.

Huebner, E. S., Drane, W., & Valois, R. F. (2000a). Levels and demographic correlates of adolescent life satisfaction reports. *School Psychology International, 21*, 281–292.

Huebner, E. S., Funk, B. A., & Gilman, R. (2000b). Cross-sectional and longitudinal psychosocial correlates of adolescent life satisfaction reports. *Canadian Journal of School Psychology, 16*, 53–64.

Layard, R. (2005). *Happiness: Lessons from a new science.* London, UK: Penguin Books.

Luttmer, E. F. P. (2005, August). Neighbours as negatives: Relative earnings and well-being. *The Quarterly Journal of Economics, 120*, 963–1002.

Ma, C. Q., & Huebner, E. S. (2008). Attachment relationships and adolescents' life satisfaction: Some relationships matter more to girls than boys. *Psychology in the Schools, 45*(2), 177–190.

Middleton, S., Ashworth, K., & Braithwaite, I. (1997). *Small fortunes: Spending on children, childhood poverty and parental sacrifice.* York, UK: Joseph Rowntree Foundation.

New South Wales Commission for Children and Young People. (2009). *Ask the children: Overview of children's understandings of well-being.* Accessed 8 March 2009. http:// www.kids.nsw.gov.au/ kids/ resources/ publications/ askchildren.cfm

Nickerson, A. B., & Nagle, R. J. (2004). The influence of parent and peer attachments on life satisfaction in middle childhood and early adolescence. *Social Indicators Research, 66*, 35–60.

Nickerson, A. B., & Nagle, R. J. (2005). Parent and peer attachment in late childhood and early adolescence. *Journal of Early Adolescence, 25*(2), 223–249.

Phipps, S. (1999). Innis lecture: Economics and the well-being of Canadian children. *The Canadian Journal of Economics, 32*(5), 1135–1163.

Prout, A. (1997). Objective vs. subjective indicators or both? Whose perspective Counts? In A. Ben-Arieh & H. Wintersberger (Eds.), *Monitoring and measuring the state of children – Beyond survival.* Vienna: European Centre for Social Welfare Policy and Research.

Qvortrup, J. (1999). The meaning of child's standard of living. In A. B. Andrews & N. H. Kaufman (Eds.), *Implementing the UN convention on the rights of the child: A standard of living adequate for development*. Westport, CT: Praeger.

Stevenson, B., & Wolfers, J. (2009). The paradox of declining female happiness. *American Economic Journal. Economic Policy 1*(2): 190–225.

Part IV
Economic Support

Assuring Child Support: A Re-assessment in Honor of Alfred Kahn

Irwin Garfinkel and Lenna Nepomnyaschy

1 Introduction

The American system of assuring child support directly affects most parents and children and indirectly affects all Americans. By child support we mean transfers to custodial parents (mostly mothers)[1] from either nonresident parents or taxpayers. More than one half of American children now spend part of their childhood living apart from one of their parents. The system indirectly affects all Americans because of its impact on transfers and taxes and on future generations.

The importance and weaknesses of child support policy are highlighted by the extraordinarily high poverty rate of single parent families. Forty percent of single mother families in the US in 2007 were poor, compared with 9% of two parent families, more than a four-fold difference (U.S. Census Bureau, 2008a).

In the past 35 years, the American system of assuring child support has changed dramatically. The public system of enforcing private child support payments from nonresident parents has moved away from local judicial discretion towards state and national administrative regularity. The public system of transferring tax-based resources to children who live apart from one of their parents has moved away from supporting mothers to stay home to raise their children towards supplementing the earnings of low-income single mothers who work.

In this chapter, written in honor of Professor Alfred Kahn, we review the extensive research on these changes and offer an assessment. In writing the chapter we are indebted to and build upon Al's many contributions. In the introduction to their 1988 edited volume, "Child Support: From Debt Collection to Social Policy," Alfred Kahn and Sheila Kamerman identify three themes related to child support that needed to be addressed. First, enforcement in the child support system was inadequate to ensure that noncustodial parents were providing support to their children. Second, the setting of support obligations was complex, arbitrary, unequal

I. Garfinkel (✉)
School of Social Work, Columbia University, New York 10027, USA

[1] Single-mother families made up 87% of single-parent families in 2007. U.S. Census Bureau. "America's Families and Living Arrangements, 2007." Table C3.

S.B. Kamerman et al. (eds.), *From Child Welfare to Child Well-Being*, Children's Well-Being: Indicators and Research 1, DOI 10.1007/978-90-481-3377-2_14,
© Springer Science+Business Media B.V. 2010

and inequitable. Third, child support can only do so much: It is imperative to consider alternative policies that will assure children in single parent families an adequate standard of living. Our assessment asks how the nation has addressed these themes. But, our intellectual indebtedness to Al goes far beyond his specific work on child support, to Al's approach to social research—rich institutional description, cross national comparative analysis, and careful, balanced evaluation of empirical evidence.

2 Evolution of the American System of Assuring Child Support

2.1 The System in the Early 1970s

Until 1974, public enforcement of private child support obligations was strictly a state and local responsibility. States had laws establishing noncustodial parents' obligation to pay support, but judges were given discretion to set obligation amounts and to enforce payments. Critics of child support enforcement policy in the 1970s concluded that the system condoned parental irresponsibility, was rife with inequity, and contributed to the poverty and welfare dependence of single mothers and their children. Only a bit more than one third of nonresident fathers paid child support (Garfinkel, Melli, & Robertson, 1994). Paternity was established in only about 19% of cases involving unwed births in 1979 (Nichols-Casebolt & Garfinkel, 1991).[2] With a few exceptions, child support awards were established on an individual and highly variable basis. In 1979, according to current child support guidelines, American nonresident fathers should have paid $24–30 billion. In fact, they owed only $10 billion and paid only $7 billion. Only a small part—$4 billion of the total payment gap of $17–23 billion—was attributable to the fathers of children on welfare (Oellerich, Garfinkel, & Robins, 1991). Nevertheless, if private child support had been perfectly enforced or assured by the government, both the poverty gap and expenditures on welfare would have been reduced by about one quarter (Meyer, Garfinkel, Oellerich, & Robins, 1992).

Public assistance to families with children in the early 1970s was limited to single parent families with low incomes. The Aid to Families with Dependent Children Program (AFDC) was established by the original Social Security Act of 1935 to provide cash assistance to families with children where one or both parents was absent, incapacitated, or unemployed. By 1975, estimates indicate that 60% of all single mothers received AFDC at some point during the course of the year (Garfinkel & McLanahan, 1986). While AFDC played an increasingly important role in the lives of single mother families during the late 1960s and early 1970s, it did nothing to prevent poverty, provided meager, below-poverty—level benefits, sharply reduced benefits when mothers earned more, and took away medical care coverage when a mother left welfare. Support for working mothers outside welfare was practically

---

[2] Earlier data for proportion of paternities established are not available.

non-existent. There was no public subsidization of low earnings and virtually no childcare subsidies. For unskilled single mothers who could not earn more than welfare or forgo health insurance, the system was akin to a poverty trap.

Dissatisfaction with both public assistance and child support enforcement was fueled by the growth of single-parenthood, the welfare explosion of the decade following the 1964 War on Poverty, and the continuing high rates of poverty of single mother families. Politicians and academics alike sought new methods for achieving the long-standing policy objectives of preventing both poverty and dependence on welfare. In 1974, Congress enacted two programs championed by Senator Russell Long that have played key roles in providing assistance to poor American families outside welfare—the Earned Income Tax Credit and the new federal/state child support enforcement program. In the years since, federal and state legislation has taken long strides on the enforcement side towards a new child support assurance system, which is akin to social insurance. Substantial changes have also been made in the public benefit system, but there has been no progress on establishing a public guarantee of a minimum level of child support.

2.2 Changes in Enforcement

Beginning in 1974, when Congress added title IV-D to the Social Security Act, thereby creating a new federal/state child support enforcement program, a spate of federal and state legislation transformed child support enforcement from a system of local, judicial discretion towards one of state and federal administrative regularity, characteristic of social insurance programs (Garfinkel, 1992, 1994; Garfinkel, Meyer, & McLanahan, 1998b; Legler, 1996). The 1974 legislation established the Federal Office of Child Support Enforcement (OCSE), required states to create similar offices, instituted a federal/state child support enforcement program, and provided federal funding for 75% of state expenditures on child support enforcement. In order to highlight what has changed, our description of subsequent legislation is organized around functions of child support enforcement.

Establishing paternity is a prerequisite to securing a child support obligation for children born out of wedlock—an increasing proportion of children who live apart from their fathers. Paternity establishment laws have their origins in the criminal law and thus prior to the 1980s, paternity establishment in most states was a difficult and costly judicial procedure, in which the rights of the accused were relatively well protected. Most courts in the 1970s admitted blood tests as evidence in paternity establishment cases *only if they excluded the putative father*. During the 1980s, states began requiring courts to admit probabilistic evidence of the putative father's paternity from blood and genetic tests. The 1988 Family Support Act (FSA) required all states to utilize blood and genetic tests in disputed cases. The Personal Responsibility and Work Reconciliation Act (PRWORA), the welfare reform bill of 1996, went much further by requiring states to give administrative agencies authority to order blood and genetic tests without the need for a court order. In perhaps the most far-reaching move away from the judicial system to state/federal administrative regularity, the 1996 PRWORA required states to have available in hospitals and birth record agencies a paternity acknowledgement form, which is voluntary, but if signed, becomes a legal finding of paternity after 60 days.

Prior to the 1980s, state laws listed factors that courts should consider in establishing how much child support should be paid. But because the factors were so general and even contradictory, all real authority was effectively delegated to local courts. The 1984 Child Support Amendments required states to adopt numerical guidelines for determining child support obligations that courts could use. The 1988 Family Support Act (FSA) required states to make these guidelines the presumptive order. Judges who departed from the guidelines were required to provide a written justification. In addition, the 1988 FSA required states to use the guidelines to review and adjust every OCSE administered child support award every three years. PRWORA gave the states greater discretion in updating awards.

To ensure that obligors pay what they owe, the 1984 Amendments required states to enact laws to require employers to withhold child support obligations of delinquent obligors. The 1988 FSA went further by requiring automatic withholding of child support obligations from the outset for all IV-D cases as of 1990 and for all child support cases as of 1994. Many states, however, failed to implement withholding for non-IV-D cases because they neither had nor wanted to develop the bureaucratic capacity to administer universal withholding of payments. The 1996 PRWORA required states to develop the bureaucratic capacity to monitor all child support payments. States were required to establish central state registries of child support orders and centralized collection and disbursement units. PRWORA also established a national directory of new hires and required each state to maintain directories of all state child support orders; the two directories are matched to facilitate the collection of orders. This federal/state directory facilitated interstate enforcement of child support obligations. PRWORA also expanded the federal role in child support collection by a requirement that states adopt the Uniform Interstate Family Support Act (UIFSA), which allowed direct withholding of child support obligations from wages between states.

PRWORA also eliminated the requirement in place since 1984 that states pass through and disregard the first $50 of child support payments in calculating benefits when child support is paid to a mother receiving cash assistance under the Temporary Assistance for Needy Families (TANF) program, the newly created welfare program that replaced AFDC. Since 1996, additional laws have imposed a series of punitive measures allowing for the revocation of the driver's and professional licenses of non-custodial parents and possible prison terms for non-payment of child support.

2.3 Changes in Public Transfer Policy

When AFDC was created in 1935 as part of the original Social Security Act, most married mothers with children did not work. As the Report of the Committee on Economic Security that designed the Social Security Act makes clear, its purpose was to enable poor single mothers to emulate the practices of the middle classes by staying home to raise their children (Committee on Economic Security, 1934).[3] But the child-rearing practices of the middle class were changing. After 60 years of steady growth in the number of women who worked outside the home, by the 1960s more than half of all married women with children worked. In 1962, President Kennedy proposed and Congress enacted amendments to the AFDC program that provided social services to help single mothers work and achieve independence from welfare. In 1967, Congress and the Johnson Administration concluded that social services had been ineffective and enacted incentives to entice welfare mothers to work. But AFDC caseloads grew substantially and work increased only trivially. By the early 1970s politicians on both ends of the political spectrum were advocating policies that included work in the marketplace for single mothers with no pre-school age children. In 1972, for the first time, Congress required mothers on welfare with no children under 6 to register for work. Because Congress never authorized enough funding for the work registration program to provide services for all the AFDC recipients who wanted them, in practice, the work requirement could not be effectively enforced. In 1988 a large bi-partisan majority led by Senator Daniel Patrick Moynihan passed the Family Support Act (FSA), which again reinforced work and gave states more flexibility to try alternative methods to increase work. During the 1980s and 1990s, states obtained waivers from federal mandates to experiment with different kinds of work requirements and supports. By 1992 several states, including most notably Wisconsin, had already enacted and successfully implemented strict work requirements.

President Clinton, pledged during his 1992 campaign to make work pay and to end welfare as we know it. One of his first major initiatives, passed by Congress in 1993, was a doubling of the Earned Income Tax Credit (EITC). The EITC is a refundable tax credit that subsidizes low-wage workers in families with children. The EITC benefit increases with work effort up to a maximum level where it plateaus, and then begins to gradually decrease as earnings increase (Holt, 2006). Continued expansions over the years have led to the EITC becoming the most important poverty reduction program for the non-elderly in the US. In 2008, for a family with two children, the maximum benefit is $4,800 for annual incomes of about $12,000–16,000 (higher for two-parent families). The benefit gradually decreases at higher levels of income and is eliminated at $38,000 ($42,000 for two-parent families). The maximum benefit reflects a 40% increase in a worker's hourly wage (Center on Budget and Policy Priorities, 2008).

In addition, over the course of the next several years Congress substantially increased child care and Medicaid funding and enacted a new child health insurance program. Clinton also proposed converting AFDC to a temporary cash assistance program to be followed by work relief for those who failed to find work on their own. But after the Republicans won control of Congress in 1994, they passed a far more restrictive bill, with lifetime limits for any kind of assistance, stringent work

---

[3] Preamble to 1938 Act, p. 34.

requirements, and the end of the federal guarantee of assistance to all who were eligible. After vetoing the bill twice, Clinton finally signed PRWORA into law in 1996. Between 1988 and 1999, welfare assistance (AFDC or TANF) fell from $24 billion to $13 billion, but federal funding to supplement the incomes of working low-income families grew from $11 to $67 billion. The increase in federal spending to supplement the earnings of low-income families dwarfed the decrease in spending on welfare assistance (Blank, 2002).[4]

3 The Effects of Strengthened Child Support Enforcement

In this section, we examine the effects of the dramatic changes in child support enforcement on child support payments and on the well-being of mothers, fathers and children.

3.1 Effects on Child Support Payments

The evidence on payments is mixed, making the story complicated. Crude trends in child support from the most reliable data, the Current Population Survey (CPS), indicate little to no improvement in support payments received by noncustodial parents. Data from the federal Office of Child Support Enforcement (OCSE) misleadingly indicate a very large increase in child support payments which is based upon an equally large increase in child support cases which get recorded by OCSE rather than an increase in payments. More sophisticated analyses of CPS and other data, suggest that strengthened enforcement has increased payments. But, bottom line, the French expression applies, "plus ca change, plus c'est la meme chose," (*the more things change, the more they stay the same*).

3.1.1 Reliable Evidence from Trends in the CPS

Every other year since 1980, the Census Bureau adds a child support supplement (CSS) questionnaire to the March Current Population Survey. The CPS-CSS questionnaire identifies all mothers (and fathers) potentially eligible to receive child support from a living absent parent and then asks the parent who lives with the child whether they are legally entitled to receive support, how much they are entitled to receive, and how much they actually received in the last year. Because the CPS-CSS is based on a nationally representative sample of all parents potentially eligible for child support and has been repeated over time since 1980, it is the best single source of data on trends in child support payments.

---

[4] Blank (2002). Includes EITC, child care, and Medicaid and SCHIP expenditures for those not receiving cash assistance.

Census Bureau reports on child support indicate no overall progress in child support outcomes between 1978 and 2003. During the entire period, the proportion of mothers eligible for child support who have a child support award has remained about 60%. Similarly, of those legally due child support, the proportion receiving any has remained about 75%. On the other hand, the proportion of child support payments received from the fathers of children on welfare doubled from a very low base of 8% in 1979 to 16% in 1999 (U.S. Census Bureau, 1989, 2007). The focus of legislators and bureaucrats has been on welfare cases. Thus a much larger improvement in child support enforcement for welfare cases over non-welfare cases is not surprising.

3.1.2 Unreliable Evidence from OCSE Data

The federal office of child support enforcement reports annually on the number of OCSE child support enforcement cases, the number and proportion of these cases with child support awards, the number and proportion of cases with child support payments, and the total and average dollar amount of child support received. The number of OCSE cases, cases with awards and payments, and the amount of child support paid have all gone up dramatically. Though OCSE can justifiably take credit for serving an increasingly large proportion of all families with children potentially eligible for child support, these data do not indicate that child support payments in the US as a whole have increased.

3.1.3 Child Support Enforcement has been Swimming Upstream

More sophisticated analyses of the CPS-CSS data indicate that child support enforcement has been more effective than the crude trends suggest. As documented in Hanson, Garfinkel, McLanahan, & Miller (1996) due to increases in the proportion of single mothers who are unwed and declines in real wages of nonresident fathers, the child support enforcement system has been forced to swim upstream. Unlike divorce and separation cases, unwed cases require that paternity be established before a child support order can be secured. Additionally, declines in real wages have reduced nonresident fathers' ability to pay support. In the absence of stronger child support enforcement, child support payments would have declined. Thus the crude trends in child support payments described above understate the effectiveness of the child support enforcement system. Though a comparable analysis has not been done for the most recent period when child support payments actually increased, it is likely that much of the improvement is due not only to strengthened enforcement, but also to the increases in wage rates and earnings of men at the bottom of the income distribution resulting from the prolonged economic boom of the 1990s.

Moreover, there are a number of academic studies that document a link between specific child support enforcement laws and increases in child support payments or in a particular component of payments. These include blood and genetic testing, laws allowing paternity to be established up to age 18, publicizing the availability of

IV-D services, establishing numerical guidelines for child support, requiring income withholding, requiring payments through a third party, and expenditures on child support enforcement (Garfinkel, Gaylin, Huang, & McLanahan, 2000).

In short, while OCSE data wildly overstate the effectiveness of child support enforcement, the crude nearly flat trends in child support payments from the CPS-CSS understate the effectiveness of enforcement. But, in retrospect, after nearly 30 years of research on the topic, correcting for the understatement does not really change the big picture. Suppose, that in the absence of stronger child support enforcement child support payments would have been 25% lower, or put differently, that strengthened enforcement increased payments by 25%. While a 25% increase resulting from policy changes is generally notable, in the context of child support enforcement where only 45% of nonresident fathers pay child support, a 25% increase, increases the proportion paying support to only 56% leaving a little less than half rather than a little more than half of nonresident fathers not paying child support. Any fair observer must conclude that there are severe limits to the enforcement of private child support.

3.1.4 The Effects of Enforcement on Informal Support and Total Support

Our recent research on the effects of child support enforcement on informal, formal, and total child support payments of unwed nonresident fathers reinforces the view that stronger child support enforcement does not lead to much larger child support payments (Nepomnyaschy & Garfinkel, 2007). We find that informal support from fathers (whether in cash or in-kind) is an important resource for mothers with non-marital births and is more prevalent than formal support for up to about 36 months after cohabitation ends and 36 months after birth for fathers who never live with the child. Over time, informal support declines, formal support increases, and the increases in formal support increasingly exceed the decreases in informal support. This pattern is consistent with declines in a father's willingness to pay child support over time as both he and the mother of his child move onto new relationships and with a positive effect of child support enforcement. States with stronger enforcement systems have bigger increases in formal support payments and somewhat bigger decreases in informal support, resulting in a statistically insignificant increase in cash support. That the results differ substantially by when parents stopped cohabiting—with negative effects in the short-run and positive effects in the long-run—suggests that child support enforcement may be more efficacious in the long run. But the effects of stronger enforcement on total (formal plus informal) payments 5 years after the birth of the child are not large.

3.2 Effects on the Well-Being of Mothers, Fathers, and Children

Research indicates that stronger child support enforcement increases the incomes of single mothers notably in percentage terms from a very low base. Garfinkel,

Heintze, & Huang (2000b) find that increases in child support payments between 1978 and 1998 increased the incomes of single mothers by 16% and the incomes of single mothers with a high school degree or less by 21%. Meyer, Garfinkel, Oellerich, & Robins (1994) estimate that perfect enforcement of private child support (or by implication, a government guarantee of private support obligations) would reduce the poverty gap among families potentially eligible for child support by 24%.

Still, even perfect enforcement would leave 1/3 to 1/2 of single mothers poor and insecure. Thirty percent of nonresident fathers earn less than $14,000 (Garfinkel, McLanahan, & Hanson, 1998a). Child support payments from fathers with low and irregular earnings, at best, will be low and irregular. To expect more is utopian.

Moreover there is evidence that stronger enforcement has negative effects on mother-father relations. There is ample evidence that parental conflict is bad for children and some evidence that strong child support enforcement increases parental conflict (McLanahan, Seltzer, Hanson, & Thompson, 1994; Seltzer & Brandreth, 1994; Seltzer, McLanahan, & Hanson, 1998). There is also some evidence from a few qualitative studies that unreasonably high child support obligations create undue strains on the relationships between mothers and fathers (Edin, 2000; Pate, 2002; Waller & Plotnick, 2001). Research on whether stronger support enforcement provokes or inhibits domestic violence is sadly lacking, though one recent study does find increased violence in strong enforcement states among mothers on welfare (Fertig, McLanahan, & Garfinkel, 2006). But, though the adverse effects of stronger enforcement on parental conflict is expected to have negative consequences for children, empirical research generally finds positive effects of child support enforcement on a number of child outcomes, including schooling, educational attainment, and behavior (Argys, Peters, Brooks-Gunn, & Smith, 1998; Graham, Beller, & Hernandez, 1994; Hernandez, Beller, & Graham, 1995; Knox & Bane, 1994). In short, research indicates stronger enforcement has benefited both mothers and children.

What about the fathers? The gains of poor mothers are far exceeded by the losses to poor fathers because most of the increases in fathers' payments have gone to reducing welfare costs rather than increasing mothers' and children's household incomes. In 2005, only 13% of child support collections for current TANF recipients and 24% for former recipients was actually distributed to families (USDHHS, 2008b).

It is possible that stronger enforcement might have beneficial effects on fathers. First, rights and responsibilities are the flip side of the same coin. By reinforcing responsibility, child support enforcement strengthens fathers' rights to be involved in their children's lives. Second, assuming greater responsibility for their children, even if at first brought about involuntarily, may be of direct benefit to fathers. Waite & Gallagher (2001) present persuasive evidence that marriage is good for men's health and well-being. Supporting one's child may well lead to some of the same kind of benefits. Unfortunately, we have no empirical evidence of these hypothetical beneficial effects of enforcement on fathers.

But, there is ample evidence that stronger child support enforcement has done damage to a large number of fathers, especially those who are poor. A serious problem with the public child support system is that at its inception, the federal Office of Child Support Enforcement viewed itself exclusively as a law enforcement agency. As a result, fathers have been viewed as lawbreakers rather than clients. Federal and state offices of child support enforcement have come a long way since the early 1980s—including co-sponsoring demonstrations to help fathers obtain access to their children and experiments such as Parents' Fair Share to help fathers meet their child support obligations (Doolitle, Knox, Miller, & Rowser, 1998). But isolated experiments are not the same as institutional change. It is particularly important for unwed and low-income fathers that child support enforcement becomes a social welfare program as well as a law enforcement agency. These fathers need the most help and suffer the most from harsh enforcement.

Only a small proportion of divorced fathers need help meeting their child support obligations. In contrast, a substantial proportion of unwed fathers need help. Whereas middle class fathers typically establish visitation rights as part of their divorce agreements, low-income fathers rarely do so. One important reason for this is because child support orders for low-income fathers are initiated by state agencies whose principal objective is to reduce welfare costs.

Offices of child support enforcement routinely impose much stiffer child support obligations (as a percentage of income) on poor fathers (Huang, Mincy, & Garfinkel, 2005). Low-income fathers are more likely to be ordered to pay amounts that exceed state guidelines than middle and upper-income fathers. Frequently the child support obligations imposed on low-income fathers are unreasonably high. A large number of these unrealistic obligations appear to arise because child support agencies or the courts base orders not on fathers' actual earnings, but on presumptive minimum earnings (e.g. the minimum wage for full time, full year work) or on how much the father earned in the past. Some fathers are required to pay back the mother's welfare or Medicaid birthing costs. Many fathers who become unemployed or incarcerated build up huge arrearages (debts) during these periods of unemployment. Such onerous child support obligations are rarely paid in full, but they do prompt fathers to avoid legitimate work where their wages are easily attached, and they breed resentment on the part of fathers and mothers towards the system and perhaps each other. Imprisonment for non-payment of support exacerbates this negative dynamic. Recent evidence from the Fragile Families and Child Wellbeing Study, which examines the lives of families with unwed births, indicates that most unwed fathers in urban areas have substantial barriers to obtaining stable jobs which would allow them to make regular child support payments. Nearly half of these fathers have a history of incarceration, many have not completed high school (40%), and more than half have children with more than one woman, suggesting multiple child support obligations (Sinkewicz & Garfinkel, 2009). Given what we know about the low earnings capacity of most unwed and virtually all poor fathers, these enforcement practices are not likely to be effective and are likely to have unintended negative consequences (Garfinkel et al., 1998a).

4 The Effects of Enforcing and Subsidizing Work

As described above, the public system of child support shifted from a system which provided unrestricted cash welfare assistance to non-workers to a system which required work in return for cash welfare assistance and subsidized earnings of low-income workers via the EITC. Between 1994 and 2000, welfare caseloads fell an unprecedented 56%, from a historic high of 5 million to 2.4 million families (USDHHS, 2008a). In the same period, single mothers' labor force participation rates increased 10% points and their poverty rates fell 11% points, from 44 to 33%. Incomes of single-mother families in all quintiles increased during both 1993–95 and 1997–99, except for the poorest fifth of single mothers, who lost income in the post-PRWORA period. Even the lowest income group experienced gains in consumption, and the share of families reporting hunger fell between 1995 and 1999 (Blank, 2002). There is, however, evidence that a small share of single mothers lost assistance because their mental health problems made them unable to comply with work requirements, or that the sanctions they received for failing to comply led to mental health problems (Reichman, Teitler, & Curtis, 2005; Reichman, Teitler, Garfinkel, & Garcia, 2004).

The dramatic declines both in welfare caseloads and in poverty rates of single-mother families were not attributable to TANF alone, but rather to a combination of three factors: (1) the enactment of TANF; (2) the increase in assistance outside welfare that made work pay; and (3) the longest peacetime economic expansion in the nation's history. Research on the decline in welfare caseloads indicates that all three factors were important in reducing caseloads. Isolating the independent effect of each is not possible because all three were moving in the same direction and reinforcing each other.[5] Blank (2002) compares the results from welfare policy experiments with work requirements only to experiments with work requirements plus earnings subsidies. Experiments that required work and supplemented earnings led to a big drop in welfare receipt and increase in employment and big gains in total income and drops in poverty whereas experiments that required work, but provided no earnings subsidy led to the big drop in welfare receipt and increase in earnings, but no increase in total income and no decline in poverty. One can infer from the experiments that TANF by itself would have reduced welfare caseloads and increased employment, but would have had no effect on poverty.

5 The US in International Context

The United States leads the rich world in the share of its children (about one half) who spend some of their childhood with a single mother. Single motherhood is experienced by approximately one third of children in the northern European rich

---

[5] See Blank (2002).

countries, and even in Italy, by one in eleven children (McLanahan, 2004). In all these countries, public policies exist to ensure that nonresident parents provide support (or maintenance) to their children living with a custodial parent.

A recent report from the UK characterized the child support enforcement regimes across 14 rich countries: Australia, Austria, Belgium, Canada (Ontario only), Denmark, Finland, France, German, Netherlands, New Zealand, Norway, Sweden, UK, and US (Wisconsin only). (Skinner, Bradshaw, & Davidson, 2007). All 14 countries allowed parents to make private agreements and had public systems in place to ratify these agreements. However, in all but two countries (Belgium and Denmark), custodial parents on public assistance (welfare) were compelled to pursue the nonresident parent through the formal system and were not permitted to make private agreements. Countries varied widely on the amount of discretion that courts or agencies had in the determination of support (or maintenance) obligations. Eight of the countries used a combination of rigid formulas and formal guidelines; with Belgium, France, Germany, Netherlands, and Sweden relying on mostly discretion and informal guidelines.

Within the formal system, in all countries, the amount of the obligation depends upon the income of the nonresident parent. In all but 4 countries (Denmark, UK, Belgium, and the US) some portion of the fathers' income is exempted for basic living expenses. However, there were large differences in what other factors are considered.

The income of the custodial parent is considered in determining the amount of the obligation in about half the countries. The exact formulas for computing obligations when both parents' incomes are taken into consideration are quite complicated and vary substantially by country (and even by localities within countries—as in the US). The simplest way of computing obligations is by taking a percentage of the noncustodial parent's income, as is done in Wisconsin in the US and Australia.

In all countries but the US, obligations to a new biological child living with the nonresident parent are considered, and in 9 out of the 14 (except for Australia, Denmark, Germany, UK and US) obligations to new partners, with or without new children, are also taken into account.

Though shared custody is much more likely in higher-income, divorce cases (vs. paternity cases) it is still uncommon even in these cases. All 14 countries took account of substantial contact time between fathers and their children in determining the obligation, with the possibility in 10 countries of fathers paying no support in shared custody cases.

The authors simulate several vignettes of family situations to examine differences in obligations across countries, using the Wisconsin formula for the US example. Considering a family where both parents are unemployed, in 8 countries, the father would not pay anything; in 5 countries, he would pay a minimal amount; while in the US this father would pay the highest amount, nearly three times that of the next closest country. In all other vignettes, including one with a working poor father and a middle-class father, the US establishes the highest obligations on noncustodial parents.

The child support enforcement tools used to collect obligations were shown to be broadly similar across countries. Commonly, deductions from earnings (or wage withholding) were the first response to noncompliance in all countries, while in the US, wage withholding is routine for all cases, not just for those in noncompliance. Other tools to deal with non-compliance included seizure of assets, passport confiscation, tax intercepts, deductions from bank accounts, interest charged on debt, revocation of drivers' license, criminal prosecution, and imprisonment (in only 5 countries).

The most important difference in child support enforcement regimes across countries was in the provision of a guaranteed minimum level of support for custodial parents and children. All the European countries (except Netherlands) had some form of a guaranteed maintenance scheme to provide support if the nonresident parent could not pay, paid only part, or would not pay child support. None of the English speaking countries have such a provision. The guaranteed maintenance schemes varied in a number of ways: whether means-tested for the custodial parent; whether the custodial parent is a lone parent; whether the nonresident parent is in non-compliance; the amount of time the guarantee has been in place; and by the amount of the guarantee. In some countries, the receipt of a guaranteed minimum affects the amount of means-tested social assistance received, while in Austria, Belgium and Denmark, this was not the case. Therefore, in these countries, mothers who received a guaranteed minimum could get more benefits than mothers who were just receiving social assistance.

Table 1 presents data on the circumstances of non-widowed single (or lone) parents in 14 rich countries. The first column shows the proportion of single parent families in each country in approximately 2000. The second column presents the proportion of lone parents receiving any child support. Fortunately, these data include both child support paid by the nonresident parent and government guaranteed/financed child support. Unfortunately, the data do not distinguish between the two. Only nations with publicly guaranteed child support payments have receipt rates over 50%, and the Scandinavian nations, with the most generous public guarantees, have by far the highest rates of receipt (69% in Finland, 78% in Norway, and 95% in Sweden). The countries that do not provide this support (Australia, Canada, Netherlands, UK, and US) have the lowest receipt rates. Germany appears to be an outlier, but their maintenance system is time-limited. The third column shows the percent of lone parent families in each country living below the poverty line (defined as less than half of median income). Given the low proportions of children receiving child support in the English-speaking countries, with no minimum guaranteed benefit, it is no surprise then that they also have the highest levels of poverty for single-parent families.

In sum, the US is not alone in its efforts to compel both parents to support their children, by encouraging resident parents to work and nonresident parents to pay support. However, the US (along with the other English-speaking countries) has taken a more punitive approach that has not taken into consideration changing demographic and economic circumstances. European countries that undergird work expectations for mothers and child support payments from fathers with a guaranteed

Table 1 Circumstances of non-widowed single parents in 14 rich countries

Country	Single/lone parent families as percent of all families	Percent receiving child support[d]	Percent in poverty[e]
Australia	14[a]	33	38
Austria	15[a]	59	33
Belgium	11[b]	40	12
Canada	19[c]	31	45
Denmark	18[c]	NA	11
Finland	15[b]	69	6
France	17[c]	56	25
Germany	21[c]	29	43
Netherlands	13[c]	28	30
Norway	17[b]	78	10
Sweden	23[c]	95	5
UK	21[c]	22	40
US	27[c]	32	57

[a]Data from Skinner (2007) from approximately 2000, except for Australia which is from 1994. Table 2.1.
[b]Data from the UNICEF Innocenti Center, Report Card No.6. Child Poverty in Rich Nations 2005, Figure 6.
[c]Data from the Clearinghouse on International Developments in Child, Youth, and Family Policies, Table 2.17a, from approximately 2000.
[d]Data from Skinner (2007) from approximately 2000, except for Australia which is from 1994. Table 2.4.
[e]Data from the Clearinghouse (Table 3.21a) from the 1990s. Poverty threshold is defined as incomes less than 50% of the median income.

minimum have much higher rates of child support receipt and much lower levels of poverty among single parent families.

6 Policy Issues and Recommendations

In this section, we discuss a few policy issues and recommendations. We begin with two issues that are not, but should be high on the US Congressional agenda for reforming the US child support system: publicly assuring child support and expressing child support orders as a percentage of the nonresident parent's income. Then we consider three other issues that are currently being discussed in the US Congress.

6.1 Publicly Assured Benefits

Children in single-parent families are disadvantaged compared with those in two-parent families precisely because there is only one parent. Just as Survivor's Insurance is a social invention to ensure that parents who die can support their children, a child support assurance system that both enforces the obligation of living parents to share income with their children and undergirds the system with a public guarantee of a minimum level of support would ensure that parents who live apart from their children nonetheless support them financially. In the United States, as we have seen, states and the federal government have already substantially strengthened enforcement of private child support. Other rich nations, learning from the U.S. experience, have also strengthened their enforcement systems. But, enforcing private support is inherently limited. Child support from fathers with low and irregular earnings, at best, will be low and irregular. The Scandinavian countries and a few of the continental European nations have advanced maintenance benefits that guarantee minimum child support payments and thereby create a floor in the child support system (Kahn & Kamerman, 1988; Kunz, Villeneuve, & Garfinkel, 2001).

Creating a child support floor—a publicly financed minimum child support benefit—that is conditional on being legally entitled to receive private child support reduces the poverty and insecurity of single mothers and their children and increases mothers' incentives to cooperate in identifying the fathers of their children, establishing paternity, and securing a child support award (Garfinkel, 1992). Assured child support, like other universal benefits, will further reduce the dependence of single mothers on TANF and other safety net programs.

Minimum benefits are common in social insurance programs. The enforcement features of the American system of assuring child support increasingly resemble social insurance. Nonresident fathers are required to pay a share of their income for child support, and the obligations are deducted from their paychecks. Adding a minimum benefit to the system is consistent with this evolution.

The Swedish advanced maintenance system began by publicly advancing private child support obligations up to a certain amount and assuming the responsibility for collecting the private obligation. To illustrate, such a system in the US would provide a $100 a month in public support if the private obligation were $100 a month and $200 a month in support if the private obligation were $200 a month. The cap could be $200 a month for one child, $300 a month for two. Such a system would be a huge step forward in providing security to single mothers and their children at minimum cost to taxpayers.

Alternatively, like the current Swedish system, the government could guarantee a minimum child support benefit independent of the nonresident parent's ability to pay support and the formal child support obligation amount. For example, the government could guarantee child support payments to all custodial parents legally entitled to receive private child support of $200 per month for one child and $300 per month for two children.

An assured child support benefit is a relatively cheap floor that would substantially reduce the poverty and economic insecurity of single mothers and their children and simultaneously strengthen child support enforcement.[6]

---

[6] So long as the guaranteed minimum benefit is conditioned on legal entitlement to support, the costs of even a very generous minimum benefit is modest—in 1985 under $5 billion (Meyer et al., 1994). If the benefit is not conditioned on entitlement to private child support, the incentive to obtain legal entitlement is eliminated and costs increase substantially.

6.2 Expressing Child Support Obligations as a Percentage of Income

Nothing would do more to simultaneously increase child support payments over time and to protect the legitimate interests of poor and unwed fathers than to require states to establish child support obligations that are expressed as a flat percentage of the obligor's income. Most nonresident father's incomes increase over time. Consequently, expressing orders as a percentage of income will increase payments over time. Oellerich et al. (1991) find that the lack of indexing of child support obligations is the biggest single factor accounting for the gap between child support guidelines and actual child support payments. At the same time, percentage expressed obligations protect poor fathers who become unemployed, ill, or incarcerated. Currently, child support obligations are not modified in response to these events. If orders were expressed as a percentage of income, obligations would automatically go down when the father was unemployed, ill, or in jail. Though child support enforcement officials continue to fear that expressing child support obligations as a percentage of the father's income will result in lower payments, the only evidence on the matter suggests that the opposite is true. Bartfeld & Garfinkel (1996) find that percentage expressed child support orders lead to substantially higher, not lower payments. As an additional protection for poor fathers, Congress should require states to revise their guidelines so that the child support obligations imposed on poor and near-poor nonresident fathers can be no higher in percentage terms that those imposed on middle-income nonresident fathers.

6.3 Taxation of Child Support Within TANF

A major problem with the child support enforcement system, as noted above, is its long-standing goal of recouping welfare costs. Mothers on welfare must sign over to the state their rights to child support payments made on their behalf. Prior to the passage of PRWORA in 1996, states were required to pass-through and disregard the first $50 of child support paid on behalf of these mothers. The cost of this pass-through was shared by the state and federal governments. But PRWORA eliminated this requirement, allowing states to choose what they wanted to do, but without federal assistance in sharing the burden of the pass-through. As of 2004: 27 states eliminated the pass through entirely; 13 states continued to pass-through and disregard the first $50 of support; 4 states increased the TANF grant for families receiving child support; 4 states passed through the entire amount of child support collected (1 also disregarded the full amount, 1 did not disregard any, and 2 disregarded the first $50); and 5 states passed through some child support under "fill-the-gap" rules (Wheaton & Sorensen, 2007). In other words, in only one state in the US (Wisconsin) could a mother on welfare receive the entire amount of child support paid on her behalf and continue to receive her entire welfare benefit.

However, even in Wisconsin, child support income is used to decrease Food Stamp benefits and impacts eligibility for other programs, such as Medicaid and public housing.

This nearly universal 100% marginal tax on child support income creates substantial disincentives for both mothers and fathers to cooperate with the child support enforcement system. Mothers are much better off making informal support arrangements with the father and refusing to pursue him through the formal system. In turn, fathers are better off working in the underground economy and contributing informally so that their payments actually benefit their children. In the long run, however, this is not a sustainable arrangement, since informal payments tend to fall off over time, fathers can be held liable for retroactive payments if they ever do come into the system, and fathers can be sent to prison for noncompliance with child support. In the states' view, this taxation of child support should compel mothers to leave welfare sooner, so they can receive the full amount of support paid on their behalf. In reality, however, poor mothers are usually associated with poor fathers, who as discussed previously have numerous barriers to stable employment and very low potential to provide a meaningful and stable amount of support. Therefore, leaving welfare for unstable child support from poor fathers is a risky move for most mothers.

In recent years, however, policymakers are revisiting this policy lever for several reasons. First, because of the time-limited nature of TANF and strict work requirements, allowing mothers to receive child support while on welfare is only a temporary disincentive to work. Second, new research based on experimental data from Wisconsin has provided evidence of positive effects of passing through child support. Cancian, Meyer, & Caspar (2008) found that a full pass-through and disregard increased the proportion of fathers who pay support, the amount of payments, and proportion of children with paternity established. And these benefits occurred with no increase in cost to the state, due to decreased eligibility for other programs. The Deficit Reduction Act of 2005, which reauthorized TANF, provides incentives for states to pass through and disregard $100 of child support paid for one child and $200 for two or more children. Given what we know about this issue, states should certainly take advantage of this provision. And, we would urge Congress to explore the benefits and costs of disregarding a very large proportion of total payments.

6.4 Obligations with Multi-Partner Fertility

An emerging issue particularly among unwed parents is that of multiple partner fertility, when either or both parents have children with other partners (prior to or following the focal relationship). Data from the Fragile Families and Child Wellbeing Study, which is representative of unwed births in urban areas, reveals that nearly 60% of unwed parents had children with prior partners at the time that the focal child in the study was born (Carlson & Furstenberg, 2006). Using administrative data on all TANF recipients in Wisconsin, Meyer, Cancian, & Cook (2005) conclude that nearly three-quarters of these families had multiple partner fertility, either on the mother's or father's side.

These complex family structures have important implications for child support enforcement, particularly for establishing the amount of child support a father must pay to children in multiple households (Cancian & Meyer, 2006). In traditional situations, fathers owe more money for more children, but the obligation is increased by a smaller amount for each additional child. For example, in Wisconsin, where obligations are expressed as a percentage of the father's income, the obligation is 17% for one child, 25% for two, 29% for three, 31% for four, and so on. This scheme takes into account economies of scale in the mother's household; however in a multiple partner fertility situation, these economies do not necessarily exist, or they exist but the children may be from different fathers. States are currently grappling with this problem. One type of response has been to deduct the amount of support the father is paying to the first child from his total income and then apply the percentage for one child to the remaining income, resulting in a smaller benefit for the second child. Another response is to calculate how much the father would owe for the number of children that he has (e.g. 25% for two) and then divide this evenly by the number of children, resulting in equal support for both children, but a smaller benefit for the first child than would have been originally ordered (e.g. 12.5% vs. 17%).

Research suggests that fathers with children in multiple households owe more support than fathers with the same number of children in one household. Ethnographic interviews with low-income fathers reveal that these obligations may be unrealistic and overwhelming and sometimes lead fathers to drop out of the regular employment system in order to avoid paying support (Pate, 2002). Meyer, Cancian, & Nam (2007) find that fathers in more complex family arrangements have higher obligations, are more likely to pay, and pay more that fathers in simple family types; but, they are also more likely to not pay the full amount owed and therefore more likely to fall behind and accrue arrears.

Currently, there is very little uniformity across states with how they decide on child support obligations in cases of multiple children in multiple households. Brito (2005) examines the complex set of laws and guidelines in every state. Her data indicate that despite the inequities currently built into the system, many states are considering a number of approaches to improve the situation. First, states are considering much more information about the circumstances of families when determining obligations, particularly considering the receipt of child support and financial resources of a new partner in the custodial parent's home. Second, states are implementing provisions to review and adjust a noncustodial parent's orders from multiple families in one proceeding. Finally, states are beginning to consider moving away from uniformity towards more discretion on a case by case basis for these complex family situations. If one believes that existing obligations to mothers and children should not be modified in response to new obligations undertaken by the nonresident parent, all three of these approaches would worsen rather than improve the situation.

6.5 *Minimizing Damage from Arrearages*

Arrearages owed to the state are increasingly recognized as a problem in child support enforcement. Based on OCSE data, national arrears reached $106 billion in 2005. In a study of arrears in 9 states, Sorensen, Sousa, & Schaner (2007) find that 70% of arrears are owed by obligors making $10,000 per year or less, and 40% are owed by those with no reported income. Vicki Turetsky, Senior Staff Attorney and expert in child support legislation at the Center for Law and Social Policy (CLASP) in a recent personal communication, reports that reforms at the state and federal level are being discussed in three policy areas. The first set of reforms focuses on preventing the build-up of arrears in the first place by: (1) setting more realistic obligations, especially for low-income fathers; (2) intervening quickly when payments stop due to periods of unemployment, disability, or incarceration; and (3) creating more linkages to community based programs which focus on responsible fatherhood, prisoner reentry, and job training. A second set of reforms being considered focuses on the long-standing policy that child support should be used to recoup welfare costs. The Deficit Reduction Act of 2005 gave states the option to pass through collected support to families on welfare; and mandates states to forward collected support to families when they leave welfare, except in cases where the support was intercepted from federal tax refunds. There is emerging bipartisan support in Congress for eliminating welfare cost recovery policies altogether and forwarding all collected payments to families. A third set of reforms focuses on reducing unrealistic arrears currently owed by low-income noncustodial parents. States are considering reducing interest on arrears and are experimenting with programs that tie debt forgiveness to stable employment and regular monthly payments of current support due.

The Responsible Fatherhood and Healthy Family Act of 2007 introduced in both houses of Congress and currently in committee would go far in addressing many of these issues as well as other disincentives for custodial and noncustodial parents to participate in the program (Turetsky, 2008). The Senate bill would prohibit TANF assignment of child support rights, mandate full distribution to families, and require states to disregard a portion of support income in calculating TANF benefits. It would ban cost recovery of Medicaid birthing costs and prohibit treatment of incarceration as voluntary unemployment—in effect stopping accrual of debt while fathers are in jail. It would also require states to deduct 20% of support income in calculating Food Stamp benefits, create an EITC-like credit for noncustodial fathers who are current on support payments, and fund grants for demonstration projects to increase employment and improve parent-child relationships for noncustodial parents.

7 Summary and Conclusion

Much has been accomplished in the last two decades, but much remains to be done. Changes in legislation have moved enforcement away from local judicial discretion towards state and national administrative regularity, characteristic of social insurance. This transformation has increased payments dramatically amongst poor and especially unwed families. Stronger child support enforcement is responsible for a modest increase in the incomes of single mothers and their children. In this regard, the US has come a long way in addressing the first two themes identified by Kahn and Kamerman: strengthening enforcement and standardizing obligations.

The final theme of providing children an adequate standard of living continues to be elusive. TANF strengthened the quarter century dramatic transformation of the US system of assuring child support. Advocates of stronger enforcement, like President Clinton, hoped that child support would reduce both poverty and welfare dependence by providing a source of income to single mothers outside the welfare system. However, large numbers of single mothers and their children remain poor and large numbers of poor fathers are affected adversely.

One of the main purposes of the Kahn and Kamerman volume was to increase awareness of and share knowledge of programs and experiences with child support in other countries. They identified the basic difference in program goals in Europe and the US. The goal of child support policies in Europe was to provide income to children in single parent families; while the goal of child support policies in the US has been to enforce support and to recoup public costs. They conclude that doing well by children and reducing public expenditures cannot work together. So long as reducing public expenditures remains the prime objective, child support policies in the US will continue to come up short.

Congress should build on the solid successes achieved to date by ensuring that low-income mothers and fathers are helped rather than hurt by our child support assurance system. This can be accomplished by establishing child support obligations that are expressed as a percentage of income, allowing mothers on TANF to receive much or all of the child support paid to them without reduction in benefits, and by publicly assuring a minimum child support payment. These steps will go a long way towards permanently moving our child support system (in the words of Kahn & Kamerman) from debt collection to an explicit social policy which improves the well-being of children in the United States.

References

Argys, L. M., Peters, H. E., Brooks-Gunn, J., & Smith, J. R. (1998). The impact of child support on cognitive outcomes of young children. *Demography, 35*(2), 159–173.

Bartfeld, J., & Garfinkel, I. (1996). The impact of percentage expressed child support orders on payments. *The Journal of Human Resources, 31*(4), 794–815.

Blank, R. (2002). Evaluating welfare reform in the United States. *Journal of Economic Literature, 9*, 1105–1166.

Brito, T. (2005). *Child support guidelines and complicated families: An analysis of cross-state variation in legal treatment of multiple-partner fertility.* Institute for Research on Poverty, University of Wisconsin, Madison.

Cancian, M., & Meyer, D. R. (2006). *Alternative approaches to child support policy in the context of multiple-partner fertility.* Institute for Research on Poverty, University of Wisconsin, Madison.

Cancian, M., Meyer, D. R., & Caspar, E. (2008). Welfare and child support: Complements, not substitutes. *Journal of Policy Analysis and Management, 27*(2), 354–375.

Carlson, M. J., & Furstenberg, F. F. (2006). The prevalence and correlates of multi-partnered fertility among urban U.S. parents. *Journal of Marriage and Family, 68*(3), 718–732.

Center on Budget and Policy Priorities. (2008). *Policy basics: The earned income tax credit.* Washington, DC: Center on Budget and Policy Priorities.

Committee on Economic Security. (1934). Report to the President of the committee on economic security. Social Security Administration. Social Security Online: History. http://www.ssa.gov/history/reports/ces/ces.html

Doolitle, F., Knox, V., Miller, C., & Rowser, S. (1998). *Building opportunities, enforcing obligations: Implementation and interim impacts of parents' fair share.* New York: MDRC.

Edin, K. (2000). Few good men: Why poor mothers don't marry or remarry. *The American Prospect, 11*(4), 26–31.

Fertig, A. R., McLanahan, S. S., & Garfinkel, I. (2006). *Child support enforcement and domestic violence among non-cohabiting couples.* Center for Research on Child Wellbeing Working Paper #02-17-FF. Princeton, NJ: Princeton University.

Garfinkel, I. (1992). *Assuring child support: An extension of the social security system.* New York: Russell Sage Press.

Garfinkel, I. (1994). The child-support revolution. *The American Economic Review, 84*(2), 81–86.

Garfinkel, I., Gaylin, D. S., Huang, C.-C., & McLanahan, S. (2000). *The roles of child support enforcement and welfare in non-marital childbearing.* Unpublished Manuscript.

Garfinkel, I., Heintze, T., & Huang, C.-C. (2000b, December 8). *Child support enforcement: Incentives and well-being.* Conference on Incentive Effects of Tax and Transfer Policies, Washington, DC.

Garfinkel, I., & McLanahan. S. (1986). *Single mothers and their children: A new American dilemma.* Washington, DC: The Urban Institute Press.

Garfinkel, I., McLanahan, S. S., & Hanson, T. L. (1998a). A patchwork portrait of nonresident fathers. In I. Garfinkel, S. S. McLanahan, D. R. Meyer, & J. A. Seltzer (Eds.), *Fathers under fire: The revolution in child support enforcement* (pp. 31–60). New York: Russell Sage Foundation.

Garfinkel, I., Melli, M. S., & Robertson, J. G. (1994). Child support orders: A perspective on reform. *The Future of Children: Children and Divorce, 4*(1), 84–100.

Garfinkel, I., Meyer, D. R., & McLanahan, S. S. (1998b). A brief history of child support policies in the United States. In I. Garfinkel, S. S. McLanahan, D. R. Meyer, & J. A. Seltzer (Eds.), *Fathers under fire: The revolution in child support enforcement* (pp. 1–13). New York: Russell Sage Foundation.

Graham, J. W., Beller, A. H., & Hernandez, P. M. (1994). The effects of child support on educational attainment. In I. Garfinkel, S. McLanahan, & P. K. Robins (Eds.), *Child support and child well-being* (pp. 317–354). Washington, DC: Urban Institute Press.

Hanson, T. L., Garfinkel, I., McLanahan, S. S., & Miller, C. K. (1996). Trends in child support outcomes. *Demography, 33*(4), 483–496.

Hernandez, P. M., Beller, A. H., & Graham, J. W. (1995). Changes in the relationship between child support payments and the educational attainment of offspring. *Demography, 32,* 249–260.

Holt, S. (2006). *The earned income tax credit at age 30: What we know.* Washington, DC: The Brookings Institution Policy Briefing.

Huang, C.-C., Mincy, R., & Garfinkel, I. (2005). Child support obligations of low-income fathers. *Journal of Marriage and Family, 67,* 1213–1225.

Kahn, A. J., & Kamerman, S. B. (1988). *Child support: From debt collection to social policy.* Newbury Park, CA: Sage.

Knox, V., & Bane, M. J. (1994). Child support and schooling. In I. Garfinkel, S. McLanahan, & P. Robins (Eds.), *Child support and child well-being* (pp. 285–310). Washington, DC: Urban Institute Press.

Kunz, J., Villeneuve, P., & Garfinkel, I. (2001). Child support among selected OECD countries: A comparative analysis. In K. Vleminckx & T. Smeeding (Eds.), *Child well-being, child poverty, and child policy in modern nations: What do we know?*. Bristol, UK: The Policy Press.

Legler, P. K. (1996). The coming revolution in child support policy. *Family Law Quarterly, 30*(3), 519–563.

McLanahan, S. (2004). Diverging destinies: How children are faring under the second demographic transition. *Demography, 41*(4), 607–627.

McLanahan, S. S., Seltzer, J. A., Hanson, T. L., & Thompson, E. (1994). Child support enforcement and child well-being: Greater security or greater conflict. In I. Garfinkel, S. McLanahan, & P. Robins (Eds.), *Child support and child well-being*. Washington, DC: Urban Institute Press.

Meyer, D., Garfinkel, I., Oellerich, D., & Robins, P. (1994). Who should be eligible for an assured child support benefit? In I. Garfinkel, S. S. McLanahan, & P. K. Robins (Eds.), *Child support and child well-being*. Washington, DC: Urban Institute Press.

Meyer, D. R., Cancian, M., & Cook, S. T. (2005). Multiple-partner fertility: Incidence and implications for child support policy. *Social Service Review, 79*(4), 577–601.

Meyer, D. R., Cancian, M., & Nam, K. (2007). Welfare and child support program knowledge gaps reduce program effectiveness. *Journal of Policy Analysis and Management, 26*(3), 575.

Meyer, D. R., Garfinkel, I., Oellerich, D. T., & Robins, P. K. (1992). Who should be eligible for an assured child support benefit? In I. Garfinkel, S. McLanahan, & P. K. Robins (Eds.), *Child support assurance: Design issues, expected impacts, and political barriers as seen from Wisconsin*. Washington, DC: Urban Institute Press.

Nepomnyaschy, L., & Garfinkel, I. (2007). *Child support and fathers' contributions to their nonmarital children*. Center for Research on Child Wellbeing Working Paper #2006-09-FF, Princeton University. http://crcw.princeton.edu/workingpapers/WP06-09-FF.pdf

Nichols-Casebolt, A., & Garfinkel, I. (1991). Trends in paternity adjudications and child support awards. *Social Science Quarterly, 72*(1), 83–97.

Oellerich, D., Garfinkel, I., & Robins, P. (1991). Private child support: Current and potential impacts. *Journal of Sociology and Social Welfare, 18*(1), 3–23.

Pate, D. J. (2002). An ethnographic inquiry into the life experiences of African American fathers with children on W-2. *W-2 Child support demonstration evaluation: Report on nonexperimental analyses: Volume II: Fathers of children in W-2 families*. Institute for Research on Poverty, University of Wisconsin-Madison.

Reichman, N. E., Teitler, J. O., & Curtis, M. A. (2005). TANF sanctioning and hardship. *The Social Service Review, 79*(2), 215–236.

Reichman, N. E., Teitler, J. O., Garfinkel, I., & Garcia, S. (2004). Variations in maternal and child well-being among financially eligible mothers by TANF participation status. *Eastern Economic Journal, 30*(1), 101–118.

Seltzer, J. A., & Brandreth, Y. (1994). What fathers say about involvement with children after separation. *Journal of Family Issues, 15*(1), 49–77.

Seltzer, J. A., McLanahan, S. S., & Hanson, T. L. (1998). Will child support enforcement increase father-child contact and parent conflict after separation. In I. Garfinkel, S. S. McLanahan, D. R. Meyer, & J. A. Seltzer (Eds.), *Fathers under fire: The revolution in child support enforcement* (pp. 157–190). New York: Russell Sage Foundation.

Sinkewicz, M., & Garfinkel, I. (2009). New estimates of unwed fathers ability to pay child support: Accounting for multiple-partner fertility. *Demography, 46*(2), 247–263.

Skinner, C., Bradshaw, J., & Davidson, J. (2007). *Child support policy: An international perspective*. Department for Work and Pensions, Research Report No. 405. Norwich, UK: Crown Copyright.

Sorensen, E., Sousa, L., & Schaner, S. (2007). *Assessing child support arrears in nine large states and the nation*. Department of Health and Human Services and Office of Child Support Enforcement, Washington, DC.

Turetsky, V. (2008). *Responsible fatherhood and healthy family Act of 2007*. Center for Law and Social Policy (CLASP) Legislation in Brief, Washington, DC.

U.S. Census Bureau. (1989). *Child support and Alimony: 1989*. Current Population Reports.

U.S. Census Bureau. (2007). *Custodial mothers and fathers and their child support: 2005*. Current Population Reports, Series P60–173.

U.S. Census Bureau. (2008a). *America's families and living arrangements: 2007*. Current Population Reports, Washington, DC.

U.S. Census Bureau. (2008b). Office of Child Support Enforcement FY 2005 Annual Report to Congress. Washington, DC: Administration for Children and Families, Office of Child Support Enforcement.

USDHHS. (2008a). *Caseload data*. US Department of Health and Human Services, Administration for Children and Families, Caseload Data. www.acf.hhs.gov/programs/ofa/data-reports/caseload/caseload_recent.html

USDHHS. (2008b). Office of Child Support Enforcement FY 2005 Annual Report to Congress. Washington, DC: Administration for Children and Families, Office of Child Support Enforcement.

Waite, L., & Gallagher, M. (2001). *The case for marriage: Why married people are happier, healthier, and better off financially*. New York: Doubleday Books.

Waller, M. R., & Plotnick, R. (2001). Effective child support policy for low-income families: Evidence from street level research. *Journal of Policy Analysis and Management, 20*(1), 89–110.

Wheaton, L., & Sorensen, E. (2007). *The potential impact of increasing child support payments to TANF families*. Assessing the New Federalism, Brief 5. The Urban Institute: Washington, DC.

Child Poverty and Antipoverty Policies in the United States: Lessons from Research and Cross-National Policies

Sandra K. Danziger and Sheldon Danziger

1 Introduction

Child poverty in the United States is higher than in most other advanced industrialized countries and has negative effects on children's development and educational attainment. We review the factors that contribute to this high rate, examine its consequences for children, and document that a number of feasible policy reforms could reduce poverty and increase opportunities for poor children.

Our chapter follows in the tradition of Alfred Kahn's research. For example, in the late 1990s, Sheila Kamerman and Kahn wrote about the role of political will in understanding differences in public investments in children and families across industrialized countries (1997). They differentiated between the "golden age" of social policy, the years from 1960 to 1975, and "the tough years" from 1975 to 1990. They concluded that "if the new and growing needs of children and their families in industrialized countries are to be met, this issue of political choice must be underscored in analyses of child and family expenditures and, more importantly, must be effectively addressed so that political effort may be transformed into political will" (p. 121). This chapter revisits their concerns about public policies towards poor children and families in the United States at a time when the recent election of President Obama seems to have signaled a significant change in political will.

Compared to nonpoor children, children who grow up in poverty, particularly if they are poor for many years, are at greater risk for problems in many domains. They are less likely to enter school ready to learn, more likely to have health and behavioral problems, and more likely to drop out of school and become teen parents (Duncan & Brooks-Gunn, 1997; Corcoran, 2001). Parents who have difficulty making financial ends meet are more likely to have emotional problems that increase stress and negatively affect their parenting styles (Gershoff, Raver, Aber, & Lennon, 2007). These families are more likely to live in neighborhoods that are

S.K. Danziger (✉)
School of Social Work and Gerald R. Ford School of Public Policy, University of Michigan, Ann Arbor, MI, USA
e-mail: sandrakd@umich.edu

S.B. Kamerman et al. (eds.), *From Child Welfare to Child Well-Being*, Children's Well-Being: Indicators and Research 1, DOI 10.1007/978-90-481-3377-2_15,
© Springer Science+Business Media B.V. 2010

dangerous and have lower quality child care facilities and schools and less healthy environments.

Holzer, Schanzenbach, Duncan, & Ludwig (2007) document that children growing up in persistently-poor households have reduced earnings as adults, are more likely to participate in criminal activities and have more health problems. They conclude that "the investment of some significant resources in poverty reduction might be more socially cost-effective over time than we previously thought" (Holzer et al., 2007, p. 31).

In this chapter, we review changes in the economy and public policies over the past five decades that have affected the extent of child poverty. We next review research on how poverty harms children and how public programs can affect the cycle of disadvantage. Then, we discuss selected poverty-reduction strategies and effective programs to "level the playing field" for poor children and provide them with greater opportunities for development and economic success.

We conclude that poverty will remain high unless the nation musters the political will to allow government to do more to reduce child poverty. President Johnson rallied Congress and the country to support the War on Poverty and Great Society in the mid 1960s; such political leadership and popular support have been absent in recent decades. In contrast, in 1999, Prime Minister Blair launched a major initiative to reduce child poverty in the United Kingdom that borrowed heavily from successful U.S. programs and policies and made progress against child poverty. Thus, if American policymakers and the public could find the political will to launch a new antipoverty initiative, we could "re-import" some of these successful policies and programs.

2 Economic Changes from the War on Poverty to the Present

The U.S. economy experienced a quarter century of sustained economic growth, rising real wages, and low unemployment rates between the end of World War II and the early 1970s. Even though the benefits of prosperity were being widely shared, concerns were raised in the early 1960s that many families, especially those headed by less-educated workers, minorities, and women, were not benefiting from the prosperous economy (Galbraith, 1958; Harrington, 1962; Lampman, 1959). Policy analysts called for government to develop new policies and programs targeted on those being left behind.

After President Johnson declared a War on Poverty, his economic advisors predicted that income poverty, as officially measured, could be eliminated by 1980. They assumed that stable economic growth would continue for the subsequent two decades much as it had for the prior two decades and that the benefits of economic growth would continue to be shared among most workers. The additional resources being devoted to the new initiatives would further reduce poverty as new employment and training programs would enhance skills and launch their graduates into an economy with low unemployment and growing wages. Human capital programs, from Head Start for pre-school children through Pell Grants for college students, would prevent the children of the poor from becoming poor workers in the next generation. Together, macroeconomic and antipoverty policies would sustain economic performance, raise the productivity of the poor and remove discriminatory barriers to participation in the education system and the labor market.

Poverty was not eliminated by 1980 or even by 2008, primarily because the optimistic economic forecasts of the 1960s could not envision the fundamental economic changes that began in the early 1970s and continue today (Danziger & Gottschalk,1995, 2005; Danziger, 2007). The labor market no longer provides rising real wages to workers across the skill distribution. Instead, real wages have fallen for the least-educated, barely kept up with inflation for the typical worker, and increased rapidly for professionals and corporate executives.

Many factors contributed to this transformation of the economy, including labor-saving technological changes that favored the most-educated workers, the globalization of markets and the deterioration in labor market institutions that help less-educated workers, such as declines in the value of the inflation-adjusted minimum wage and declines in the percentage of workers covered by union contracts. Unemployment rates were high for most years between the early 1980s and the mid 1990s, and again starting in 2008; growth in median earnings (adjusted for inflation) has been very slow and wages and access to employer-provided health insurance and pensions have fallen for many workers.

As a result of these labor market changes, progress against poverty has been very slow. The poverty rate remains very high for children who are African American, Native American and Hispanic, who do not live with both parents, and whose parents have completed no more than a high school degree. Child poverty in the U.S. is higher than it is in many advanced economies, even though U.S. living standards on average are higher than living standards in most other countries (Gornick & Jäntti, "Child Poverty in Upper-Income Countries: Lessons from the Luxembourg Income Study" of this book).

Poverty is also higher than in other advanced economies because the U.S. social safety net provides smaller benefits to fewer low-income families. Smeeding (2006a) shows that the U.S. spends only about 3% of GDP on social expenditures for the nonelderly, compared to about 12% in the Scandinavian countries and more than 6% in Australia, Canada and the United Kingdom.

Smeeding (2006b) compares the U.S. poverty rate around the year 2000 with that in eight other advanced economies by converting each country's currency into U.S. dollars and utilizing a poverty line that is similar to the official Census Bureau measure. He finds that U.S. per capita GDP in 2000 was about 20% higher than that in the other countries, but the U.S. child poverty rate, 12.4%, was higher than their 9.1% average. The rate in Canada, for example, was 9.0%; that in Sweden, 5.8%.

Figures 1 and 2 present cross-national data from years around 2000 for eleven advanced industrialized countries and indicate that the greater are government income transfers to single-mother and two-parent families, the lower are the proportion of children in these families that have disposable income below 50% of

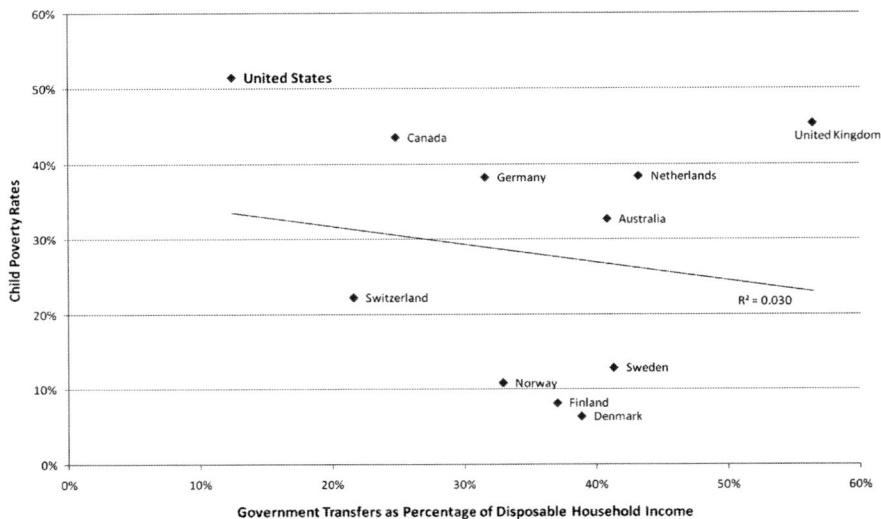

Fig. 1 Relationship between cash transfers and child poverty rates, eleven industrialized countries, single-mother families
Source: Data provided by M. Jäntti of the Luxembourg Income Study. Child poverty rate is based on disposable household income being less than 50% of the country's median.

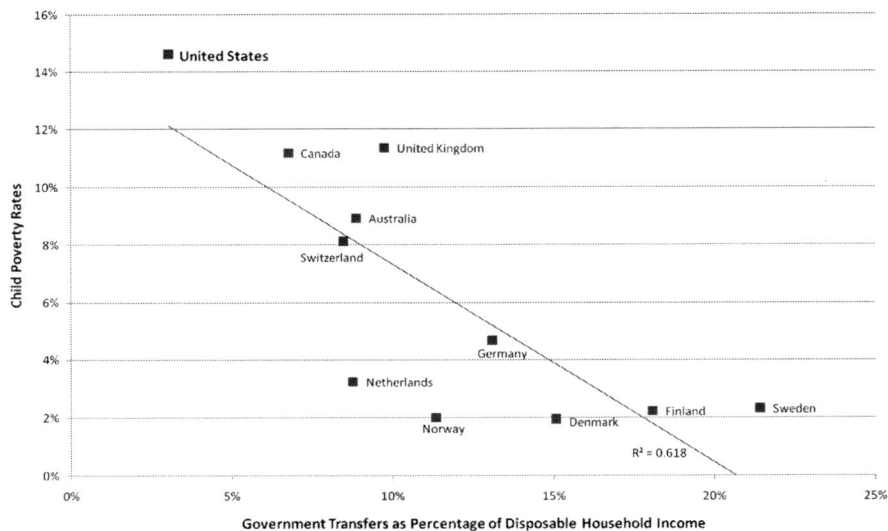

Fig. 2 Relationship between cash transfers and child poverty rates, eleven industrialized countries, two-parent families
Source: Data provided by M. Jäntti of the Luxembourg Income Study. Child poverty rate is based on disposable household income being less than 50% of the country's median.

the country's median disposable household income.[1] In the U.S., the percent of government disposable income that comes from government transfers for single parent families and two-parent families, 12.4 and 3.0% respectively, is lower than in any of the other ten nations. In contrast, 56.4% of disposable household income for single-mother families in the United Kingdom comes from government transfers; government transfers account for 22.3% of disposable income for two-parent families in Sweden. Relative child poverty is highest in the U.S.—51.5% for those living in single-mother families and 14.6% in two-parent families, compared to rates around 10% for children in single-mother families and around 2% among two-parent families in the four Scandinavian countries.

3 Trends in Poverty by Age: The Role of Economic and Policy Changes

Since the late-1960s, the U.S. has made substantial progress in reducing poverty among the elderly, and the economic status of the elderly has increased relative to that of children and nonelderly adults. Figure 3 shows trends in the U.S. poverty rate (an absolute poverty measure) for these three groups and highlights the dramatic reduction in poverty among the elderly compared to that among adults and children.[2] In 1959, the poverty rate for elderly persons was 35.2%, more than twice the 17.0% rate for adults ages 18–64. By 2006, the elderly poverty rate had fallen to 9.4%, lower than the adult rate, 10.8%, and much lower than the child poverty rate, 17.4%.

Government assistance for the elderly increased dramatically after the War on Poverty-Great Society era, and is the major reason elderly poverty rates have fallen so much. Between 1965 and 1973, there were seven across-the-board increases in social security benefits (Derthick, 1979). Then, Congress indexed social security benefits to the inflation rate, beginning in 1975. Because the earnings of workers have not kept up with inflation after the mid 1970s, social security benefits increased relative to earnings, relative to the poverty line, and relative to the government benefits available to adults and children.

The Supplemental Security Income Program (SSI), enacted in 1972, provides a minimum monthly cash payment to all poor elderly persons (as well as poor disabled and blind persons). Benefits are indexed for inflation, and SSI is available to the elderly who did not work in enough years to qualify for social security benefits. It also supplements income for those elderly who had very low earnings and hence low

---

[1] The data in Figures 1 and 2 were provided by Markus Jäntti of the Luxembourg Income Study.

[2] The U.S. measures poverty using an absolute poverty line that was established in the late 1960s. The poverty line for a family, which varies with its size, is compared to the money income received by the family members. Unlike the poverty rates based on disposable income in Figures 1 and 2, the U.S. measure does not reflect non-cash transfers received or taxes paid or tax credits received. The poverty line increases each year only to account for inflation. Because income has increased over the last four decades, the official poverty line for a family of four persons fell from 48 to 30 percent of median family income for a family of that size between 1960 and 2004 (Smeeding, 2006b).

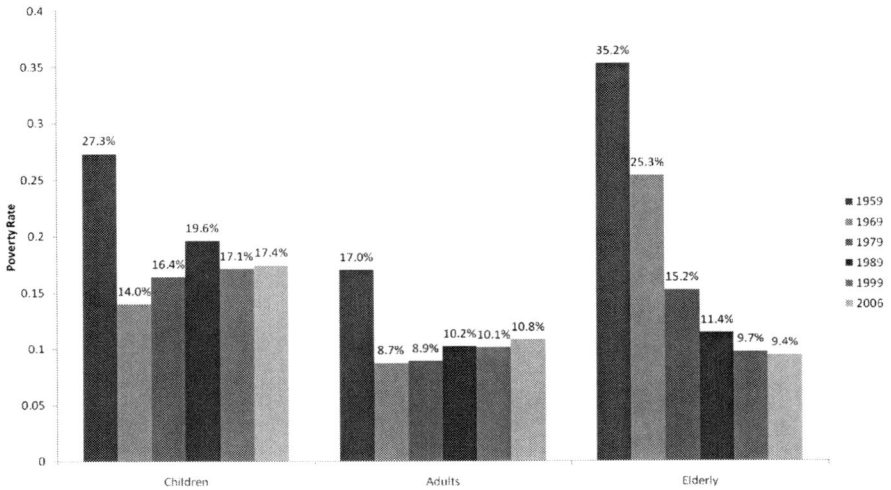

Fig. 3 Official U.S. poverty rates, by age, selected years 1959–2006
Source: Census Bureau (March CPS Historical Poverty Table 3).

social security benefits. As a result, all of the poor elderly, but not all poor children or adults, are eligible for cash assistance.

Between 1969 and 2006, there was little progress against poverty for children and adults, largely because of labor market difficulties that eroded the real wages of less-educated workers and because government income support for children whose parents did not work eroded after the late 1970s. Cash welfare payments for families with children did not keep up with inflation and the 1996 welfare reform dramatically reduced the percentage of poor children whose families are eligible to receive cash welfare. Also, a smaller percentage of unemployed workers received unemployment insurance in the early 2000s compared to the 1970s (Levine, 2006).

In addition, after 1980, the minimum wage fell relative to the average wage and failed to keep up with inflation. In the 1960s and early 1970s, the minimum wage was about half of the average wage of private nonsupervisory workers; by 2006, it had fallen to only 31% of this average (Bernstein & Shapiro, 2006). The minimum wage was increased to $5.85 in July 2007, to $6.55 in July 2008 and to $7.25 in July 2009. However, in inflation-adjusted terms, it will still be low by the historical standards of the late 1960s and early 1970s.

4 Exception to the Declining Support for Poor Children: The Earned Income Tax Credit

The primary exception to the pattern of declining government income support for low-income parents and children is the dramatic increase in the earned income tax credit (EITC), enacted in 1975. The value of the EITC is not included in the official poverty rates shown in Fig. 3 because that measure is based on pre-tax money income. The EITC is reflected in the relative poverty rates shown in Figs. 1 and 2. If the EITC were counted as money income, poverty rates for children and adults would be somewhat lower than the rates shown. For example, according to the U.S. House Committee on Ways and Means (2004), in 2002, if the EITC were included as income and other taxes were subtracted from income, the child poverty rate would have been reduced by 2.2 percentage points.

Since the mid 1970s, the EITC has provided income supplements to working poor and near-poor parents at the same time that access to cash welfare and unemployment insurance has declined. Unlike a welfare program that provides benefits to nonworkers, EITC payments are zero for nonworkers and reach a maximum for minimum-wage workers who work year-round full-time. EITC payments rise with earnings until the maximum benefit is reached, and then fall as incomes rise beyond some amount before phasing out at income levels about twice the poverty line. The EITC is available to both one- and two-parent families with children and provides a benefit level that is constant across the nation. (About half of the states supplement the federal EITC with their own EITC.)

The maximum federal EITC for a family with two or more children (in current dollars) was $400 in 1975, $953 in 1991 and $4824 in 2008. The number of families receiving credits increased from between 5 and 7.5 million families a year between 1975 and 1986 to about 23 million by 2005. The EITC increases each year with inflation. Because the EITC is available only to families with earnings, it has benefitted from bipartisan political support.

5 The 1996 Welfare Reform and Reductions in Cash Assistance for Poor Children

The Personal Responsibility and Work Opportunity Reconciliation Act (PRWORA) of 1996 decisively "ended welfare as we knew it." The Act eliminated the entitlement to cash assistance for single mothers that had been in place for 60 years. A single mother is no longer allowed to reject a job offer and remain on cash assistance; a recipient who refuses to search for work or co-operate with the welfare agency is sanctioned by having her benefits reduced or ended. Together, welfare reform and the economic boom of the late-1990s contributed to a sharp decline in welfare caseloads and a substantial increase in the employment of single mothers. In a single decade, the national welfare rolls fell by almost 70%. Because the 1996 reform has been so popular among politicians and the public, there is little reason to expect that cash assistance to nonworking, nondisabled parents will be expanded. Indeed, welfare reform furthered a profound shift in social welfare spending away from the nonworking poor and toward the working poor that began in the early 1980s (Scholz, Moffitt, & Cowan, 2009).

6 Disparities in Child Poverty by Race and Ethnicity

Figure 4 shows trends in the official Census Bureau (2006) child poverty rates for
all children between 1959 and 2005 and for white non-Hispanic, African American,
Hispanic and Asian children starting at different years. The Census Bureau did not
gather information on large enough numbers of families to publish an annual poverty
rate for Hispanic children until the early 1970s or the rate for Asian children until
the mid-1980s.

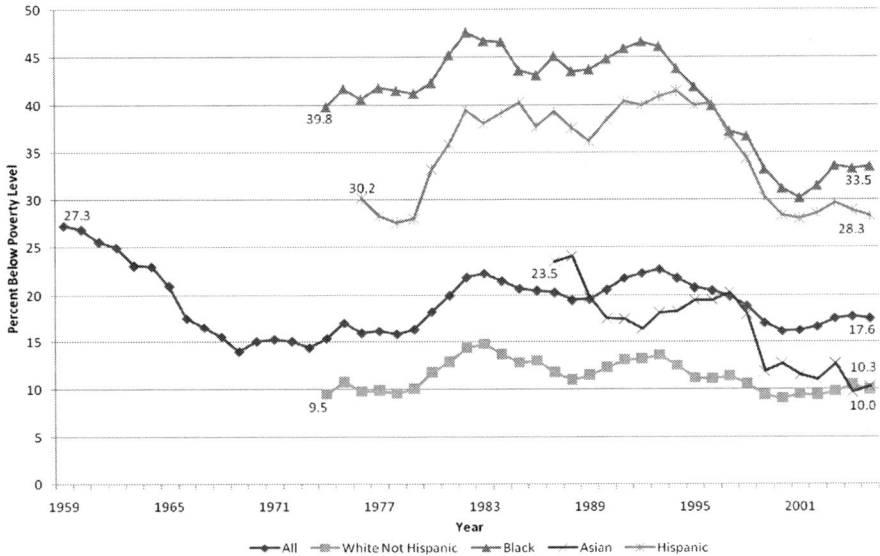

Fig. 4 Child poverty by race & ethnicity, 1959–2005
Source: U.S. Census, Bureau (2006).

For all children, poverty fell from 27.3% in 1959 to 14.4% in 1973. After that
year, economic growth faltered and in 1983, the national unemployment rate reached
its highest levels since the Great Depression of the 1930s—about 10%. As a result,
child poverty rose to 22.3% in 1983. During the economic boom of the late 1980s
poverty fell a bit, but rose again to 22.7% in 1993, following the 1990–1991 recession. The economic boom of the 1990s reduced child poverty rate to 16.2% in 2000,
before rising to 17.6% by 2005. The official child poverty rate in 2005 was about
the same as it was in 1966, just after the War on Poverty was declared. If the value
of noncash transfers and the earned income tax credit are counted as income (data
not shown), the child poverty rate in 2005 is about 14%, the same as the official rate
in 1973. The severe economic recession that began in late 2007 will lead poverty
rates for all groups to be higher in 2010 than they were in 2005.

Trends in child poverty are similar for children of each race/ethnic group. White
non-Hispanic children and Asian children have much lower poverty rates than

African American and Hispanic children in every year. The rates for all race/ethnic groups were highest during the recession of the early 1980s and fell substantially during the economic boom of the late 1990s. The poverty rate for white non-Hispanic children rose from 9.5% in 1974 to 14.8% in 1983 and then fell to 10% in 2005. The rate for Asian children fell from 23.5% in 1987 to 10.3% in 2005, just about the same level as that of white non-Hispanic children.

Even though poverty fell dramatically for African American and Hispanic children in the 1990s, they remain about three times as likely to be poor as white and Asian children. For African Americans, child poverty peaked at 47.6% in 1982 and fell to 33.5% in 2005; Hispanic child poverty peaked at 41.5% in 1994 and fell to 28.3% in 2005.

Welfare reform contributed to increased maternal employment which led to reduced child poverty even though cash welfare was reduced. Nonetheless, poverty among children living with single mothers remains very high. Welfare reform also produced a small, but increasing, group of mothers who are disconnected from regular sources of economic support—they have no work, no cash assistance and do not live in households that have other earners (Turner, Danziger, & Seefeldt, 2006). Economic hardship for this group increased after welfare reform.

Child poverty would be lower if a greater percentage of children lived in two-parent families. This is particularly the case for African-American children, who are much more likely than other children to live with only their mothers. However, there is a complex relationship between parental economic status and the likelihood that a child will live with both parents. For example, many low-income single mothers do not marry the fathers of their children because they have poor labor market prospects—their wage rates are low and they are frequently unemployed (Edin & Kefalas, 2005).

The administration of President G.W. Bush sought to reduce poverty by encouraging states to adopt marriage-promotion programs. These initiatives aimed to increase the likelihood that single mothers married the fathers of their children and to reduce the likelihood of divorce. The results of randomized evaluations of these programs are not yet available. However, the high child poverty rate implies the need for programs that can increase employment and earnings of parents regardless of marital status (Cancian & Reed, 2009).

7 Why Poverty Matters for Children

A substantial body of research documents that poverty has negative effects on many aspects of a child's development (Haskins, 2008; Neuman, 2008; Duncan & Brooks-Gunn, 1997; Corcoran, 2001). Magnuson & Votruba-Drzal (2009) review research on the negative effects of childhood poverty in the domains of health; emotional well-being and mental health; and educational achievement and economic attainment. They specify three theoretical processes through which poverty disadvantages children—family and environmental stresses, lack of resources and investments, and the interplay of social class/cultural patterns and poverty.

Each mechanism can operate on multiple levels of the child's environment from intra-personal processes, such as predisposing deficiencies in infant health from lack of mother's prenatal medical care, to low income neighborhoods' increasing social contact with juvenile criminal activity. Poverty's influence on child well-being theoretically can operate across the most proximal to the most distal levels, as shown in Fig. 5. Conceived as a series of concentric circles, this model allows us to posit the pathways from poverty to child effects at multiple levels and to consider their simultaneous, interactive, and multi-directional relationships.

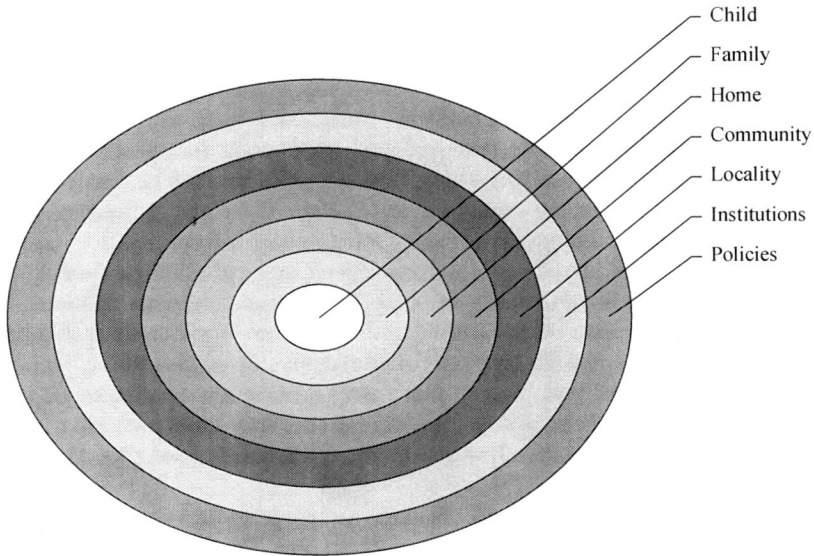

Fig. 5 Circles of influence: multiple processes through which poverty affects children

At the most direct level of influence, poverty can reduce the level and types of parental and family supports that enhance child development and well-being. For example, poor parents are likely to be less-educated about what helps children and to be less able to buy child-safe and enriching goods and services. At the next level, poverty can reduce the quality of a child's housing and create health risks through problems such as lead paint or asbestos. Or, overcrowded housing can hurt children by increasing the chances of accidents and by increasing parental stress that reduces their ability to nurture. Neighborhood or community-level poverty reduces access to neighbors with resources, and is associated with more health hazards or crime in public spaces where children play. Local area poverty in a rural area or large urban area may mean greater distance from high quality children's services and lack of economic and employment opportunities for parents. At the institutional level, poor families, especially if they live in impoverished communities, have less access to high-quality schools, medical care, police and fire protection. Differences at the policy level across countries determine the extent of public resources that are provided to poor children (see data in Figs. 1 and 2).

To document how Fig. 5 relates to the literature, we first illustrate how some of these multiple pathways influence child well-being and then highlight successful interventions that attempt to disrupt the cycle of poverty and disadvantage. The concentric circle model suggests that even if disadvantage can be countered successfully at one level, it may continue to reduce child well-being if it operates at multiple levels.

Gershoff et al. (2007) examine how poverty reduces young children's socio-emotional competence and cognitive skills using data from the Early Childhood Longitudinal Study (ECLS), a nationally-representative sample of parents and their kindergarten children. They find that material hardships, such as food insecurity, residential instability, financial troubles and inadequate medical care, in addition to low income, can contribute to marital conflict or parental depression, and, in turn, negatively affect a child's emotional or cognitive well-being. These hardships also lead some parents to reduce investments in their children, whether money, time, energy, or emotional support.

Gershoff et al. also find that greater material hardship negatively effects a child's socio-emotional development by raising parental stress and reducing positive parenting behaviors. Low income also negatively affects child well-being. They endorse comprehensive intervention policies aimed at proximate levels (raising parental investments in enrichment activities) and at environmental levels (raising income and lowering material deprivation). However, most policies operate in only one domain and families may not have access to the full range of assistance that would benefit their children. For example, early childhood intervention programs, such as Head Start, address primarily the child's cognitive and emotional development, but do not address financial hardships.

Caspe & Lopez (2006) review the results of numerous intervention programs and find that 13 programs that offered training to high-risk parents who resided in inner-city neighborhoods improved parenting skills, increased the quality of parent-child relationships, improved family functioning, and improved child well-being, especially school readiness. However, the programs did not address other parental needs, such as financial strains and educational and skill deficits.

A poverty-reduction strategy that sought to help both children and their families was the New Hope Program (Duncan, Huston, & Weisner, 2007) which featured a contractual promise to raise a family's income above the poverty line if the parent worked at least 30 hours per week. A cafeteria-style package of benefits included access to subsidized jobs for the unemployed, health insurance, and child care. The program reduced poverty, boosted work and earnings for some participants, increased access to health insurance, increased enrollment in child care centers, and improved children's school performance and behavior (Duncan, 2007). It is a unique program that improved both family economic well-being and the cognitive and socio-emotional well-being of their children.

Another successful program that provides benefits to both parents and children is the Nurse Family Partnership Program, developed by Olds (2002; Nurse Family

Partnership Program, 2009). Replicated in several randomized clinical trials and in many sites in the U.S. and in other countries (Olds, 2002), the program provides structured home visits by nurses for first-time high-risk mothers from early pregnancy through the child's second birthday. The program has improved outcomes for both child and parent, including healthier birth outcomes, improved child health and functioning, reduced risk of child abuse, and improved parental education and employment. For example, at the 15-year follow up of the Elmira, NY sample, nurse-visited poor unmarried mothers compared to the comparison group had 0.11 verified child abuse reports vs. 0.53, fewer subsequent pregnancies, 1.5 vs. 2.2, and fewer months on welfare, 60 vs. 90 (pp. 162–163).

8 How the 1996 Welfare Reform Affected Children

The 1996 welfare reform stimulated substantial research on its effects on child well-being. The results suggest few direct effects on child well-being, but some subgroups experienced improvements and some showed declines in child outcomes. Chase-Lansdale et al. (2003) analyzed early child and young adolescent cognitive, psychological and behavioral outcomes and the effects of mothers' transitions in and out of work and welfare over a 16-month period from 1999 to 2001. They did not find significant effects on the well-being of preschool children. They found mixed effects for 10–14 year olds. For example, mental health improved for these children if their mothers increased their employment. In some models, the young adolescents whose mothers lost welfare, but did not work, had declines in reading skills and/or increases in drug and alcohol use.

A recent special issue of *Children and Youth Services Review* (29, 2007) examined child well-being post welfare reform. The articles present analyses from five non-experimental panel studies conducted in numerous states. They documented that the transition to work itself did not directly affect child behavior, but operated through mediators such as parental stress and experiences of economic hardship. The mothers' stress and hardship levels in many studies remained high regardless of employment and welfare status, indicating that increased employment raised income but improved neither mothers' well-being nor child outcomes.

Johnson, Kalil, & Dunifon (2010) analyzed panel data from Michigan and examined how welfare mothers' post-1996 work behavior and history affected child behavior problems. They found that the children of mothers who experienced job instability, who worked full time in poor quality jobs, and who had irregular, fluctuating schedules had increased behavior problems and reduced academic progress. If mothers worked full time in jobs requiring cognitive skills and offering opportunities for wage growth, their children benefited.

Cook et al. (2002) found that families whose welfare benefits were terminated or reduced, as opposed to those whose benefit status remained constant, had greater odds of child hospitalization, of being food insecure, and of having children admitted to the hospital after being seen in emergency care. On the other hand, Deleire &

Lopoo (2006) found that restrictions in the availability of welfare benefits for teen mothers contributed to a decline in births among 15–17 years olds between 1992 and 1999.

9 A Post-welfare Reform Antipoverty Agenda

Policies to reduce child poverty and its negative effects on child development can reduce financial hardship directly by raising a family's income or improving its access to resources. Examples include cash welfare, food assistance programs, the minimum wage and the earned income tax credit. Other policies seek to reduce poverty's negative consequences by, for example, expanding access to health care or increasing child care subsidies or placing more poor children in early enrichment programs such as Early Head Start and Head Start. Based on our review of what works to reduce poverty and promote the development of poor children, we first discuss selected policies that would reduce poverty by raising earnings and expanding income support and access to health care. Then, we discuss interventions that would improve a child's early familial environment, and increase access to programs that would foster child development.

9.1 Raising Wages, Employment, and Income and Expanding Access to Health Insurance

If the U.S. is to reduce poverty in a post-welfare reform world, additional public policies are needed to supplement low earnings of former welfare recipients and other less-educated workers and to increase their access to subsidized health care. We focus on four examples—raising the minimum wage, subsidizing health insurance for low-income families not covered by Medicaid or the State Child Health Insurance Program (SCHIP), reforming the unemployment insurance program to cover more low-wage workers, and providing transitional jobs of last resort for those who want to work but cannot find steady employment.

Raising the minimum wage is the simplest example. In inflation-adjusted terms, the minimum wage was above $6.00 per hour in every year between 1962 and 1983, reaching a maximum of $8.67 (in 2006 inflation-adjusted dollars) in 1968. In 2007, Congress increased the minimum wage in three steps to $7.25 by July 2009. During the 2008 Presidential campaign, Candidate Obama called for raising the minimum wage to $9.50 by 2011 and indexing it for inflation.[3] Such a change would restore

---

[3] It is not likely that a minimum wage that is 45 percent of the average wage, as it was in the U.S. in the late-1960s, would have a large negative effect on the employment of low-wage workers. Card & Krueger (1997) conclude that the minimum wage increase of the early 1990s had only modest employment effects. And, there has been little concern expressed by employers following the minimum wage increases that were phased in between 2007 and 2009.

the minimum wage relative to the average wage to the level of the 1960s and 1970s and would be likely to reduce child poverty.

A second example is the State Child Health Insurance Program (SCHIP) enacted in 1997. Together with a series of Medicaid expansions from the late 1980s to the mid 1990s, all poor and near poor children now have access to subsidized health care coverage. In 2004, the uninsurance rate was 11.2% for children, 31.4% for those ages 18–24, and 25.9% for those 25–34. Wisconsin, under Republican Governor Tommy Thompson, adopted Badger Care, a program that allows low-income adults to purchase SCHIP coverage at a subsidized rate. This experience shows that government can do more to help offset the fact that fewer firms today offer subsidized insurance to workers. Lack of insurance has fallen for children because government has done more to help them; at the same time, lack of insurance has increased for adults because of labor market changes.

In January, 2009, Congress passed and President Obama signed an SCHIP expansion that will cover an additional 4 million children who would otherwise be uninsured. States are allowed to increase the program's income eligibility ceiling from 200 to 300% of the poverty level and cover children of legal immigrants (Swartz, 2009). The expansion was financed by an increase in the federal tobacco tax.

The third example is that labor market changes, especially the increase in part-time and low-wage employment, has reduced the likelihood that unemployed workers receive unemployment insurance benefits (UI). In the 1950s, about half of the unemployed received benefits; about three-quarters received benefits during the recession of the mid-1970s when Congress provided a federal extension of unemployment insurance for up to 39 weeks in addition to the traditional 26 weeks of coverage. In recent years, only about one-third of the unemployed have received benefits.

One solution is to mandate that all states provide UI coverage to part-time workers; less than half the states now do so. Another is to raise the UI replacement rate for low-wage workers. A minimum-wage worker who is laid off from a 30-hour per week job, for example, would, if she met other eligibility requirements, receive only about $75 per week in most states (National Employment Law Project, 2004).

The American Recovery and Reinvestment Act of 2009 (ARRA) provides states with additional federal funds if they modernize their unemployment insurance programs. States must adopt at least two of the following four provisions in order to qualify for additional fiscal relief under the Act: allow part-time workers to qualify for benefits; allow workers who leave a job for compelling reasons (such as a child's illness) to qualify for benefits; allow UI recipients to engage in approved training; pay dependents' allowances of at least $15 per week per dependent (National Employment Law Project, 2009).

A fourth, more ambitious policy to help those who have been negatively affected by the changing economy and changing safety net of the last quarter century and those affected by the very high unemployment rates due to the severe recession that began in late 2007, is transitional jobs of last resort. Many among the poor want to work and are willing to work, but do not have the labor market skills and experiences that firms demand when the unemployment rate is low and who are even less likely to be hired when the unemployment rate is high.

Access to a transitional job is especially important for single mothers who have been terminated from welfare and men with felony records. The federal government, for example, might pay 80% of the total employment costs—but the positions would be administered by non-profit or community-based organizations or by state and local governmental agencies that would pay the remaining costs. Workers would be expected to perform socially-beneficial tasks for which there is little effective labor demand. For example, they might provide labor-intensive public services in poor areas that are generally provided in affluent communities, such as monitoring of playgrounds, neighborhood maintenance and assisting the elderly.

Wages could be somewhat lower than the minimum wage, providing an incentive to take an available private sector job. Employees who did not meet performance standards would be dismissed. Those hired might be limited to a year to two years of the transitional job, after which time they should have acquired the experience and skills needed to get a private sector job. Transitional jobs of last resort would provide a post-welfare reform safety net to those who want to work but cannot find a regular private or public sector job.

9.2 Expanding Successful Child and Family Programs

In addition to policies that would raise wages, employment and family income and increase access to health care, other programs can directly promote child development in low-income families. These include expansions of two programs discussed above—the Nurse Family Partnership and New Hope that benefit both parents and children. Here, we highlight exemplary programs that target different levels of influence. First, some policies can help parents with young children balance work and family obligations. Second, successful early childhood enrichment programs can promote learning and developmental opportunities in the child's home and local community. Third, institutional changes in schools show promise for expanding educational opportunities for poor children.

First, Waldfogel (2006) advocates expanding access to affordable and high-quality child care and after school programs as a means to both increase investment in child well-being and increase parent's productivity. The Family Medical Leave Act now provides unpaid leave for childbirth. Waldfogel advocates a paid leave program, based on the experiences of many European countries, to support parents after childbirth and for extended family illness or other exceptional family responsibilities. She would also give workers the ability to request part-time or flexible hours in order to meet job and family needs, without loss of job security or reduced wages. She notes that extensive maternal employment and nonparent care in early infancy can negatively affect child health, cognitive and socio-emotional development.

Second, the child care subsidy voucher program benefits both parents and young children. It is funded by the federal Child Care and Development Block Grant

(CCDBG) and by the states with their own or with TANF funds. As cash welfare benefits declined after the 1996 welfare reform, states increased spending on subsidies, in part, to facilitate employment of women leaving welfare for work (Danziger, Ananat, & Browning, 2004). Between 1996 and 2005, federal block grant funding doubled from $2.2 to $4.8 billion; together, state and federal funding in 2005 provided 2.4 million vouchers per month (Child Care Bureau, 2006).

Child care subsidy use is associated with increased maternal employment (Schaefer, Kreader, & Collins, 2006; Blau & Tekin, 2007) and parents who use child care centers are more likely to receive subsidies (Schaefer et al., 2006). The ARRA expands funds for child care subsidies and for quality improvements in child care services. However, it is unclear whether simply providing subsidies leads to higher quality care (Antle et al., 2008). One way to encourage parents to choose higher quality care would be to have reimbursement rates increase as the quality of care increases (National Research Council, 2001; Burchinal, 2006).

Third, high quality early enrichment programs for at-risk children and families promote child development (Waldfogel, 2006; Currie, 2006). Intensive preschool programs, such as the Perry Preschool for 3–4 year-olds for part day for two years and the Carolina Abecedarian Project, which provided home visits and full-day high-quality chare care from early infancy through age 5, showed long term positive effects on children. Abecedarian children showed higher educational attainment and tests scores relative to controls as teens and young adults (Currie, 2006). The Perry preschool had its largest effects on social outcomes, reducing crime and welfare use through middle adulthood (Waldfogel, 2006). The Early Head Start and Head Start programs, which received additional funding from the ARRA could try to replicate some aspects of these programs.

Fourth, at the institutional level, there is some evidence that K-12 educational reforms can reduce some the disadvantages of poverty. Jacobs & Ludwig (2009) call for changes that would decrease the link between low-income neighborhoods and poor-quality schools. They would reform the No Child Left Behind legislation and target additional supports to at risk youth. They suggest, for example, that higher pay for teachers in disadvantaged schools can reduce teacher turnover rates and attract better teachers to these schools. They would also create incentives and give bonuses to low-income or low-performing schools that adopt successful instructional practices. They also would encourage wider public school choice through the expansion of magnet and charter schools.

10 Successful Strategies: Prime Minister Blair's Pledge to End Child Poverty

The United Kingdom has demonstrated that the kinds of policies we have discussed can reduce child poverty and promote child development. In 1999, Prime Minister Tony Blair pledged—"Our historic aim will be for ours to be the first generation to end child poverty, and it will take a generation. It is a 20 year mission but I believe it can be done" (Blair, 1999). The policies and programs put into place by the Blair government were based to a significant extent on the U.S. experience and research evidence on successful programs; they represented a significant increase in funding for investments in children. For example, universal preschool for 4-year olds was expanded to 3-year olds and some 2-year olds; there were extensions of paid maternity leave, a new Sure Start program for 0–3 year-olds in the poorest communities, and a national child care improvement strategy. In response to these programs, a rising minimum wage, a Working Families Tax Credit modeled on the EITC, expansions of child benefits and other income support benefits, child poverty in the UK fell dramatically (Hills & Waldfogel, 2004).

11 Conclusion

The reforms we have suggested would increase the wages, employment and family incomes of those who work for low wages and receive few fringe benefits. These antipoverty strategies and expansions in supports for poor families and children would be particularly beneficial for the groups of children with the highest poverty rates—those living with single parents, African Americans, Hispanics, and those who live in inner cities. Although a combination of economic, demographic, and policy changes that began in the 1970s have kept child poverty high, effective policies to reduce economic hardships and disparities and promote the well-being of poor children are available and are more common in other countries. What has been absent in the U.S. is the political leadership and public support to take bold actions to commit the public funds needed to reduce poverty and promote child development.

In our view, the high child poverty rates should be viewed as an unnecessary waste of human resources that is amenable to policy interventions. Children growing up in poor households typically have parents who both lack sufficient resources and lack the education and skills needed to find and hold good jobs in the 21st century labor market. Many poor children do not have access to enrichment programs and safe living environments; many still lack access to health care. Many of their parents have health and mental health problems that exacerbate the stresses of poverty and compromise parenting skills. Deficits in their families, homes, neighborhoods and communities negatively affect children's cognitive, socio-emotional, and academic well-being. Poor children are more likely to be poor as adults and raise poor children in the next generation than are children who grow up with greater resources and supports.

In other advanced economies, a wider range of government programs provide a greater proportion of low-income children with quality health care, early childhood education and child care, housing subsidies, and access to higher education and training. The research reviewed here and the experiences of other countries have, to date, not made much of an impression on U.S. policymakers and the public. There is a need for presidential leadership, as there was during the "golden age" of social policy, to convince Congress and the public that expanded public policies can improve the lives of poor children.

Some of the program expansions we have recommended were included in the American Reinvestment and Recovery Act of 2009 or were proposed in President Obama's budget for FY2010 or have been cited as Administration policy priorities. It remains to be seen if the Obama Administration can move further in this new direction and reverse the social policy trends that have been dominant since the early 1980s.

References

Antle, B. F., Frey, A., Barbee, A., Frey, S., Grisham-Brown, J., & Cox, M. (2008). Child care subsidy and program quality revisited. *Early Education and Development, 19*, 560–573.

Bernstein, J., & Shapiro, I. (2006). *Nine years of neglect: Federal minimum wage remains unchanged for ninth straight year, falls to lowest level in more than half a century*. Washington, DC: Center on Budget and Policy Priorities. Available at: http://www.cbpp.org/8-31-06mw.htm

Blair, T. (1999). Beveridge revisited: A welfare state for the 21st Century. In R. Walker (Ed.), *Ending child poverty: Popular welfare for the 21st century?* (pp. 7–18). Bristol, UK: Policy Press.

Blau, D., & Tekin, E. (2007). The determinants and consequences of child care subsidies for single mothers in the USA. *Journal of Population Economics, 20*, 719–741.

Burchinal, M. (2006). Child care subsidies, quality and preferences among low-income families. In Cabrera, N., Hutchens, R., & Peters, H. E. (Eds.), *From welfare to child care: What happens to young children when mothers exchange welfare for work* (pp. 261–266). Mahwah, NJ: Lawrence Erlbaum Associates.

Cancian, M., & Reed, D. (2009). Family structure, childbearing, and parental employment: Implications for the level and trend in poverty. In M. Cancian & S. Danziger (Eds.), *Changing poverty, changing policies* (pp. 92–121). New York: Russell Sage Foundation.

Card, D., & Krueger, A. (1997). *Myth and measurement: The economics of the minimum wage*. Princeton, NJ: Princeton University Press.

Caspe, M., & Lopez, M. (2006). *Lessons from family-strengthening interventions: Learning from evidence-based practice*. Cambridge, MA: Harvard Family Research Project.

Chase-Lansdale, P.L., Moffitt, R.A., Lohman, B.J., Cherlin, A.J., Coley, R.L., Pittman, L.D., Roff, J., Votruba-Dzal, E. (2003). Mothers' transitions from welfare to work and the well-being of preschoolers and adolescents. *Science*. 299:1548–1552.

Childcare Bureau, Administration for Children and Families, U.S. Department of Health and Human Services. (2006). *Child care and development fund (CCDF) report to congress for FY 2004 and FY 2005*. Washington, DC.

Cook, J.T., Frank, D.A., Berkowitz, C., Black, M.M., Casey, P.H., Cutts, D.B. Meyers, A.F. Zaldivar, N. Skalicky, A., Levenson, S. & Heeren, T. (2002). Welfare reform and the health of young children: A sentinel survey in 6 US cities. *Archives of Pediatric & Adolescent Medicine 156*: 678–684.

Corcoran, M. (2001). Mobility, persistence, and the consequences of poverty for children: Child and adult outcomes. In S. Danziger & R. Haveman (Eds.), *Understanding poverty*, (pp. 127–161). Cambridge, MA: Harvard University Press.

Currie, J. M. (2006). *The invisible safety net: Protecting the nation's poor children and families*. Princeton, NJ: Princeton University Press.

Danziger, S. (2007). Fighting poverty revisited: What did researchers know 40 years ago? What do we know today? *Focus: The newsletter of the Institute for Research on Poverty*. Madison, WI: University of Wisconsin-Madison. Available at: http://www.irp.wisc.edu/ publications/focus.htm

Danziger, S., & Gottschalk, P. (1995). *America unequal*. Cambridge, MA: Harvard University Press.

Danziger, S., & Gottschalk, P. (2005). Diverging fortunes: Trends in poverty and inequality. In R. Farley & J. John Haaga (Eds.), *The American people: Census 2000* (pp. 49–75). New York: Russell Sage Foundation.

Danziger, S. K., Ananat, E., & Browning, K. (2004). Child care subsidies and the transition from welfare to work. *Family Relations, 53*(2), 219–228.

Derthick, M. (1979). *Policy making for social security.* Washington, DC: Brookings Institution.

Duncan, G. J., & Brooks-Gunn, J. (1997). *Consequences of growing up poor.* New York: Russell Sage Foundation.

Duncan, G., Huston, A., & Weisner, T. (2007). *Higher ground: New hope for the working poor and their children.* New York: Russell Sage Foundation.

Edin, K., & Kefalas, M. (2005). *Promises I can keep: Why poor women put motherhood before marriage.* Berkeley: University of California Press.

Galbraith, J. K. (1958). *The affluent society.* New York: New American Library.

Gershoff, E., Raver, C., Aber, T. L., & Lennon, M. C. (2007). Income is not enough: Incorporating material hardship into models of income associations with parenting and child development. *Child Development, 78*(1), 70–95.

Harrington, M. (1962). *The other America: Poverty in the United States.* New York: MacMillan.

Haskins, R. (2008). *A plan for reducing poverty.* Washington, DC: Brookings Institution.

Hills, J., & Waldfogel, J. (2004). A 'Third Way' in welfare reform? Evidence from the United Kingdom. *Journal of Policy Analysis and Management, 23*(4), 765–788.

Holzer, H. J., Schanzenbach, D. W., Duncan, G. J., & Ludwig, J. (2007). The economic costs of poverty in the United States: Subsequent effects of children growing up poor. Ann Arbor: Michigan National Poverty Center Working paper series #07-04.

Jacobs, B., & Ludwig, J. (2009). Improving education outcomes for poor children. In M. Cancian & S. Danziger (Eds.), *Changing poverty, changing policies* (pp. 266–300). New York: Russell Sage Foundation.

Johnson R.C., Kalil A., & Dunifon, R. (2010). *Work after welfare reform and the well being of children.* Kalamazoo, MI: W.E. Upjohn Institute for Employment Research.

Kamerman, S. B., & Kahn, A. J. (1997). Investing in children: Government expenditures for children and their families in western industrialized countries. In G. A. Cornia & S. Danziger (Eds.), *Child poverty and deprivation in the industrialized countries 1945–1995* (pp. 91–121). New York: Oxford University Press.

Lampman, R. (1959). *The low-income population and economic growth.* U.S. Congress, Joint Economic Committee: Study Paper no. 12. Washington, DC: USGPO.

Levine, P. (2006). Unemployment insurance over the business cycle: Does it meet the needs of less-skilled workers? In R. Blank, S. Danziger, & R. Schoeni (Eds.), *Working and poor: How economic and policy changes are affecting low-wage workers* (pp. 366–395). New York: Russell Sage Foundation.

Lopoo L.M., DeLeire T. (2006). Did welfare reform influence the fertility of young teens? *Journal of Policy Analysis and Management 25*(2): 275–298.

Magnuson, K., & Votruba-Drzal, E. (2009). Enduring influences of child poverty. In M. Cancian & S. Danziger (Eds.), *Changing poverty, changing policies* (pp. 153–179). New York: Russell Sage Foundation.

National Employment Law Project. (2004). *Changing workforce, changing economy: State unemployment insurance reforms for the 21st century.* New York. Available at: http://www.nelp.org/docUploads/ChangingWorkforce.pdf

National Employment Law Project. (2009) *Concise guide to assistance for jobless workers in the American Recovery and Reinvestment Act.* NewYork. Available at: http://www.nelp.org/page/-/UI/ARRAConcise.pdf?nocdn=1

National Research Council. (2001). *Working families and growing kids.* Washington, DC: The National Academies Press.

Neuman, S. B. (Ed.). (2008). *Educating the other America: Top experts tackle poverty, literacy, and achievement in our schools.* Baltimore, MD: Paul H. Brookes Publishing Co.

Nurse Family Partnership Program (http://www.nursefamilypartnership.org/)

Olds, D. L. (2002). Prenatal and infancy home visiting by nurses: From randomized trials to community replication. *Prevention Science, 3*(3), 153–172.

Schaefer, S., Kreader, J. L., & Collins, A. M. (2006). *Parent employment and the use of child care subsidies*. Child Care and Early Education Research Connections. Available at: www.childcareresearch.org

Scholz, K., Moffitt, R., & Cowan, B. (2009). Trends in income support. In M. Cancian & S. Danziger (Eds.), *Changing poverty, changing policies* (pp. 203–241). New York: Russell Sage Foundation.

Smeeding, T. M. (2006a). Government programs and social outcomes: Comparison of the United States with other rich nations. In A. J. Auerbach, D. Card, & J. Quigley (Eds.), *Poverty, the distribution of income, and public policy* (pp. 149–218). New York: Russell Sage Foundation.

Smeeding, T. M. (2006b). Poor people in rich nations: The United States in comparative perspective. *Journal of Economic Perspectives, 20*(1), 69–90.

Swartz, K. (2009). Health care for the poor: For whom, what care, and whose responsibility? In M. Cancian & S. Danziger (Eds.), *Changing poverty, changing policies* (pp. 330–363). New York: Russell Sage Foundation.

Turner, L., Danziger, S., & Seefeldt, K. (2006). Failing the transition from welfare to work: Women chronically disconnected from work and cash welfare. *Social Science Quarterly, 87*(2), 227–249.

U.S. Census Bureau (2006). *Historical poverty tables*. Available at: http://www.census.gov/hhes/www/poverty/histpov/hstpov3.html

Waldfogel, J. (2006). *What children need*. Cambridge, MA: Harvard University Press.

Income Support for Families and the Living Standards of Children

Peter Saunders

1 Introduction

The term income support generally refers to government programs that provide income assistance in circumstances where income would otherwise not exist because of factors such as unemployment or disability that prevent people from earning. It can also be interpreted to include programs that supplement incomes that already exist, a view that acknowledges that families often receive a combination of government income transfers and market incomes. The circumstances that determine eligibility for income support and the level of support provided vary greatly across different systems and change over time within them as priorities shift. But all income support systems provide income transfers (or tax offsets) that support those who would otherwise have no or little income for reasons that are largely outside of their immediate control. These systems play an important role in all countries in providing an income safety net that maintains living standards and reduces poverty and inequality.

The programs that deliver income support differ within and between countries in terms of their underlying structure, the degree of reliance on cash transfers, tax reliefs or specific subsidies (e.g. for food or housing), the parameters that shape coverage and generosity, and the methods used to deliver, administer and monitor benefits. These components determine the impact of income support provisions, and affect the interaction between the income support system the labour market and the tax system. There is great interest in understanding how income support is structured in different countries, how much is spent, how specific programs are designed and administered, what interactions exist with other parts of the system and the overall effects on the incomes and living standards of different groups. Detailed and systematic study of overseas experience can provide important lessons for domestic policy, by highlighting success stories but also by identifying potential pitfalls and unintended consequences.

P. Saunders (✉)
Social Policy Research Centre, University of New South Wales, Sydney, Australia

S.B. Kamerman et al. (eds.), *From Child Welfare to Child Well-Being*, Children's
Well-Being: Indicators and Research 1, DOI 10.1007/978-90-481-3377-2_16,
© Springer Science+Business Media B.V. 2010

Nowhere are these issues more important than in relation to the provision of income support for children or, more accurately, for families with children. Family benefits have been a central feature of the welfare state for many decades, reflecting the importance attached to protecting children from poverty and promoting their healthy development. In recent years, the importance of these provisions has increased as research has shown that the early years are important for the longer-term development of children: the experience of poverty in ones early years can often leave permanent scars. However, this realization has been accompanied by a more nuanced understanding of the complexity of some of the issues, particularly those relating to the interaction between the income support system and the labour market. There is increasing awareness of the need to ensure that when parents are able to work, they are supported to do so. This has implications for the kinds of income support they receive, including whether an increase in hours worked (or earnings) leads to an increase ("making work pay") or reduction ("targeting on the most needy") in family benefits. Underlying these debates is a growing acceptance of the importance of avoiding joblessness within households with children, particularly young children, because of the inappropriate signals that passive parental dependence on income support can send to children. "Work is the best form of welfare" has become a popular (and populist) mantra in some liberal welfare states, where it has been used to tighten eligibility or reduce benefits for those unwilling to participate in workfare and related schemes. The success of these schemes in promoting parental employment may conflict with the goal of providing the most intensive support for children in their early years, or produce time pressures on parents (particularly sole parents) that reduce the time spent with, and caring for, their children.

Many of the issues highlighted in this discussion have featured prominently in research conducted by Al Kahn, some of it stretching back many decades. Much of that work has adopted a comparative approach and although this is a normal feature of contemporary research, it was far less common when Al and his colleagues first employed it. The advantages of the comparative approach, set out in his Introduction (with Sheila Kamerman) to *Child Support. From Debt Collection to Social Policy*, are as compelling today as they were when they were written 20 years ago:

> In a world increasingly described as a *global village* and a *world economy*, it is difficult, if not impossible, to deny the potential for learning that the experiences of other countries provide. In the social policy arena, the worldwide development of social security is the prime example of how countries can learn and adapt from one another (Kahn & Kamerman, 1988, p. 16; italics in the original).

That particular study, which focused on international developments in child support policy, was significant because it represented a shift of focus in income support analysis away from issues of cost, efficiency and effectiveness that are primarily focused on the impacts on *adults*, onto the implications of income support provisions for *children* (in this instance after parental separation). In this sense, the study was an important forerunner to what has since become the mainstream approach that involves placing the impacts on children at the centre when examining programs designed for families.

Another example of the prescient value of Al Kahn's work can be found in the even earlier comparative study of income transfers for families with children. This was one of the first studies to apply a "national informants" approach in which a common framework is developed and applied to analyse individual country experience with the assistance of experts from each participating country, who provide the national pieces from which the cross-national jigsaw is assembled. This method is now widely used to examine the design and impact of social policy in a range of areas, including by researchers examining policy-driven outcomes for children (Bradshaw, Hoelscher, & Richardson, 2006) and by agencies like the OECD when examining poverty and income distribution trends (Förster & d'Ercole, 2006). What is striking about this study are its conclusions, which Kahn and Kamerman (1983) identify as being: that policy makes a difference; that children are an expense; and that it usually pays to work. All three remain highly relevant today, despite the enormous social upheavals and seismic policy shifts that have occurred in the 30 years that have elapsed since the study was conducted.

The remainder of this chapter reviews the evidence from recent comparative studies and draws out some of the lessons learnt about the impact of income support provisions on the well-being of children. Section 2 provides a brief review of the methods used in comparative studies and the data sources to which they have been applied. As will become clear, the estimates presented draw heavily on studies conducted by two of the leading international agencies working on child well-being, the OECD and UNICEF. Section 3 compares two of the most important contributors to the living standards of children, public spending on family benefits and parental employment rates. Section 4 focuses on child outcomes, comparing child poverty rates and broader indicators of child well-being. Section 5 draws on recent Australian research to show that (as in many other countries) child poverty in Australia does not overlap with living standards measures that seek to identify the economic and social circumstances of children more directly. The main conclusions are briefly summarised in Section 6.

2 Methods and Data

The fact that child-rearing predominantly takes place within a family setting places boundaries around what state intervention can achieve. It cannot directly guarantee specific outcomes for children in terms of their actual functioning (Sen, 1985), although it can provide support to parents in the form of income transfers or information, advice and counseling services. It can also fund, subsidize or provide services that meet the needs of children (e.g. health care services and child care) and enact legislation that requires children to utilise certain services (e.g. primary and basic secondary schooling). These services promote children's capabilities by expanding their capacity to set their own objectives and act as autonomous agents to achieve them. Although the state can, as a last resort, remove children into state care when families become dysfunctional, its impact on child outcomes will generally be mediated (as it should be) by the influence of parents.

Income support represents a crucial sphere of state influence because it improves the ability of parents to meet the current consumption needs of children and thus provides more scope for future investment in them. It is common to direct such support to the parent who has primary responsibility for the child (usually the mother) and the available evidence indicates that child benefits paid to mothers are more likely to be spent on items that meet the needs of children (Lundberg, Pollak, & Wales, 1997). Even so, there may be a gap between the money spent by governments and the benefits received by children and this can limit their impact. The gap is unlikely to be large (or persistent) enough to distort the use of spending levels to capture impacts, but it is important not to lose sight of its existence—particularly when support is provided through the tax system to primary earners (often the father).

Income support may replace earnings for those parents who are unable to engage with the labour market, or it may supplement the earnings of those who are employed. The relationship between earnings and income support is complex and controversial, with some arguing that provision of the latter can cause a compensating decline in the former, with little net income effect, aside from a switch from financial independence (earnings) to financial dependence (welfare) that is underwritten by taxpayers. To counter these effects, some governments have introduced in-work benefits that are only paid when the parent is employed and increase as the number of hours worked rises (at least over certain ranges). One way of assessing the net impact of these countervailing forces is to examine the participation rates, hours worked and earnings of parents (both partners in couples, and sole parents) and try to link the observed differences to variations in policy parameters. This is a complex exercise, and far beyond the scope of this chapter. Instead, the simpler task of comparing parental employment rates within and between countries is undertaken in order to illustrate that income support (and employment support) policies vary in ways that can have potentially large effects on the incomes of parents and the living standards of children.

Thus far, the discussion has focused on inputs (income support, paid to parents) and intermediate outputs (parental employment rates). In terms of the outcomes for children, two indicators are examined. The first is child poverty, defined as the number of children living in families or households (these two concepts are different, but are used interchangeably to limit the discussion) with incomes below a poverty line. Comparative studies generally adopt a relative poverty line, fixed as a percentage of median income. This measure implies that those identified as poor in rich countries may have a higher absolute standard of living than those identified as poor in less rich countries, although this is not inevitable. Thus, Smeeding (2006) has shown in relation to the United States, for example, that not only is the relative child poverty rate above that in most other rich countries, the absolute living standards of American children are also below those of children in many other countries.

One important limitation of the way that child poverty is measured is that it actually measures family poverty and thus can equally be described as a measure of parental poverty. In the standard poverty literature, children are treated as passive agents with "needs" expressed (through the equivalence adjustment of family income) as a proportion of those of adults, and with the issue of intra-family redistribution assumed away (or ignored) under the equal sharing assumption. There is evidence that low-income mothers often put their children's needs before their own, and direct their limited resources disproportionately towards their children. When this happens, the conventional approach can lead to an over-estimate of poverty among children and an under-estimate of poverty among parents (particularly mothers).

Another limitation is that income is an imperfect metric on which to base the identification and measurement of poverty. Having an income below the poverty line is neither a necessary nor a sufficient condition to guarantee that poverty exists—in the sense of living standards falling below some level of acceptability. Some families with incomes below the poverty line will be able to draw on other resources (savings or access to credit) to meet their needs, while some families with incomes above the poverty line may face exceptional costs (e.g. relating to their health needs, or the presence of a child with a disability) and be forced into poverty. In order to establish that poverty exists, we need to look beyond income, to the actual living conditions experienced and establish whether or not these conditions—and the associated living standards—are representative of poverty. As Ringen (1987, p. 162) has argued:

> To ascertain poverty we need to identify directly the consequences we normally expect to follow from low income. . . . We need to establish not only that people live as if they were poor but that they do so because they do not have the means to avoid it

The conceptual imperfections of using income alone to identify poverty are compounded by the practical difficulties surrounding the measurement of income. People are notoriously reluctant to provide information about their incomes in surveys and often when they do, what is provided is incomplete or inaccurate.

These issues and problems have seen the emergence of alternative approaches that seek to locate the identification of poverty within a framework that measures living standards more directly. One such approach is based on the concept of deprivation, first developed for this purpose by Townsend (1979) and subsequently refined and defined as "an enforced lack of socially perceived necessities" by Mack & Lansley (1985, p. 39). Deprivation studies proceed in three stages: they first identify whether each of a list of items is necessary or not, and then whether people have each item and, if they do not, whether this is because they cannot afford it or because they do not want it. Those who do not have and cannot afford the items regarded as necessities by a majority are then identified as deprived, and the extent of deprivation can be measured by summing the number of items of which they are deprived.

One advantage of the deprivation approach is that it can be used to examine the circumstances of children more directly than income poverty studies. It is possible to specify deprivation indicators that relate directly to the living standards of children (e.g. access to new school clothes, or the ability to participate in school outings and activities that may involve out-of-pocket costs), and countries like Britain and

Ireland that have established child poverty reduction targets include such indicators in the suite of measures used to monitor progress (Department for Work and Pensions, 2003; Whelan, Nolan, & Maître, 2006). Even though the existence of child deprivation may be based on information provided by parents, the focus is placed more on how children are faring in terms of outcomes as opposed to their presumed share of family income. In this way, deprivation studies allow the living standards of children to differ, in certain dimensions, from those of their parents—a possibility that is not possible under conventional income-based poverty studies.

Collecting the data required to identify and measure deprivation is a difficult and expensive task. However, an increasing number of countries have recognized the value of such data in supplementing income poverty studies by showing whether low-income is accompanied by deprivation and an inadequate standard of living. A recent OECD study, for example, identifies four European-wide surveys that collect comparative information on aspects of deprivation, in addition to the national surveys being undertaken in three European and six other OECD countries (Boarini & d'Ercole, 2006, Annex 2). Although not without their limitations, deprivation studies provide new evidence on the living standards and well-being of families, and of children. As noted in the OECD study cited above:

> measures of material deprivation add important information to that provided by conventional income measures, permitting an assessment of poverty from a longer-run perspective and furthering understanding of the causal mechanisms at work (Boarini & d'Ercole, 2006, p. 6).

3 Public and Parental Support for Children

Governments support children through a wide variety of programs although the focus here is on those that provide income support, either directly in the form of cash benefits paid to parents, or indirectly in the form of child-related tax concessions. The comparisons in Table 1 indicate that in 2003, the combined value of these measures exceeded 2% of GDP in several countries, and averaged 1.3% of GDP across the OECD. The predominant form of assistance in most countries is cash benefits, although tax concessions are important in several countries, including Germany, France, the United States, Belgium, Netherlands and the Slovak Republic. The United States and Japan are the only countries where the value of tax concessions exceeds spending on cash benefits, and in both cases this reflects the fact that spending on cash benefits is very low.

Despite important differences in the way these schemes are structured in each country (specifically the criteria used to determine eligibility for tax concessions) these aggregate comparisons provide an initial insight into the role of government in providing income support to families with children and the importance attached to different policy instruments in different jurisdictions. The fact that more than half of all OECD countries spend over 1.5% of their GDP support family incomes illustrates the important role that government plays in assisting families when they are raising children.

Table 1 Spending on cash benefits and tax concessions for families in OECD countries in 2003 (percentage of GDP)

	Cash benefits	Tax Concessions	Total
Luxembourg	3.5	–	3.5
Australia	2.6	0.0	2.6
United Kingdom	2.2	0.4	2.6
Austria	2.5	0.0	2.5
Ireland	2.3	0.1	2.4
Belgium	1.7	0.5	2.2
France	1.4	0.8	2.2
Germany	1.2	1.0	2.2
Hungary	2.1	–	2.1
Norway	1.9	0.1	2.0
New Zealand	1.9	0.0	1.9
Slovak Republic	1.3	0.5	1.8
Czech Republic	1.3	0.4	1.7
Sweden	1.6	0.0	1.6
Denmark	1.6	0.0	1.6
Finland	1.6	0.0	1.6
Iceland	1.5	0.0	1.5
Netherlands	0.8	0.5	1.3
Switzerland	1.1	–	1.1
Poland	1.0	–	1.0
Canada	0.9	0.1	1.0
Greece	0.9	–	0.9
United States	0.1	0.7	0.8
Japan	0.3	0.5	0.8
Portugal	0.7	–	0.7
Italy	0.6	0.0	0.6
Spain	0.4	0.1	0.5
Mexico	0.3	0.0	0.3
Korea	0.1	0.0	0.1

Source: OECD (2007a, Chart 4.1)

Comparative data on parental employment rates is not easy to come by and that which is available focuses on mothers (primarily because fathers' employment rates vary little from male employment rates generally). Table 2 provides information on employment rates of women generally, of mothers differentiated by the age of the youngest child, and of sole parents (the vast majority of whom are women). The differences need to be interpreted with care because they embody and reflect a number of factors that are likely to distort the comparisons. One such factor is age: mothers are on average younger than women overall and this implies that the figures will reflect the increasing tendency of younger cohorts of women to participate in the labour market—a reflection of the decline of the "male breadwinner" model of family finances. Another important determinant of parental employment is the availability and cost of child care, and these both vary considerably across OECD countries (OECD, 2007b).

With these effects in mind, the first point that emerges from Table 2 is that in overall terms, mothers tend to have similar employment rates to women generally.

Table 2 Employment rates of all women, mothers and sole parents

	All women (2006)	Mothers (by age of youngest child, 2005)				Sole parents (2005)
		0–16	0–2	3–5	6–16	
Australia	65.5	63.1	48.3	–	70.5	49.9
Austria	63.5	64.7	60.5	62.4	67.5	75.0
Belgium	53.6	59.9	63.8	63.3	56.9	62.0
Canada	69.0	70.5	58.7	68.1	71.1	67.6
Czech Republic	56.8	52.8	19.9	50.9	67.6	63.0
Denmark	73.2	76.5	71.4	77.8	77.5	82.0
Finland	67.3	76.0	52.1	80.7	84.2	70.0
France	57.1	59.9	53.7	63.8	61.7	70.1
Germany	61.5	54.9	36.1	54.8	62.7	62.0
Greece	47.5	50.9	49.5	53.6	50.4	82.0
Hungary	51.2	45.7	13.9	49.9	58.3	–
Iceland	81.6	84.8	83.6	–	86.5	81.0
Ireland	58.8	57.5	55.0	–	59.9	44.9
Italy	46.3	48.1	47.3	50.6	47.5	78.0
Japan	58.8	52.4	28.5	47.8	68.1	83.6
Luxembourg	53.7	55.4	58.3	58.7	52.7	94.0
Netherlands	66.0	69.2	69.4	68.3	69.4	56.9
New Zealand	68.4	64.6	45.1	60.6	75.3	53.2
Portugal	62.0	67.8	69.1	71.8	65.4	77.9
Slovak Republic	51.9	48.4	23.1	46.6	60.4	–
Spain	54.0	52.0	52.6	54.2	50.9	84.0
Sweden	72.1	82.5	71.9	81.3	76.1	81.9
Switzerland	71.1	69.7	58.3	61.7	77.0	83.8
United Kingdom	66.8	61.7	52.6	58.3	67.7	56.2
United States	66.1	66.7	54.2	62.8	73.2	73.8

Source: OECD (2007a, Tables 1.1 and 3.2)

The main exceptions are in Finland and Sweden, where mothers have above-average employment rates, and the Czech Republic, Germany, Hungary, Japan, New Zealand and the United States, where mothers' employment rates are well below those of women generally. In virtually all countries, mothers are less likely to be in employment when their youngest child is under 2, although employment rates increase along with the age of the youngest child, aside from declines among mothers of older children in Belgium, Luxembourg, Portugal and Sweden.

The cross-national differences in the employment rates of sole parents are greater than those for all mothers, although in most countries sole parents are more likely to be employed than mothers generally. There are, however, several cases where the employment rate of sole parents lies well below that of all mothers, particularly in Australia, Finland, Ireland, Netherlands, New Zealand and the United Kingdom. It is noteworthy that most of these countries have transfer systems that target assistance to those with lowest incomes, and these schemes tend to produce high effective marginal tax rates (or "poverty traps") that lower the financial rewards from working and thus reduce labour supply. This is an example of how the structure of income support provision for parents can indirectly affect family income and hence the living standards of children, by reducing the willingness of parents to be employed.

The results in Tables 1 and 2 show that there is considerable variation in government direct and indirect financial support for families and in employment rates of those who are the main carers of most children. The links between the level and structure of support and the willingness of parents to join the labour force are varied and complex and cannot be identified in aggregate statistics like those presented. Nevertheless, the interactions between state support for families and parental labour supply behavior and hence family market incomes imply that it is important to adopt a broad view when thinking about how income support provision by the state influences decisions made within families that can have profound effects on the well-being of children.

4 Outcomes for Children

As noted earlier, the most common indicator of child outcomes used in the social policy literature has been the child poverty rate. Poverty studies can be used to assess the impact of government programs within countries by comparing poverty rates before and after taking account of state benefits and taxes, and these comparisons can also be used to assess the relative effectiveness of policy packages between countries. Despite their limitations, such studies can have an important impact on the public discourse about the extent of disadvantage and put pressure on governments to take action to reduce poverty. It is also clear from research that the experience of poverty in the childhood years—particularly in the early years—can have a lasting impact on the ability of children to realise their full potential in later years. As Brooks-Gunn and Duncan (1997) concluded after reviewing the findings from US longitudinal studies:

> ... family income can substantially influence child and adolescent well-being [and] incomes policies ... can have immediate impact on the number of children living in poverty and on the circumstances in which they live. Most important ... would be efforts to eliminate deep and persistent poverty, especially during a child's early years (Brooks-Gunn and Duncan, 1997, pp. 67–68).

Although the authors acknowledge that the links between income and child outcomes are "complex and varied" the evidence provides overwhelming support for the view that government action can prevent and reduce child poverty as well as mediating its effects (Plotnick, 1997).

Table 3 summarises recent evidence on the extent of child poverty in OECD countries. Poverty has been estimated using a poverty line equal to 50% of each country's overall median disposable income, after adjusting for differences in household size using an equivalence scale equal to the square root of household size. The estimates in the first column relate to individuals (in this case children) while those in the remaining four columns relate to households with children. Several features of these results are worthy of emphasis. First, there is considerable cross-country variation in the child poverty rate, which ranges from below 5% in Finland, Norway and Sweden to over 20% in Italy, Mexico, Switzerland and the United States. And

Table 3 Poverty rates in OECD countries around 2005 (percentages)

				All households with children	
	All children	Sole parent households	Couple households	After taxes and transfers	Impact of taxes and transfers (%)
Australia	11.8	38.3	6.5	10.1	57.8
Austria	8.5	22.1	6.5	7.8	51.0
Belgium	11.6	27.9	8.6	10.4	43.8
Canada	15.1	44.7	9.3	12.6	38.0
Czech Republic	10.2	42.3	6.9	9.2	47.2
Denmark	5.0	16.0	2.3	4.0	69.2
Finland	4.2	13.7	2.7	3.8	72.5
Germany	16.3	41.5	8.6	13.1	41.7
Greece	13.2	26.5	11.7	12.1	30.3
Hungary	8.7	25.2	6.8	6.8	58.8
Ireland	16.3	47.0	10.1	13.8	51.4
Italy	26.2	29.3	23.4	23.6	−3.5
Korea	10.7	18.9	8.6	9.6	8.6
Luxembourg	12.4	41.2	9.7	11.0	45.9
Mexico	22.2	32.6	18.7	19.5	5.7
Netherlands	11.5	39.0	6.3	9.3	46.6
New Zealand	15.0	39.1	9.4	12.5	45.5
Norway	4.6	13.3	2.1	3.7	68.3
Portugal	17.4	35.8	14.9	15.5	6.4
Slovak Republic	10.9	33.5	9.2	10.0	36.1
Spain	17.3	40.5	13.9	14.7	18.6
Sweden	4.0	7.9	2.8	6.2	68.5
Switzerland	24.6	39.4	20.0	–	–
United Kingdom	11.0	24.5	6.1	8.9	58.5
United States	20.6	47.5	13.6	17.6	25.5

Source: OECD (2007b, Tables 3 and 14)

as this latter grouping of countries illustrates, the level of national income is not the main factor driving differences in child poverty outcomes: increased national affluence does not automatically translate into lower poverty among children. In most countries, poverty among children in sole parent households is between three and six times higher than in couple households—in large part because couples have greater opportunity to participate in employment and hence receive earnings. The fact that the household poverty rate (column 4) is below the child poverty rate (column 1) indicates that the poverty rate tends to be higher in households containing more children. So two of the main poverty risks facing children are living with only one parent, and having a large number of siblings, neither of which the children themselves have any influence over.

The figures in the last column of Table 3 estimate the impact of taxes and transfers by comparing the difference between poverty rates based on income before the receipt of transfers and payment of taxes (market income) and after taking account of transfers received and taxes paid (disposable income). These estimates show, for example, that in Australia transfers and taxes reduce the poverty rate by 57.8% from 23.9% (on the basis of market income) to 10.1% (on the basis of disposable income).

The difference captures the impact of all transfer payments and the (direct) taxes that fund them, and indicates that the removal of these benefits and taxes would produce a huge rise in poverty. Even though such a change would lead to significant offsetting second-round effects, the estimates provide a valuable indication of the powerful effects of transfer systems on child poverty (and adult poverty).

These effects vary so greatly across countries because of two main factors: the level of family transfers, and the way in which they are structured. The former factor determines how much is received by the average recipient and thus determines the average impact on poverty for a given initial distribution. The latter determines which families receive a transfer (or are liable for tax) and how much they receive (or pay) as a result of targeting and other measures. Heavily targeted systems tend to concentrate assistance on those households with low incomes and/or low attachment to the labour force, but this does not guarantee that the impact on poverty is high because this also depends on the amount of income that is transferred through the system. Countries like Finland, Norway and Sweden that provide generous levels of assistance on a universal basis have a bigger impact on poverty and end up with less of it than countries like Australia, Ireland and the United Kingdom that target more effectively but provide less generous levels of support overall (see Table 1). Countries that rely heavily on targeted assistance also tend to have greater inequality in market incomes—particularly wages (Bradbury & Jäntti, 1999)—and thus face a tougher challenge in reducing poverty. This is a highly simplified account of what is a very complex set of interactions, but it reinforces the point made earlier about the need to take account of how the income support system interacts with other forms of income when examining its impact on poverty.

Income is one among many factors that affect the standard of living. In relation to children in particular, the tenuous link between the income of their family and their own standard of living is likely to make (equivalised) income an even more imperfect measure. For some time, UNICEF has been publishing a regular series of Report Cards that compare rich countries in terms of the well-being of children using a broader range of indicators than income alone. Early reports in the series used income poverty as a proxy measure of well-being (e.g. UNICEF, 2006) but in 2007, for the first time, a composite measure was developed that summarized available data across six broad dimensions of well-being. Although the limitations of the new measure were acknowledged, the bold claim that *Report Card 7*

> ... breaks new ground by bringing together the best of currently available data and represents a significant step towards a multi-dimensional overview of the state of childhood in a majority of the economically advanced nations of the world (UNICEF, 2007, p. 7).

is borne out by the wealth of information it contains and the new perspectives it has opened up.

The six dimensions of well-being identified in the report are shown in Table 4, which ranks each country on each dimension and across all six dimensions (by averaging the six separate rankings). The figures indicate that no single dimension of well-being is a reliable proxy for overall well-being and, as a consequence, country rankings vary greatly across the different dimensions. The UNICEF report notes that

Table 4 Child well-being and poverty rankings in OECD countries

	Dimension of well-being							
	Material well-being	Health and safety	Educational well-being	Family and peer relationships	Behaviours and risks	Subjective well-being	Average ranking	Child poverty ranking
Netherlands	10	2	6	3	3	1	4.2	9
Sweden	1	1	5	15	1	7	5.0	4
Denmark	4	4	8	9	6	12	7.2	1
Finland	3	3	4	17	7	11	7.5	2
Spain	12	6	15	8	5	2	8.0	17
Switzerland	5	9	14	4	12	6	8.3	6
Norway	2	8	11	10	13	8	8.7	3
Italy	14	5	20	1	10	10	10.0	19
Ireland	19	19	7	7	4	5	10.2	18
Belgium	7	16	1	5	19	16	12.7	5
Germany	13	11	10	13	11	9	11.2	10
Canada	6	13	2	18	17	15	11.8	14
Greece	15	18	16	11	8	3	11.8	11
Poland	21	15	3	14	2	19	12.3	15
Czech Rep.	11	10	9	19	9	17	12.5	7
France	9	7	18	12	14	18	13.0	8
Portugal	16	14	21	2	15	14	13.7	16
Austria	8	20	19	16	16	4	13.8	13
Hungary	20	17	13	6	18	13	14.5	12
United States	17	21	12	20	20	–	18.0	21
United Kingdom	18	12	17	21	21	20	18.2	20

Source: UNICEF (Report Card 7, p. 2 and Figure 1.1)

there is no obvious relationship between levels of child well-being and measures of economic prosperity such as GDP per capita, and the final column of Table 4 shows that this is equally true of the relationship between child well-being and child poverty rankings. Children in some countries (e.g. Netherlands, Italy and Ireland) fare much better in terms of well-being than in terms of income poverty, but the reverse is also the case in several instances (e.g. Norway, Belgium and France). This does not mean that reducing child poverty by raising levels of income support is not an important element of any campaign to improve the well-being of children. On the contrary, such a move will not only raise well-being directly by improving performance in the material well-being dimension (because the child poverty rate is an indicator), but also because this is likely to produce flow-on improvements in other dimensions of well-being.

These results highlight the fact that seeking to improve well-being through income support improvements *alone* will achieve only limited success unless accompanied by other measures that tackle the other dimensions of child well-being. The varied rankings shown in Table 4 thus reflect the real world complexities that must be addressed in order to produce significant and sustainable improvements in the well-being of children in different countries.

5 Some Australian Evidence

Australia has one of the most targeted income support systems in the OECD, with government cash benefits paid on a categorical means-tested basis. Benefits are subject to income and assets tests, and are financed from general revenue. There are no earmarked social security contributions. Poverty relief has been a high priority, although concern over poverty measurement issues and policy shifts has seen greater attention being paid to the issue of welfare dependence, particularly when it persists over a sustained period. This is part of a broader move away from Australia's traditional reliance on a dual income support strategy which combines targeted but extensive income support provision with centralised wage determination aimed at protecting minimum wage levels (Castles, 1985; Whiteford & Angenent, 2002). Deregulation of the labour market and a reduction in the power of the wage fixing body (the Industrial Relations Commission) has introduced a degree of flexibility into minimum wages, although they remain under the independent control of the newly-established Fair Pay Commission.

Australian poverty research has a long history and has exerted a crucial impact on policy at critical junctures. Interest in the issue is increasing, driven in part by the availability of new data that is providing important new insights into the living standards of Australian households, including those with children. One important new source of such data is the *Household, Income and Labour Dynamics in Australia* (HILDA) Survey, a government-backed longitudinal panel study which began interviewing people in almost 8,000 households in 2001 (Headey & Warren, 2008). Just under 14,000 adults (aged 15 and over) were interviewed in wave I and

Table 5 The impact of government transfers and taxes on poverty in Australia in 2005 (percentages)

Household type	Pre-government poverty rate	Post-government poverty rate	Change due to government (%)
Prime age (<65) single person	18.8	16.0	–14.9
Older (65+) single person	75.6	44.7	–40.7
Older couples	60.1	24.4	–59.4
Prime age couples, no children	7.6	4.0	–47.4
Prime age couples, with children	14.3	6.4	–55.2
Lone parents	52.7	26.1	–50.5
All households	26.4	12.9	–51.1

Source: Headey and Warren (2008, Tables 1 and 2, p. 57)

almost 10,400 of these completed an interview in the fifth wave, conducted in 2005. Analysis of the latest wave of HILDA data, summarized in Table 5, allows the impact of income support payments (including family benefits) on the "static" (single year) poverty rate to be estimated.

In aggregate terms, government cash benefits and personal taxes reduced the national poverty rate (assessed using a poverty line set at 50% of median income) by just over half (51.1%), from the assumed (no government transfers or taxes) counterfactual level of 26.4% to the observed rate of 12.9%. The reduction was largest (at between 55 and 60%) among older couples and prime age couples with children and lowest (15%) among prime age single people. These different impacts cause a marked decline in the post-government poverty relativities facing different household types and an associated narrowing of post-intervention income inequalities. The differential effects shown in Table 5 reflect the structure and targeting of income support provisions, but they also illustrate the impact of the minimum wage in protecting the vast majority of those in work (and their families) from poverty. Thus, the pre-government poverty rates of all prime age households except lone parents are not only well below the overall pre-government rate, they are also below the post-government rate of 12.9% for couples without children and only just above it for couples with children. Income support in the form of minimum wages has thus allowed working families to avoid poverty if they have a job—particularly a full-time job (Saunders, 2006).

A second survey has allowed the circumstances of Australian households to be examined using a metric other than income. The *Community Understanding of Poverty and Social Exclusion* (CUPSE) Survey was conducted by the author and colleagues at the Social Policy Research Centre in mid-2006 (see Saunders, Naidoo, & Griffiths, 2008; Saunders, 2008 for further details). The three concepts that are the focus of much of the information collected in the survey are poverty—defined as having an income below a poverty line, deprivation—defined earlier as "an enforced lack of socially perceived necessities", and social exclusion—defined by the LSE's Centre for the Analysis of Social Exclusion as existing when "an individual . . . does not participate in key activities in the society in which he or she lives" (Burchardt,

Le Grand, & Piachaud, 2002, p. 30; see Kahn & Kamerman, 2002, for an extended discussion of social exclusion and children).

Space limitations prevent a comprehensive discussion of the research findings, and attention is thus focused on showing how deprivation indicators can shed light on the adequacy of income support payments. This issue is normally addressed by comparing benefit levels with a poverty line or some other income benchmark (e.g. a budget standard—see Bradshaw, 1993). The deprivation approach avoids some of the problems involved in using income, including the need to specify an equivalence scale and the equal sharing assumption referred to earlier. As explained earlier, deprivation exists when people cannot afford to purchase items that are regarded as necessary or essential by a majority of the community in which they are living, following the methods developed in other deprivation studies (Townsend, 1979; Callan, Nolan, & Whelan, 1993; Nolan & Whelan, 1996; Pantazis, Gordon, & Townsend, 2006).

The CUPSE survey included 61 items, of which 48 were seen as essential by a majority of respondents. Not all of these are items that can be bought by individuals: some are provided free by government and others do not reflect material needs (e.g. to be treated with respect by other people). When these are omitted the number of purchasable essentials declines to 26. Three of these items are used for illustrative purposes to examine the adequacy of three of the most important forms of income support in Australia: the age pension, the disability support pension and Newstart Allowance (or unemployment benefit). Together, these three payments account for almost 3.1 million income support recipients in June 2007, or 67% of all beneficiaries (excluding those receiving family payments) (Harmer, 2008, Table 1). The CUPSE survey includes a question asking people to identify their main source of income in the previous week and this is used to identify four groups of respondents: wage and salary earners; age pension recipients; disability pension recipients; and unemployment beneficiaries.

Rather than focus on the complete list of 26 essential items (which would require a process for aggregating them, about which there is some controversy in the literature—see Halleröd, Bradshaw & Holmes, 1997; Halleröd, 2006; Van den Bosch, 2001), attention is focused on three items. The items (and the percentage who said they are essential) are: a substantial meal at least once a day (99.6%); up to $500 in savings for use in an emergency (82.3%); and being able to buy medicines prescribed by a doctor (99.4%). Table 6 compares the incidence of deprivation of these three items according to the principal source of income of respondents. Recipients of disability pension and unemployment benefit are most deprived on all four dimensions, while age pensioners appear somewhat better-off on average than wage and salary earners. This latter finding reflects the higher savings of older people and their better access to free medical services under the Medicare system, although it may also be a consequence of the lower needs of older people, or their reluctance to admit that they cannot afford items that they do not have (a feature of many deprivation studies: see McKay, 2004).

When the deprivation patterns are compared with the income levels of the three groups, some interesting implications are suggested. First, the incomes of most age

Table 6 Incidence of deprivation by principal source of income (percentages)

Principal source of income	No substantial daily meal	No emergency savings	Cannot afford prescribed medicines
Wages and salaries	0.6	17.0	3.7
Age pension	0.7	10.1	2.0
Disability pension	10.6	42.2	11.4
Unemployment benefit	10.3	53.8	16.7

Source: CUPSE survey (see text)

pensioners are well below those of most workers, as a consequence of the means-testing of payments described earlier. Second, whereas income support payments for older people and people with a disability are the same, those for unemployed people are around 20% lower. Thus, if measured deprivation is capturing the inability to meet current needs with existing income levels, the results in Table 6 suggest that the needs of older people are on average lower than those of working people, that people with a disability have higher needs than those who receive an age pension, and that income support payments for unemployed people are inadequate—more so than payments for age and disability pensioners, possibly considerably so.

Of course, these conclusions are based on a limited set of findings and apply on average to relatively small samples of families. They also reflect the circumstances of the adults who provided the responses, although they have clear implications for the children in many of the families covered by the analysis. The results thus have their limitations, but even so, they highlight the role that deprivation (and other non-monetary indicators) can play in shedding new light on important questions surrounding the adequacy of income support provisions and their impact on the living standards of families, and of children.

6 Conclusions

This chapter continues a tradition of comparative analysis of the nature of income support policies for children and their impact on child well-being that was pioneered by Al Kahn and his collaborators (most notably Sheila Kamerman) several decades ago. The impact of that work on the development of the comparative method to examine policy issues relating to children has provided many valuable insights for researchers and policy makers, not to mention stimulating the collection of better comparative data without which the kind of analysis reported here would not have been possible.

Income support provides assistance to large numbers of families in the rich countries that belong to the OECD and thus plays a crucial role in affecting the living standards of children. The size of the impact depends upon how benefits are structured, how generous they are and how they affect the willingness and ability of parents to participate in the labour market. What matters for children's financial security is the combined impact on the family income package, and how much of it is redistributed within the family to meet their needs. This chapter has explored some of the factors that determine this impact, drawing on a variety of data, much of it comparative. What it has not done is examine some of the other impacts (not all beneficial) of parental employment on child development from a broader perspective than one that focuses merely on income and economic well-being.

The results presented cannot be claimed to be definitive, but they do raise important issues about how income support affects the incomes of parents and thus the living standards of children. Children rarely have access to incomes of their own, but are dependent on the actions of others to ensure that their needs are met and their well-being is maximized. To fully understand how these mechanisms operate, and their effects, it is necessary to look beyond income to alternative frameworks that capture living standards more directly. However, this should not detract attention from the importance of income support as a vehicle for promoting the well-being of children and raising their standard of living.

References

Boarini, R., & d'Ercole, M. M. (2006). *Measures of material deprivation in OECD Countries.* Working Paper No. 37, Directorate for Employment, Labour and Social Affairs. Paris: OECD.

Bradbury, B., & Jäntti, M. (1999). *Child poverty across industrialized nations.* Innocenti Occasional Paper No. 71. Florence: UNICEF International Child Development Centre.

Bradshaw, J. (Ed.). (1993). *Budget standards for the United Kingdom.* Avebury: Aldershot.

Bradshaw, J., Hoelscher, P., & Richardson, D. (2006). *Comparing child well-being in OECD countries: Concepts and methods.* Innocenti Working paper IWP-2006-03. Florence: Innocenti Research Centre.

Brooks-Gunn, J., & Duncan, G. (1997). The effects of poverty on children. *The Future of Children, 7*(2), 55–71.

Burchardt, T., Le Grand, J., & Piachaud, D. (2002). Degrees of exclusion: Developing a dynamic, multidimensional measure. In J. Hills, J. Le Grand, & D. Piachaud (Eds.), *Understanding social exclusion* (pp. 30–43). Oxford: Oxford University Press.

Callan, T., Nolan, B., & Whelan, C. T. (1993). Resources, deprivation and the measurement of poverty. *Journal of Social Policy, 22*(2), 141–172.

Castles, F. G. (1985). *The working class and welfare. Reflections on the political development of the welfare state in Australia and New Zealand, 1890–1980.* Sydney, Australia: Allen & Unwin.

Department for Work and Pensions. (2003). *Measuring child poverty.* London: DWP.

Förster, M., & d'Ercole, M. M. (2006). *Income distribution and poverty in OECD countries in the second half of the 1990s.* Working Paper No. 22, Directorate for Employment, Labour and Social Affairs. Paris: OECD.

Halleröd, B. (2006). Sour grapes: Relative deprivation, adaptive preferences and the measurement of poverty. *Journal of Social Policy, 35*(3), 371–390.

Halleröd, B., Bradshaw J., & Holmes, H. (1997). Adapting the consensual definition of poverty. In D. Gordon & C. Pantazis (Eds.), *Breadline Britain in the 1990s* (pp. 213–234). Ashgate: Aldershot.

Harmer, J. (2008). *Pension review. Background paper.* Department of Families, Housing, Community Services and Indigenous Affairs, Canberra.

Headey, B., & Warren, D. (2008). *Families, incomes and jobs, Volume 3: A statistical report on waves 1 to 5 of the HILDA survey.* Melbourne Institute of Applied Economic and Social Research, University of Melbourne.

Kahn, A. J., & Kamerman, S. B. (1983). *Income transfers for families with children: An eight-country study*. Philadelphia: Temple University Press.

Kahn, A. J., & Kamerman, S. B. (Eds.). (1988). *Child support: From debt collection to social policy*. Newbury Park, CA: Sage Publications.

Kahn, A. J., & Kamerman, S. B. (Eds.). (2002). *Beyond child poverty: The social exclusion of children*. Institute for Child and Family Policy, Columbia University.

Lundberg, S. J., Pollak, R. A., & Wales, T. J. (1997). Do husbands and wives pool their resources? *Journal of Human Resources, 32*, 463–480.

Mack, J., & Lansley, S. (1985). *Poor Britain*. London: George Allen and Unwin.

McKay, S. (2004). Poverty or preference: What do 'Consensual deprivation indicators' really measure? *Fiscal Studies, 25*(2), 201–223.

Nolan, B., & Whelan, C. T. (1996). *Resources, deprivation and poverty*. Oxford: Clarendon Press.

OECD. (2007a). Babies and bosses: Reconciling work and family life (Volume 5): A synthesis of findings for OECD countries. www/oecd.org/els/social/family, OECD, Paris.

OECD. (2007b). *Child poverty in OECD countries: Trends, causes and policy responses, document DELSA/ELSA/WP1(2007)17*, OECD, Paris.

Pantazis, C., Gordon, D., & Townsend, P. (2006). The necessities of life. In C. Pantazis, D. Gordon, & R. Levitas (Eds.), *Poverty and social exclusion in Britain. The millennium survey* (pp. 89–122). Bristol: Policy Press.

Plotnick, R. (1997). Child poverty can be reduced. *The Future of Children, 7*(2), 72–87.

Ringen, S. (1987). *The possibility of politics*. Oxford: Clarendon Press.

Saunders, P. (2006). A perennial problem: Employment, joblessness and poverty. In B. S. Grewal & M. Kumnick (Eds.), *Engaging the new world: Responses to the knowledge economy* (pp. 306–325). Melbourne: Melbourne University Press.

Saunders, P. (2008). Measuring well-being using non-monetary indicators: Deprivation and social exclusion. *Family Matters, 78*, 8–17.

Saunders, P., Naidoo, Y., & Griffiths, M. (2008). Towards new indicators of disadvantage: Deprivation and social exclusion in Australia. *Australian Journal of Social Issues, 43*(2), 175–194.

Sen, A. K. (1985). *Commodities and capabilities*. Ámsterdam: North-Holland.

Smeeding, T. M. (2006). Poor people in rich nations: The United States in comparative perspective. *Journal of Economic Perspectives, 20*(1), 69–90.

Townsend, P. (1979). *Poverty in the United Kingdom*. Harmondsworth: Penguin Books.

UNICEF. (2006). *Child poverty in rich countries 2005*. Report Card 6. Florence: Innocenti Research Centre.

UNICEF. (2007). *An overview of child well-being in rich countries. A comprehensive assessment of the lives and well-being of children and adolescents in the economically advanced nations*. Report card 7. Florence: Innocenti Research Centre.

Van den Bosch, K. (2001). *Identifying the poor. Using subjective and consensual measures*. Ashgate: Aldershot.

Whelan, C. T., Nolan, B., & Maître, B. (2006). *Measuring consistent poverty in Ireland with EU SILC data*. Working Paper No. 165. Dublin: The Economic and Social Research Institute.

Whiteford, P., & Angenent, G. (2002). *The Australian system of social protection – An overview* (2nd ed.). Occasional Paper No. 6. Canberra: Department of Family and Community Services.

An International Perspective on Child Benefit Packages

Jonathan Bradshaw

1 Background

Alfred Kahn was the father of comparative studies of family policies (and of course Sheila Kamerman is the mother). I was one who has followed their footsteps, initially inspired by *Family Policy: Government and Families in Fourteen countries* (Kamerman & Kahn, 1978) and *Income Transfers for Families with Children: An eight Country Study* (Kahn & Kamerman, 1983) and later their multi-volume multi-country study *Family Policies and Family Change in the West* (Kamerman & Kahn, 1997). I was honoured to be one of their many contacts on their frequent visits to Europe as they kept up to date on family policy.

Their notions of family policy were much wider than the subject of this chapter.

> Explicit family policies may include population policies (pro or anti natalist), income security policies designed to assure families with children a certain standard of living, employment-related benefits for working parents, maternal and child health policies, child-care policies, and so forth. Implicit family policy includes actions taken in other policy domains, for no family related reasons, which have important consequences for children and their families as well (Kamerman & Kahn, 1997, p. 6).

The Kahn & Kamerman (1983) study of ten countries was, I think, the first to use national informants to write descriptive chapters on the arrangements (in 1979) in their countries and then to publish a comparative analysis based on it.

Without doubt K and K were the inspiration for a stream of comparative studies from the University of York which used similar methods. Most of these (but not all—see Bradshaw et al., 2006; Eardley et al., 1996) have sought to compare the structure and level of child benefit packages as a way of getting a handle on the financial contribution that the state was making in different countries to the, mainly, private financial burden of child rearing. Our first study of this kind (Bradshaw & Piachaud, 1980) was actually motivated by an anxiety that the government of

J. Bradshaw (✉)
Department of Social Policy and Social Work, University of York, York, UK
e-mail: jrb1@york.ac.uk

S.B. Kamerman et al. (eds.), *From Child Welfare to Child Well-Being*, Children's Well-Being: Indicators and Research 1, DOI 10.1007/978-90-481-3377-2_17, © Springer Science+Business Media B.V. 2010

Margaret Thatcher elected in 1979 was going to abolish financial support for children. We thought that if we demonstrated that every country had such support, the Government might be dissuaded. In the event Mrs Thatcher did not abolish child benefits, rather they were left to "wither on the vine" while means-tested Family Credit was extended.

We called the subject matter of that study "child support systems". In the next study of packages in 15 countries (Bradshaw, Ditch, Holmes, & Whiteford, 1993) we called them "child support packages". But by the third study (Bradshaw & Finch, 2002), the UK, Australia, New Zealand and the USA had Child Support schemes—arrangements to ensure that absent parents provided financial support for caring parents and so our language changed to "child benefit packages". We have also undertaken a comparative study of Child Support regimes (Skinner, Bradshaw, & Davidson, 2007).

I do not remember where the language of packages came from but I am sure it must have been influenced by Rainwater, Rein, and Schwartz (1986) in their book *Income packaging in the welfare state*. Certainly welfare states, for a variety of different motives (Wennemo, 1992), have developed packages of tax benefits, cash benefits and other elements that help parents, and to compare just one part of the package is misleading.

The most recent comparison we have undertaken was initially of eight countries in 2004 (Bradshaw & Mayhew, 2006) and later increased to fifteen countries (Bradshaw, 2006) and this chapter presents some data on 19 countries. The data is available on line.[1]

We have certainly not been the only people doing this kind of work. Since the end of the 1970s, the European Commission has published comparative descriptive information on social security systems, including child benefits. Since 1990 this series has developed into The Mutual Information System on Social Protection (MISSOC). The MISSOC series is now on line.[2]

Also the OECD has had the *Taxing Wages* series since at least 1972 (OECD, 1978) and a report is produced annually (OECD, 2008b). The data on which it is based is published on line.[3]

Now there is a new study using model family methods emerging from at University of British Columbia directed by Dr Paul Kershaw (Kershaw, 2007) and the method has also been used in Japan (Tokoro, 2003).

This chapter will discuss the methods involved in using model families and national informants to compare child benefit packages. It will then present the results of recent comparisons, some based on our own studies, and some based on the analysis of OECD data. At the time of writing that is the most up to date available. First however we present the results of one other approach to comparing child benefit packages.

---

[1] http://php.york.ac.uk/inst/spru/research/summs/welempfc.php

[2] http://ec.europa.eu/employment_social/spsi/missoc_en.htm

[3] http://www.oecd.org/document/29/0,3343,en_2649_34637_39618653_1_1_1_1,00.html

2 Comparison of National Accounts

One technique that can be used to compare the overall effort made by countries on behalf of children is to compare how much of national resources they spend on families with children. This usually requires international bodies to collect national accounts data on public spending directed to families with children. There are a number of difficulties in doing this. It is not always possible to identify how much of insurance, assistance or other cash benefits go to families with children, or to disaggregate what proportion of services expenditure goes to services for families with children. Housing benefits, child support (alimony), and the value of exemption from health charges and education charges and benefits, for families with children may not be included. Occupational benefits (important in Japan) are excluded. In the past, national accounts have also failed to take into account the value of tax expenditures (the OECD calls them tax breaks). This is a problem because tax expenditures have been becoming an increasingly important part of the child benefit package. The ESSPROS series published by the European Union contains quite up to date data on expenditure on families with children but does not include tax expenditures. The OECD, thanks to the work of Adema (2001), has begun to publish a series on family spending which does take account of tax expenditures. The most recent data is for 2005 and is reproduced in Fig. 1

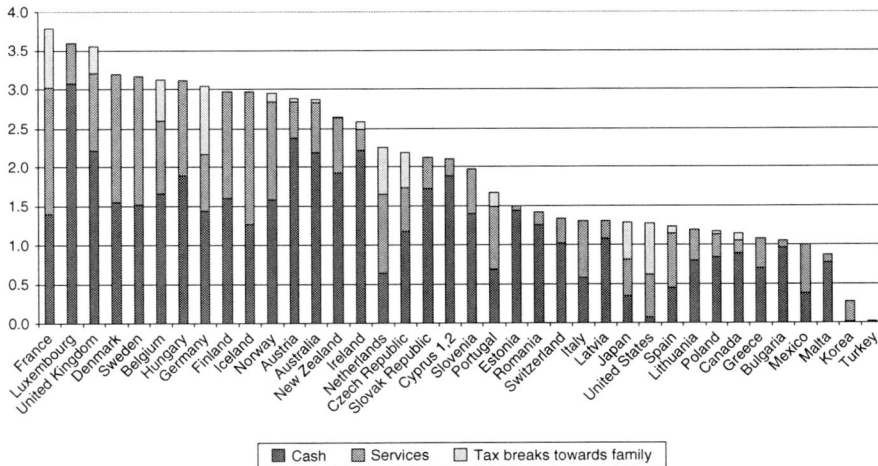

Fig. 1 Family spending in cash, services and tax measures, in percentage of GDP, in 2005
Source: OECD Family Data Base, http://www.oecd.org/dataoecd/55/58/38968865.xls

On average in 2005 the OECD countries spent 2.3% of GDP on family benefits, services and tax breaks (it was 2.5 in 2003) and this proportion varied from 3.8% in France to 0.02% in Turkey. There were differences in how the expenditure was structured between countries—between cash benefits, services and tax breaks. Services are a more important part of the package in the Nordic countries and France. But tax breaks were an important component of the package in a number of countries especially in France, Germany, the Netherlands and the United States. There are perhaps some surprising results in this figure: Sweden does not come top of the league, the UK comes third (up from eighth in 2003), Hungary seventh, New Zealand fourteenth (up from seventeenth in 2003), the Netherlands sixteenth.

3 Model Family Methods

This analysis of public expenditure as a proportion of GDP data gives us an overall picture of effort made by welfare states on behalf of families with children. The model family method enriches that information. This method uses national informants to provide information on the tax/benefit system in their own countries. In order to compare like with like, they estimate what a set of standard model families would receive, at a specified set of earnings levels, in the way of a specified set of taxes and benefits that make up the child benefit package. The information is entered into a set of data matrices and these are used to explore the level and structure of the child benefit package, converted to a common currency or expressed as a proportion of average earnings. The package that the York studies have taken into account includes tax benefits for children, income related and non income related child benefits, housing benefits, exemptions from local taxes, direct childcare subsidies, the value of health charges and benefits, the value of education charges and benefits, child support (where it is guaranteed), and other benefits such as food stamps or social assistance. The OECD series covers tax breaks, cash benefits, housing benefits and social assistance. What has not generally been incorporated into the model family method is parental leave and indirect subsidies for example childcare.

Each element of the package is given a separate line on the data matrix so its contribution to the overall value of the package can be calculated. By comparing the net incomes of couples or lone parents with children with the net income of single people or childless couples on the same earnings it is possible to isolate the value of the support paid specifically in respect of children. It is more difficult to establish what the child specific elements are in national accounts or survey micro data. Another advantage over national accounts and the analysis of micro data is that account can be taken of the charges that families have to pay for services—health services, education and childcare. In this way we can get at the net value of the package. National accounts and survey data may show that a country provides a generous gross package but it does not show what people have to spend their package on.

There are other advantages to the model family method. It enables comparisons of like with like to be made, and the results can be produced quite quickly. It also enables comparisons of the level and structure of the benefit package and how it varies by family type, earnings, number and ages of children and before an after housing and childcare costs. It is also possible to use the data to make estimates of notional marginal tax rates and replacement rates (and the OECD use their Benefits and Wages series mainly with the latter in mind).

There are also a number of problems with the method (discussed more fully in Eardley, Bradshaw, Ditch, Gough, & Whiteford, 1996). There are limits to the number of model families, income levels and parental employment permutations that can be covered. This means that the comparisons have to be illustrative rather than representative. We have made attempts to build a sample of family types and take the average as representing a common picture, but family types vary greatly in their composition between countries and a sample that would be representative for one country cannot be representative for all countries.

The method also gives a picture of the situation that should exist given the existing formal rules and laws. It does not represent how these rules and laws operate in practice and, although it can, it does not often attempt to take account of the non take-up of cash benefits. Nevertheless there is value in taking account of what the state seeks to do—it represents the intention of public policy.

Also there are particular problems in representing the education and health benefit elements of the package. But by far the most difficult problem is the treatment of housing costs and benefits (Bradshaw & Finch, 2004). Housing costs vary by tenure, age, size and location of the dwelling, and in the case of some countries, by the length of occupancy. In the case of owner occupiers they also vary by the age of the mortgage and the interest rate. In our earlier studies using this method we asked national informants to specify a "typical" housing cost for their country, but found that it was too variable to compare like with like. So we eventually followed the OECD method of taking rent as 20% of national average earnings and then estimating housing benefit payable on that rent. This is not a very satisfactory solution because it means that rent does not vary with the size of the dwelling or income—20% of average income is far too low for better off families and far too high for poorer families. This is a problem without an adequate solution, but there is no denying that it is a serious one, given that housing benefits are such an important part of the child benefit package in many countries.

The estimates of gross earnings can be problematic. OECD uses its own estimates of average production workers wages for full-time work, not seasonally adjusted, no over-time and with no account of gender. The York studies have tended to rely on national informants to determine gross male and female earnings for full-time work and then taken variations of the average (either mean or median) for different cases and combinations of workers including a case of someone working full-time on the minimum wage or half average earnings whichever is higher.

4 Comparisons of Child Benefit Packages

At the time of writing the most up to date comparisons of the child benefit package are derived from the OECD Taxing Wages series for 2007. Figure 2 compares the overall level of the package for a couple with two children with two earners (one on average earnings and the other on a third of average earnings). The vertical axis shows the percentage extra that this family gets over what a childless couple on the same earnings would get. It varies from nothing in Turkey and Mexico to 20% extra in the Czech Republic and 16% extra in Hungary. To find these countries at the top

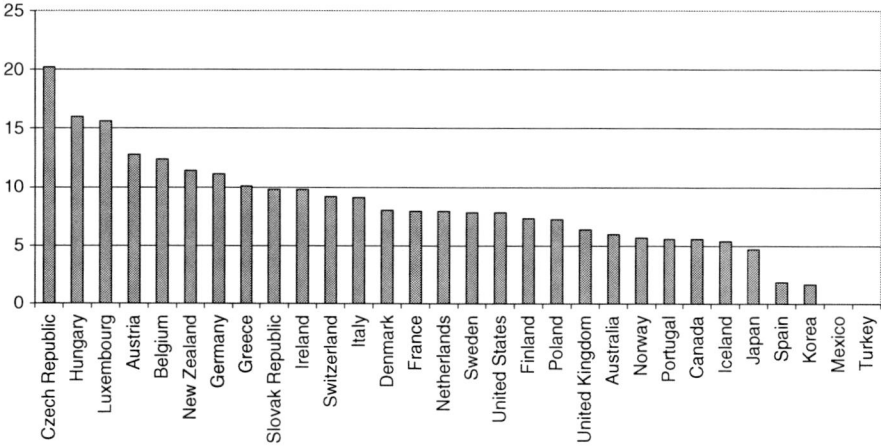

Fig. 2 Child benefit package Couple plus 2 (average and third average earnings) 2007. Percentage more than a childless couple on the same earnings
Source: Own analysis of OECD Taxing Wages (2008a)

of the league may be quite unexpected—also the fact that the USA is not at the bottom of the league, Sweden and France are in the middle and the New Zealand near the top.

This is a standard two earner family in 2007. However, it can be seen in Fig. 3 that the rankings of countries changes considerably with the level of earnings assumed for the model family. At low earnings Ireland, the USA, Denmark, the UK and Australia have the most generous child benefit package in 2005. All countries except

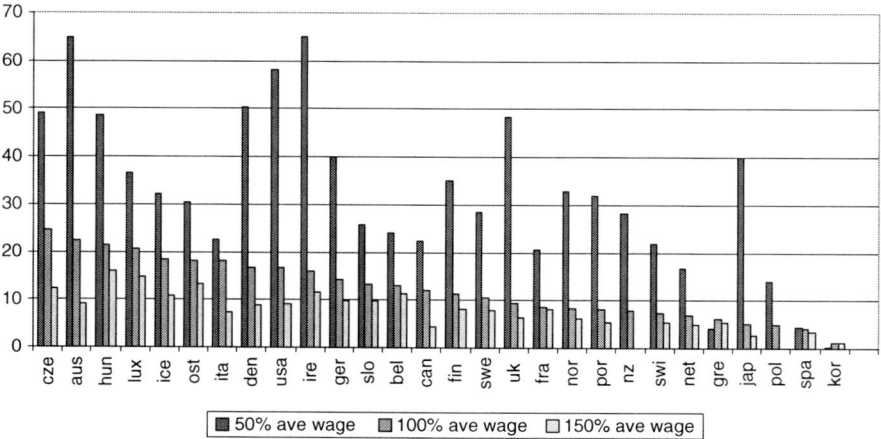

Fig. 3 Child benefit package couple with two children one earner by level of earnings 2005. Ranked by average earnings: percentage extra over a childless couple on the same earnings
Source: Own analysis of OECD Taxing Wages (2006)

Greece and Korea have progressive child benefit packages—that is they are more generous to low paid families. But some are more progressive then others. New Zealand does not pay any family benefits beyond a given income level.

So the level of the child benefit package varies with the level of earnings. It also varies by family type. Figure 4 shows the level of the package paid to couples and lone parents with the same number of children and the same earnings. There is a very mixed picture—some countries pay a higher package to lone parents—much higher in Sweden and Poland. Other countries pay higher child benefits to couples—much higher in Luxembourg and Germany. Other countries pay the same, or roughly the same including Denmark, the UK, Austria and France.

The OECD only collects data for lone parents and couples with two children, and childless couples and singles (and from 2006 it (annoyingly) changed the parental employment assumptions so that we have had to use 2005 data in Figs. 3 and 4).

However in the York studies we have collected data on a wider range of families with children. This data enables us to compare how the child benefit package varies with family size. It can be seen in Fig. 5, where we compare the variation in the child benefit package for a one earner couple on average earnings by family size, that New Zealand only provided any package for the third child at this earnings level. Australia, Belgium, the Czech Republic were more generous to the second and subsequent child. France and Austria were much more generous to the third child. The other countries provided more or less equal amounts per child. The UK is unique in having a higher child benefit package for the first child in the family. This reflects the priority given to poverty relief in its package—most poor families are small families, though larger families have a higher risk of poverty (Bradshaw et al., 2006).

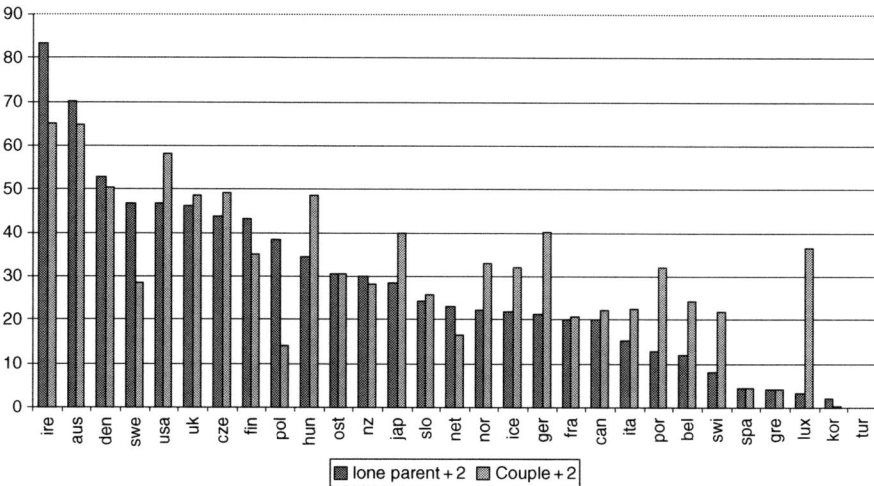

Fig. 4 Child benefit package at half average earnings, lone parents and couples with two children. Percentage more than a childless couple on the same earnings
Source: Own analysis of OECD Taxing Wages (2006)

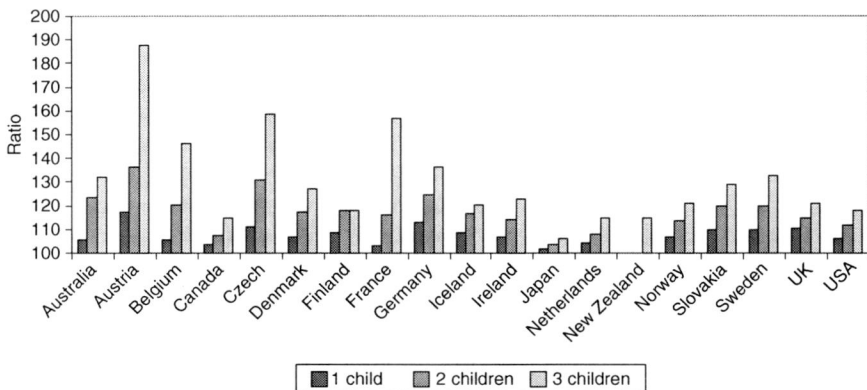

Fig. 5 Child benefit package for a couple by number of children, one earner average earnings in Jan 2004. Childless couple = 100

It is also possible to use the York data to explore variations in the structure of the child benefit package between countries. Figure 6 compares the structure of the package for a low earning lone parent with one child. The bars above the line are what she would receive per month more than a childless couple on the same earnings, and the amounts below the line are what she would have to pay more than a childless couple (in childcare costs, income tax and net rent). So, for example, in the UK a lone parent would receive Child Benefit, Child Tax Credit and Housing Benefit and together they are the most generous of any country in the comparisons.

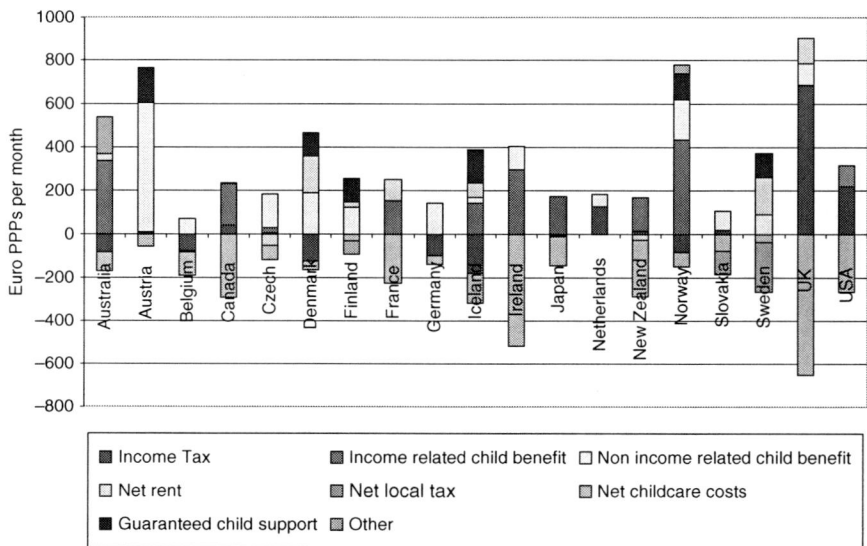

Fig. 6 Structure of the child benefit package for a lone parent with one preschool aged child on half average earnings in Jan 2004 in Euros purchasing power parities per month

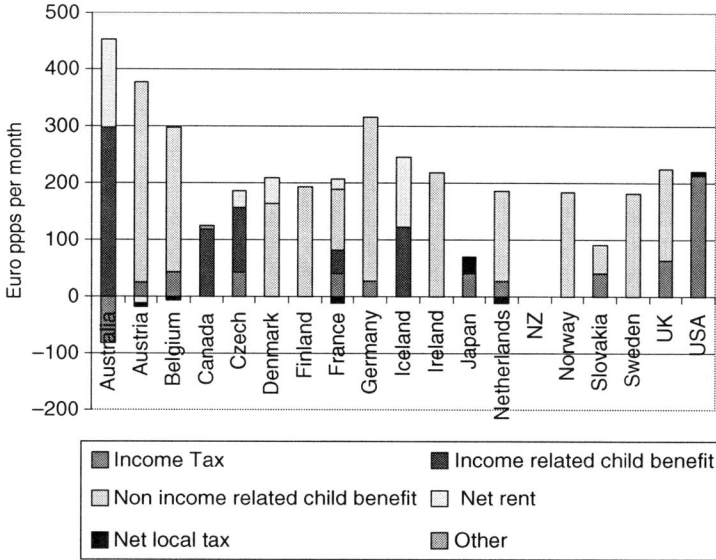

Fig. 7 Structure of the child benefit package. Couple with two children with one earner on average earnings in Jan 2004 in Euros purchasing power parities per month

However in the UK the lone parent would have to pay childcare costs[4] which effectively would wipe out most of the value of the package. Overall the figure shows the importance of direct and indirect subsidies for childcare costs in the child benefit package.

Figure 7 shows that structure of the package for a couple with two children with one earner on average earnings. Because there is one earner the child benefit package (difference form a childless couple on the same earnings) is mainly positive and mainly made up of non income related child benefits and housing benefits, and in the USA, Earned Income Tax Credit. In Australia income related child benefit and housing benefit make up the positive elements of the package, but curiously the couple with two children pay more income tax than a childless couple on the same earnings.

Model family data can also be used to compare replacement rates (the proportion of net income in work that is replaced by out of work benefit income). The OECD publishes replacement rates for various stages of unemployment. Figure 8 provides comparisons of replacement rates for families with two children who have been out of work recently and for five years (no childcare taken into account) in 2006. For some countries short-term replacement rates are higher—notably Canada, the USA, Portugal and Spain. Most countries are more generous to the long term unemployed families. Replacement rates tend to be higher in the Nordic countries than they are

---

[4] The York model assumes childcare costs are what a parent with a child under 3 would have to pay in the most prevalent type of full-time formal childcare in the country.

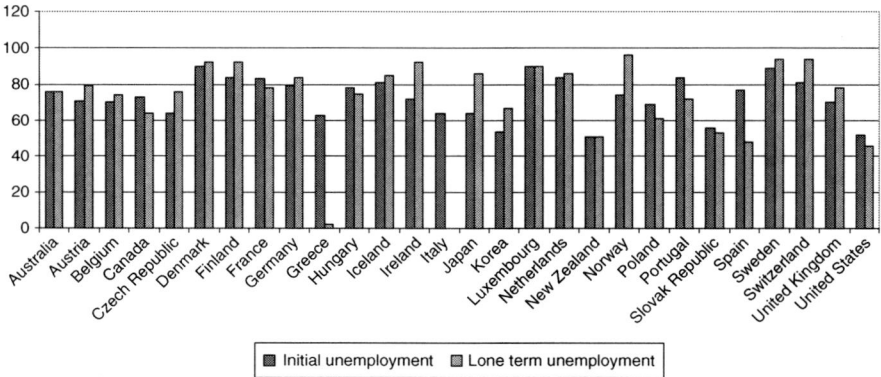

Fig. 8 Replacement rates for couples with two children who had been earning 67% of average wage. Initial and long term unemployment 2006
Source: OECD, http://www.oecd.org/dataoecd/17/21/39720238.xls; http://www.oecd.org/ dataoecd/17/19/39720308.xls

in most Anglophone and southern European countries – probably because in these countries there is not so much anxiety about work incentives. Replacement rates are particularly low in the USA, and Greece and Italy do not have long term out of work benefits.

We have used our York data to make estimates of the notional marginal tax rates that families would experience by increasing earnings, working more or having a spouse in employment. Figure 9 shows the effective average marginal tax rate on one

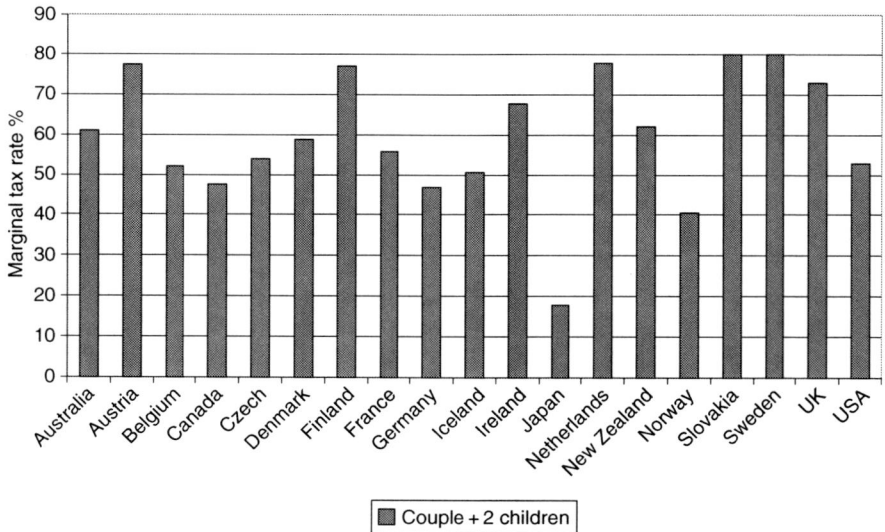

Fig. 9 Effective average marginal tax rates for a couple with two children on increasing earnings from half average to average in Jan 2004

earner increasing earnings from half average earnings to average earnings. Marginal tax rates tend to be highest in those countries with strongly income related child benefit packages, because as well as paying extra income tax and social security contributions, they suffer the loss of income related child and other benefits. For couples with two children they are highest in Slovakia and Sweden where 80% of additional earnings is taken in extra taxes and loss of benefits. Obviously the marginal tax rates would be different for second earners and be influenced by whether there is joint rather than separate taxation.

5 Overall Child Benefit Package

As discussed earlier it is difficult to summarise the overall effort that welfare states are making on behalf of families with children using model family methods. The child benefit package varies by earnings, employment status, number of earners, and by family type, the number and ages of children, and whether child care, housing costs and the value of services are taken into account. In an attempt to take account of all that variation we have produced an average package for 32 different family types/earnings levels. The resulting league table is presented in Fig. 10 in purchasing power parity terms. Out of our nineteen countries, Austria is a clear outlier with an average package of 475 Euros per months more than a childless couple on the same earnings. It is interesting that Austria does not appear to be an outlier in the league table of spending on family benefits in Fig. 1. Austria has a generous child benefit package across the board, but particularly for large families, lone parents and out of work families, and the package is universal—hardly varying with income. The position of the UK is quite surprising—this is a substantial improvement in the relative position from the previous York study, and reflects the impact of the improvements in the package made by the Labour Government, some time after it came to power. It is also reflected in the UK's improved position in the OECD expenditure league table in Fig. 1.

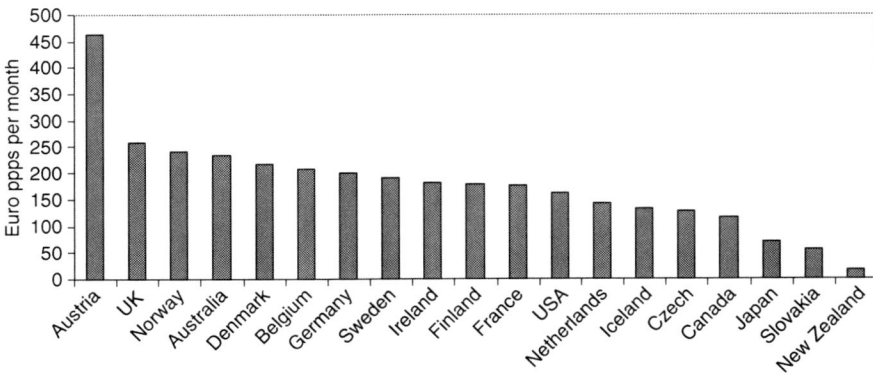

Fig. 10 Overall "average" child benefit package after taxes, benefits, childcare and housing costs (difference from childless couple) Euro ppps per month, Jan 2004

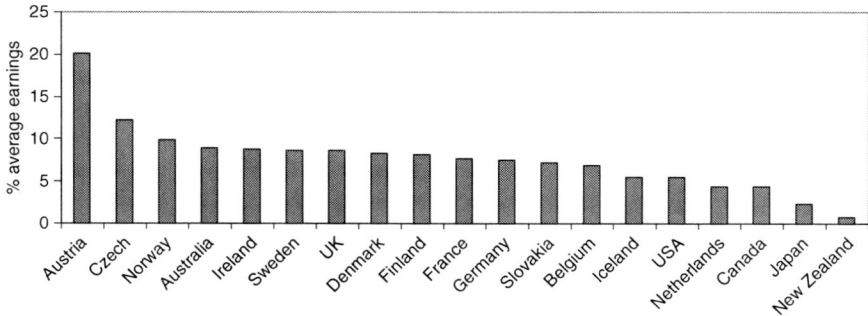

Fig. 11 Overall "average" child benefit package after taxes, benefits, childcare and housing costs (difference from childless couple) Euro ppps per month, Jan 2004

However it makes a difference how the package is measured. In Fig. 11 we present the same league table but with the average child benefit package expressed as a proportion of average earnings in each country. Austria is still an outlier at the top of the table but the Czech and Slovak Republics move up the league table using this more relative indicator.

6 Poverty Reduction

There is one other technique that is used to evaluate the impact of child benefit packages. Survey data can be used to evaluate the extent to which transfers reduce poverty rates and (close poverty gaps). Of course transfers are only part of the child benefit package and this kind of analysis does not take account of the contribution of services in kind. Nor do these analyses include tax benefits in the transfer package. Poverty rates are assessed on the basis of net market (after tax) income and then reassessed after having added cash benefits. Figure 12 is based on an analysis of EU Statistics of Income and Living Conditions (SILC) data. It shows that the league table of child poverty rates in the EU would be very different if child poverty was measured before transfers—just on the basis of market incomes. The Nordic countries have much lower after transfer poverty rates than the southern and eastern European countries because their family policies are much more effective in reducing poverty.

7 Conclusion

The OECD (2008b) found that between the mid 1990s and the mid 2000s child poverty rates increased in the majority of rich countries (the exceptions were Mexico, UK, Italy, USA, Hungary, Australia and Belgium). The OECD also found that the poverty rates in the mid 2000s for children were higher than the population poverty rates in most countries (the exceptions were all the Nordic countries, Cyprus, Slovenia, Austria, Korea, Australia and Japan). Reducing child poverty is not the only objective of child benefit packages, but it is certainly an outcome of them. If children have a higher risk of child poverty and child poverty is increasing, then it is a strong indication that welfare states are not investing enough in benefits and services for families with children.

At present the existing evidence base is not really good enough. The OECD series is really rather limited given that it only models the package for two types of families—lone parents and couples with two children. The EU MISSOC series does not compare packages—only individual benefits. There has been a major investment in Euromod,[5] the micro-simulation project based at the University of Essex and this has some advantages over model family methods. With Euromod policies and the impact of policy changes can be assessed on their impact on a fairly up-to-date (2005) representative samples of the population. But micro simulation is not really an alternative to model family comparisons. At present Euromod only covers the EU 15 and four new EU countries and it has not yet been used to explore the structure and compare the level of the child benefit package. However it is being extended in a big new project directed by Professor Holly Sutherland at the University of Essex.

Euromod is "big science". Model family methods are smaller science and is needed if we are to keep up to date with the constant changes in child benefit packages, explore their consequences and learn from other countries experiences. There is a need for a new institutional framework for assessing family policies in

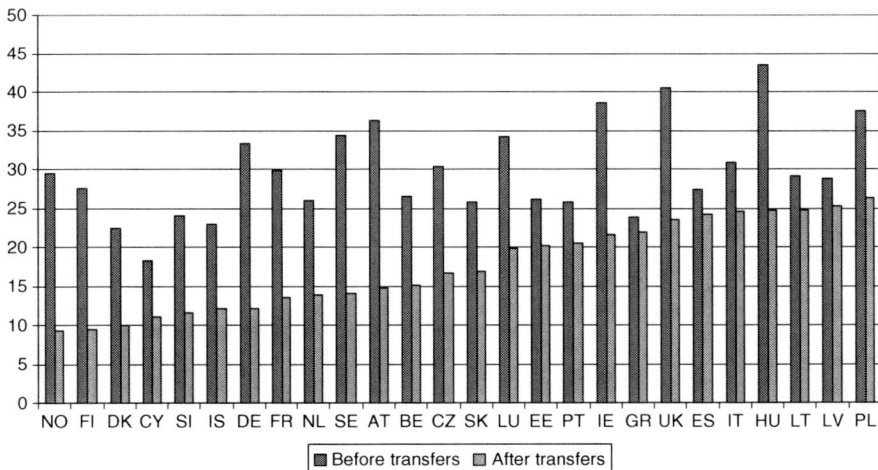

Fig. 12 Child poverty rates before and after transfers: own analysis of EU SILC (2006)

---

[5] http://www.iser.essex.ac.uk/research/euromod

the EU and elsewhere, that could undertake model family studies on a regular basis. This was the challenge set by Al Kahn with Sheila Kamerman in their early work and it remains a challenge for comparative studies.

References

Adema, W. (2001). *Net social expenditure* (2nd ed.). OECD Labour Market and Social Policy Occasional Papers, No. 52. OECD Publishing. doi:10.1787/426352083452

Bradshaw, J., & Finch, N. (2004). Housing benefits in 22 countries. *Benefits, 12*(2), 87–94.

Bradshaw, J. R., & Piachaud, D. (1980). *Child support in the European community.* Occasional Paper in Social Administration No. 66. Bedford Square Press: London.

Bradshaw, J. R., Ditch, J., Holmes, H., & Whiteford, P. (1993). *Support for children: A comparison of arrangements in fifteen countries.* Department of Social Security Research Report No. 21. London: HMSO.

Bradshaw, J., & Finch, N. (2002). *A comparison of child benefit packages in 22 countries.* Department for Work and Pensions Research Report No. 174. Leeds: Corporate Document Services.

Bradshaw, J., Finch, N., Mayhew, M., Ritakallio, V.-M., & Skinner, C. (2006). *Child poverty in large families.* Policy Press/Joseph Rowntree Foundation. http://www.jrf.org.uk/ book-shop/eBooks/9781861348777.pdf. Accessed 11 May 2009.

Bradshaw, J., & Mayhew, E. (2006). Family benefit packages. In J. Bradshaw & A. Hatland (Eds.), *Social policy, family change and employment in comparative perspective* (pp. 97–118). Cheltenham, MA: Edward Elgar.

Bradshaw, J. (2006). Child benefit packages in 15 countries in 2004. In J. Lewis (Ed.), *Children, changing families and the welfare state* (pp. 69–89). Cheltenham, MA: Edward Elgar.

Eardley, T., Bradshaw, J., Ditch, J., Gough, I., & Whiteford, P. (1996). *Social assistance in OECD countries: Synthesis report.* Department of Social Security Research Report No.46. London: HMSO.

Kamerman, S., & Kahn, A. (Eds.). (1978). *Family policy: Government and families in fourteen countries.* New York: Columbia University Press.

Kahn, A., & Kamerman, S. (1983). *Income transfers for families with children: An eight country study.* Philadelphia: Temple University Press.

Kahn, A., & Kamerman, S. (Eds.). (1983). *Essays on income transfers and related programs in eight countries.* New York: Columbia University, School of Social Work, Cross-National Studies.

Kamerman, S., & Kahn, A. (Eds.). (1997). *Family change and family policies in Great Britain, Canada, New Zealand and the United States (and seven other volumes).* Oxford: Clarendon Press.

Kershaw, P. (2007). Measuring up: Family benefits in British Columbia and Alberta in international perspective. *IRPP Choices, 13*(2), 1–42.

Rainwater, L., Rein, M., & Schwartz, J. (1986). *Income packaging in the welfare state.* Oxford: Oxford University Press.

Skinner, C., Bradshaw, J., & Davidson, J. (2007). *Child support policy: An international perspective.* Department for Work and Pensions Research Report 405. Leeds: Corporate Document Services. http://www.dwp.gov.uk/asd/asd5/rports2007-2008/rrep405.pdf

Tokoro, M. (2003). Social policy and lone parenthood in Japan: A workfare tradition? *The Japanese Journal of Social Security Policy, 2*(2), 45–58.

OECD. (1978). *The tax/benefit position of selected income groups in OECD member countries 1972–1976.* Paris: OECD.

OECD. (2006). *Taxing wages 2004/5.* Paris: OECD.

OECD. (2008a). *Taxing wages 2006/7*. Paris: OECD.

OECD. (2008b). *Growing unequal?. Income distribution and poverty in OECD countries*, Paris: OECD.

Wennemo, I. (1992). The development of family policy: A comparison of family benefits and tax reductions in families in 18 OECD countries. *Acta Sociologica, 35*, 201–217.

Canadian Policies for Families with Very Young Children in International Perspective

Shelley Phipps

1 Introduction

In this chapter, Canadian policies for families with children under the age of three are compared with those available in eight other affluent countries (i.e., Finland, France, Germany, Italy, Norway, Sweden, the UK, and the US), three from each of Esping-Andersen's "three worlds" of welfare capitalism (Esping-Andersen, 1990). The focus on policies for families with very young children seems an appropriate choice for a book in honor of Alfred Kahn, who, with co-author Sheila Kamerman, has contributed enormously to international comparative research on the "under-three's."

For families with very young children, cash maternity and/or parental benefits are particularly important and are thus the focus of this chapter which provides, in the first section, a survey of what is available in each of the countries studied. Specific features that are important to consider include: (1) what determines eligibility; (2) what is the total duration of benefits available to an eligible claimant; (3) what is the level of compensation (paying attention to potential ceilings on benefits as well as nominal replacement rates); what are the provisions for fathers? Since maternity and parental benefits are only part of an over-all package offered to families with infants/young children, a shorter description of other cash transfers available to families with very young children is also provided.[1]

A comparative policy discussion in the second section of the chapter is focused around calculated benefit entitlements for the same five "sample" new parents in each country: (1) a mother working full-time with average Canadian female earnings; (2) a mother working full-time but with low earnings; (3) a new mother

S. Phipps (✉)
Canadian Institute for Advanced Research and Department of Economics, Dalhousie University, Halifax, Nova Scotia, Canada
e-mail: Shelley.Phipps@dal.ca

[1] Public provision of healthcare during the pre- and post-natal periods also varies considerably across the 9 countries studied here as does public provision of daycare. Both are critical to the well-being of very young children, but are beyond the scope of the present chapter.

S.B. Kamerman et al. (eds.), *From Child Welfare to Child Well-Being*, Children's Well-Being: Indicators and Research 1, DOI 10.1007/978-90-481-3377-2_18,
© Springer Science+Business Media B.V. 2010

working full-time with high wages; (4) a self employed new mother; (5) a new father with average male wages.

The third section of the chapter uses the most recent microdata available from the Luxembourg Income Study (LIS) to compare the relative contributions of markets and states to the *over-all* financial well-being of families with infants, including both maternity/parental benefits as well as other cash transfers for families with very young children. If, for example, one country offers lower maternity benefits though all families with newborns will at the same time receive a very generous child allowance, this will be important for understanding the economic well-being of very young children in that country. LIS data are also used to compare labor market participation rates for parents of very young children. Conclusions are provided in the final section of the chapter.

2 Institutional Survey

Countries included in this study offer a variety of different combinations of programs to help new parents either by providing time to stay at home with their newborns (or newly adopted children) and/or by providing money to help with the financial costs associated with a new child.[2] "Maternity leave" provides new mothers with job-protected time away from paid work before/after the birth of a child; cash benefits are not necessarily provided. "Paternity leave" provides fathers with some time off paid work when a new child is born. "Maternity benefits" provide new mothers with cash benefits while they are away from paid work before/after childbirth; "paternity benefits" provide the equivalent to men at or near the time their wife/partner gives birth. "Parental" or "child-rearing" benefits provide cash benefits to parents who remain at home to care for a young child, though not necessarily immediately after the child is born. Such benefits can usually be shared by the mother and the father. Finally, some countries offer "birth grants"—lump sum cash transfers to new parents to help with associated extra costs. Programs described below reference the most recently available documentation (i.e., generally, October, 2008).

2.1 Canada

Eligibility

The Canadian maternity/parental benefits system is unique among the 9 studied here in being considered part of the unemployment insurance system rather than

---

[2] The institutional survey is drawn principally from "the Mutual Information System on Social Protection (MISSOC) 2007" for EU member countries and from "*Social Security Programs Throughout the World, 2006*" for all countries. Additional material is drawn from Gornick & Meyers (2003), and from Phipps (1994, 1998 and 2006) as noted in the text.

part of health or family benefits. Maternity and parental benefits claimants require 600 hours of eligible paid employment in the last year. Self-employed workers are not eligible for benefits.

Duration

Maternity benefits are available for 15 weeks; parental benefits, which can be shared by mother and father, are available for a further 35 weeks. A 2-week waiting period before benefits can begin is unique to Canada, perhaps as a legacy of being part of the unemployment (employment) insurance program. Note, however, that since 2001, only one parent is required to serve the 2-week waiting period if they share parental benefits. Adoption benefits are offered on the same terms as parental benefits. No additional benefits are available for multiple births. In the event of medical complication associated with the pregnancy/delivery, a mother can receive up to 15 weeks of EI sickness benefits without penalty to her total entitlement, resulting in a maximum period of 65 weeks.

Benefit Levels

Maternity or parental benefits are compensated at a basic rate of 55% of previous earnings to a weekly maximum of $435, though the 2-week waiting period effectively reduces this nominal replacement rate. Beneficiaries from lower-income families (i.e., total net income less than $25,921) can receive a "family supplement" to their benefits. The supplement can raise effective replacement rates to as high as 80%; total payments can never exceed the maximum of $435. Parental benefits claimants are now entitled to earn up to 25% of their weekly benefits or $50 without a deduction in benefits. Benefits are taxable.

Maternity and Parental Benefits in Quebec

In January of 2006, the province of Quebec began to offer its own system of maternity/paternity and parental benefits. Two options are available. In the first "basic plan," eligible biological mothers can receive 18 weeks of maternity benefits with 70% replacement of previous earnings, 7 weeks of parental benefits again with a 70% replacement rate, plus an additional 25 weeks with a 55% replacement rate which can be divided between mother and father. Five weeks, with a 70% replacement rate are available exclusively for fathers. Under the second "special plan," duration is shorter but replacement rates are higher. Mothers are entitled to 15 weeks of maternity benefits at 75% replacement, 25 weeks of parental benefits compensated at 75% of past earnings can be split between mother and father, 3 weeks of benefits with 75% replacement are available only to fathers. Under both plans, maximum insurable earnings are higher under the Quebec plan ($57,000 compared to $39,000 under EI). A final difference between the EI and Quebec plans is that self-employed workers are covered in Quebec if they have had more than $2,000 of earnings in the year prior to the birth.

Other Benefits for Which Families with Infants may be Eligible

Families with children less than 18 are eligible for the Canada Child Tax Benefit which is intended to help with the cost of raising children. Although CCTB amounts decline as family income increases, positive benefits are paid until family net income exceeds $103,235 (for one child). CCTB benefits are paid monthly to the "primary care-giver" (usually the mother), and are non-taxable. The maximum annual value of the benefit in 2008 is $1,307 for each child (with a supplement of $7.58 per month for third and subsequent children).

In addition to CCTB, lower-income families may be eligible for the National Child Benefit Supplement (NCBS). Maximum NCBS of $2,025 for a first child is available to families with net income less than $21,287. Benefits are phased-out at a rate of 12.2% for incomes higher than $21,287; some provinces also reduce social assistance payments for recipients of NCSB.

Finally, since 2006, each child under the age of six receives a $100 per month Universal Child Care benefit intended to help with the cost of child care. The benefit is taxable and paid to the parent with the lower income. No advance maintenance payments are available.

2.2 Finland

Eligibility

All employees, self-employed persons or students aged 16–64 are eligible for cash benefits if they are residents of Finland; immigrants are required to complete a 180-day waiting period.

Duration

Maternity benefits are available from 50 to 30 days before the due date for a period of 105 days (15 weeks). Paternity benefits are available for a maximum of 18 days. "Parents' allowance," payable to either parent, are available immediately following the maternity benefits for a further 158 days, excluding Sundays (i.e., 26 weeks). As an incentive to encourage fathers to take some of this allowance, they are entitled to an additional 1–12 days if they have taken at least 12 days of the parents' allowance. Parents' allowance is available for 60 extra days for multiple births and from 100 to 234 days for adoption. Finally, a "child home care allowance" is available for parents opting to remain home or to reduce work hours below 30 per week to care for a child aged less than 3 years.

Benefit Levels

Cash maternity and parental benefits are paid at the rate of 70% on annual earnings less than € 28,403 ($32,928); plus 40% of earnings between € 28,404 and € 43,698 ($32,928 and $50,655); plus 25% of earnings above € 43,698 ($50,655).

Maternity benefits are calculated on a daily basis; the minimum benefit is € 15.20 ($18) per day.[3]

The child home care allowance is € 3,027 ($3,509) per year for one child with an increase of € 600 ($696) for each additional child under the age of 7. A means-tested supplement up to € 135 ($156) per month is available to lower-income families. Parents who continue to work for pay but reduce hours to less than 30 per week receive € 70 ($81) per month. All of the above benefits are subject to taxation. A birth grant of € 140 ($162) is often paid in kind (e.g., a package of baby-care necessities); receipt of the birth grant is conditional upon having obtained pre-natal medical care.

Other Cash Benefits for Which Families with Infants may be Eligible

All families with children under 17 receive family allowances (€ 1,200 a year or $1,391) for one child; € 2,526 ($2,928) for two children; € 4,098 ($4,750) for three children; € 5,917 ($6,859) for four children and € 2,064 ($2,393) for each additional child. This benefit is paid to the mother. Single-parent supplements of € 439 ($509) per year for each child are available; the state advances mainte-nance payments to a maximum of about € 130 ($151) per month in the event no child support payments are received from the non-custodial parent. Supplements to unemployment benefits for recipients with dependant children are available.

2.3 France

Eligibility

To be eligible for maternity or paternity benefits, a woman/man must have been "registered" for at least 10 months and have worked 200 hours in the 3 months prior to certification of pregnancy. To be "registered" means contributing premiums to the social insurance program which covers sickness, disability, survivor, medical and maternity benefits. Note that the general program is also available for job-seekers who are receiving or who have received unemployment benefits during the last 12 months. Except in the case of farmers who hire replacement workers, maternity benefits are not available for the self-employed.

To be eligible for the "income supplement for reduced work," a parent must have stopped or reduced paid work to care for a child aged less than 3 years. Either parent may claim this benefit. Eligibility is easier as number of children increases. That is, a parent must have had 2 years of paid work in the 2 years prior to the child's birth

---

[3] Throughout this report, currency values are reported both in the country's own currency as well as in Canadian dollars. Conversions to Canadian dollars are made using purchasing power parities for individual household consumption (ICP, 2008) to adjust for differences in cost-of-living across the countries.

for a first child, in the past 4 years if there are 2 children in the family; in the past 5 years if there are more than 2 children.

Duration

For first and second children, maternity benefits are available for a total of 16 weeks (6 weeks prior to the birth and 10 following the birth). However, in keeping with a long-standing French tradition of designing social programs with a "pro-natalist" flavor, a longer duration is available for third and subsequent children (26 weeks, 8 prior to the birth and 18 weeks after the birth). Additional weeks are also available in the case of medical complication or multiple births.

Paternity benefits are available for 11 days within the 4 months following the birth (18 days for multiple births). Adoption benefits correspond with post-natal maternity benefits (i.e., 10 weeks for a first child; a birth mother is entitled to 16 weeks of maternity benefits in total, but 6 of these weeks must be taken prior to the birth). Adoption benefits can be split between mother and father if both are eligible.

The "income supplement for reduced work" (i.e., child-rearing or parental benefit) is available for 6 months from the month after childbirth, adoption, or from the end of maternity, paternity or adoption leave for a first child; the benefit is available until the child reaches 3 years for second and subsequent children.

Benefit Levels

Maternity/paternity benefits are paid at 100% of earnings (net of social insurance contributions) with a minimum daily benefit of € 8.48 ($11) and a maximum daily benefit of € 74.24 ($94); these benefits are taxable. The monthly "income supplement for reduced work" is € 538.72 ($720) for the complete suspension of paid work activity, less if the parent elects to work part-time, more if the family is not eligible for the "base allowance" described below. Funds for birth allowances, the child-rearing grant and family allowances are obtained through a 5.4% payroll tax on employers and a government contribution of 1.1% of total tax revenues.

Other Benefits for Which Families with Infants may be Eligible

A universal family allowance is available for families with at least two children aged less than 20 (€ 120.92 per month for two children ($162); € 275.84 ($368) for three children; € 430.76 ($575) for four children, etc.). The family allowance is paid to the mother. Lone-parent families receive an additional € 85 ($114) per month.

Several additional benefits are available to families with young children:

1. A means-tested birth grant of € 868.13 ($1,159) is paid at the start of the 7th month of pregnancy (or at the time of adoption).
2. A means-tested "base allowance" (€ 173.63 or $232 per month) is paid from the month of the child's birth until he or she is 3 years old.

3. An additional means-tested "single-parent" allowance provides up to € 735.75 ($983) for single parents with at least one child (or, € 551.81 for pregnant lone mothers).
4. A supplement for childcare that varies with number of children and family income is paid to help cover costs of accredited child care. If parents work part time, they can combine the child care supplement with the child-rearing supplement.

The state also provides advance maintenance payments to single-parent families not receiving child support from a non-custodial parent (to a maximum of € 85 ($114) monthly. Annual "school starting grants" of up to € 268 ($358) are provided on a means-tested basis.

2.4 Germany

Eligibility

To be eligible for cash maternity benefits in Germany, a woman must be a member of a sickness insurance fund (or be co-insured through a husband or father). Benefits are not available for self-employed workers (MISSOC, 2007).

Parental allowance is also available to fathers or mothers who stay home or reduce work hours (to below 30 hours per week) in order to care for a young child under the age of 14 months.

Duration

Maternity benefits are available for a total of 14 weeks (6 weeks prior to the birth and 8 weeks after; 12 weeks after the birth are available in the case of multiple or pre-mature birth).

Parental allowance is available until the child reaches 14 months. For two-parent families, one parent can claim at most 12 months; at least 2 months are reserved for the other parent.

Benefit Levels

For women who are members of a sickness fund and who have an employment contract, the maternity benefit is 100% of average earnings during the past 3 months. The state sickness fund will pay up to € 13 ($18) per day; employers of higher-wage women are required to top up this benefit so that an eligible woman receives 100% of her past average net earnings. The maternity allowance for uninsured employees is a fixed grant of € 210 per month ($291). Maternity benefits and allowances are not subject to taxation.

Parental allowance is worth between, at a minimum, € 300 per month ($415) and, at a maximum, € 1,800 per month ($2,492). Within these limits, the benefit is, in general, calculated as 67% of the net income of the parent making the claim. However, if net income prior to confinement was less than € 1,000 per month

($1,385), the replacement rate is increased by 0.1% for each € 2 short of € 1,000 to a maximum of 100%. Families with multiple children receive a 10% "sibling bonus" (worth at least € 75 per month ($104)).

Other Benefits for Which Families with Infants may be Eligible

A universal, government financed family allowance benefit is available in Germany, so all families with children will receive a benefit (€ 154 or $213) per month for first, second and third children; € 179 ($248) per month for each subsequent child. Families decide whether the benefit should be paid to the mother or the father (where applicable). Low-income families may be eligible for a supplementary child allowance of up to € 140 per month ($194). And, the state also provides advance maintenance (up to € 170 or $235 per month) for single-parent families with children under 12 in the event of default by non-custodial parent.

2.5 Italy

Eligibility

To be eligible for maternity benefits, a woman must currently be covered by the sickness/maternity program. Self-employed workers can qualify if they have made contributions. There is not, however, a minimum work requirement to establish eligibility as in some other countries.

Parental leave is also available beyond the maternity leave period and can be shared by the mother and father. The father is allowed to take any weeks the mother does not wish to use; no benefits are specifically reserved for the father only.

Duration

Eligible women receive maternity benefits for a total of 5 months (either 2 months before the birth and 3 after or 1 month before and 4 after). Eligible self-employed women can also receive maternity benefits for 5 months.

The parental benefits are then available for an additional 6 months, to be taken by either the mother or father at any time before the child is 3. A further 6 months of income-tested benefits are available before the child is 8 years old. (The self-employed are eligible for a 3-month leave before the child is one.)

Benefit Levels

Maternity benefits are paid at a rate of 80% of earnings in the month before the leave (with no ceiling). Self-employed workers are compensated at the same rate. The first 6 months of parental leave is compensated at 30% of earnings. The additional 6 months are also compensated at 30% of earnings, but are only available on an income-tested basis (monthly income must be less than 2.5 times the minimum pension of € 412 or $570). A birth grant of € 1,000 ($1,385) is available for second and subsequent children. All benefits are subject to income taxation.

Other Benefits for Which Families with Infants may be Eligible

Family allowances in Italy are employment-related and means-tested. To be covered, parents must be employees or social insurance, welfare or unemployment beneficiaries; employers are required to make pay-roll contributions to help fund the program. Benefit amounts vary with income and family structure, with higher benefits for larger, lower-income, and single-parent families; families with a disabled member also receive more. The monthly benefits vary from a low of € 10.33 ($15) and a high of € 965.26 ($1,336). Benefits disappear entirely when annual family income exceeds € 67,000 ($92,768). An additional means-tested "family support" benefit is available in the case of 3 or more children. These benefits are not subject to income taxation. No advance maintenance benefits are available.

2.6 Norway

Eligibility

To be eligible for cash parental benefits, individuals must have 6 months of employment or self-employment during the preceding 10-month period.

Duration

A total of 44 weeks of benefit are available at the highest replacement rate; parents can opt to take 54 weeks at a lower replacement rate.

Benefit Levels

Parental benefits are paid at a rate of 100% of covered earnings (65% of assessed earnings for self-employed workers) if the individual chooses the shorter benefit duration of 44 weeks. Alternatively, it is possible to receive benefits for 54 weeks, but recompensed at a rate of 80% of covered earnings. The mother is required to take 3 weeks of benefit prior to the birth and at least 6 weeks immediately following the birth. Six weeks of the total is *only* available for the father (the "father quota"); otherwise, the benefits can be divided between the parents as they choose. Benefits can be received at a reduced rate for up to 3 years if parents opt to work part-time and collect benefits part-time. The annual maximum on total benefits that can be received is NOK 377,352 ($48,516). Parental benefits are subject to normal social security contribution and income taxation.

A maternity grant of 33,584 kroner ($4318) is available to anyone not receiving the maternity benefit described above (including women who do not participate in paid work). If the total value of parental benefits to which the individual is entitled is less than the maternity grant, the difference is made up. The maternity grant is not subject to taxation or social security contribution.

Other Benefits for Which Families with Infants may be Eligible

All families in Norway receive a family allowance (of NOK 11,640, or $1497 per year, paid monthly to the mother, for each child. Families living in the Arctic receive a per child supplement worth NOK 3,840 or $494). Families with children aged between 1 and 3 who are not attending state-subsidized day care receive an additional cash benefit of NOK 39,636 ($5,096) each year per child. If the child attends daycare part-time, a reduced small child benefit is paid. This benefit is not taxable.

Single parents receive family allowance benefits for one more child than is actually present. Single parents are also entitled to income tested "transitional benefit" valued at NOK 116,350 (or $14,959) per year for 3 years (or up to 5 years if they are taking training). Transition benefits begin to be taxed back when income exceeds NOK 31,446 ($4,043). Single parents with children under 3 entitled to the transitional benefit also receive an infant supplement of NOK 7,920 ($1,018) per year; this is in addition to the small child benefit received by all families with children under 3. Single parents engaged in paid work can receive a cash transfer valued at up to 64% of child-care costs (the child-care subsidy is no longer available after income reaches NOK 377,352 or $48,516). Finally, the state pays "advance maintenance" to single parent families in the event of default on child support payments by the non-custodial parent. That is, a single parent receiving no support from the other parent would receive NOK 1,250 per month (or, $161) from the state.

2.7 Sweden

Eligibility

All Swedish residents earning at least 9,600 kronor ($1,265) per year are entitled to parents' cash benefits; the involuntarily unemployed are also entitled to benefits provided they are registered with the employment service. The self employed are covered.

Duration

Parents share a total duration of 480 days of parental insurance with at least 60 days reserved for each. These days can be taken at any point from 60 days before expected delivery until the child reaches the age of 8 years.

As well, 50 days of pregnancy benefits are also available if a pregnant woman has a physically demanding job that cannot accommodate or is forced to take time away from paid work during her pregnancy. These benefits are available between 60 and 11 days prior to the expected delivery date. Fathers are entitled to 10 days around the time of childbirth.

Benefit Levels

The guaranteed minimum level of parental insurance is SK 180 ($24) per day. For those with at least 240 days of paid work prior to delivery date and with earnings exceeding the minimum guarantee level, earnings are replaced at 80% for 390 days. However, the maximum daily benefit cannot exceed SK 652 ($86). An additional 90 days are payable at the "basic level" of SK 60 ($8) per day. These benefits are subject to taxation.

Other Benefits for Which Families with Infants may be Eligible

General revenue financed family allowances of SK 1,050 ($138) per child per month are available to all families with children under age 18; benefits are typically paid to the mother. Larger families receive supplements (e.g., SEK 100 for the second child ($13); SEK 354 for the third child ($47); SEK 860 for the fourth child ($113). Advance maintenance payments for single-parent families not receiving child support from the non-custodial parent are available (SEK 1,273 per month or $168).

2.8 United Kingdom

Eligibility

To be eligible for the first-tier "statutory" maternity benefits, a woman must have been continuously employed for at least 26 weeks by the *same employer* by the 15th week before the expected delivery date and must have average weekly earnings of at least £84 ($160) per week. Men whose partners are expecting a baby can receive "statutory paternity benefits" if they satisfy the same eligibility rules.

To be eligible for the flat-rate "maternity allowances," a woman must have worked (as an employee or in self employment) for at least 26 weeks in the 66-week period before the expected week of delivery and have had average weekly earnings of at least £30 ($57) in a 13-week period. She must not be eligible for statutory benefits, nor be receiving maternity benefits from her employer. Birth grants of £500 ($955) are available to women in receipt of social assistance benefits (who would thus be low-income and not in paid work).

Duration

Both statutory maternity benefits and maternity allowances are available for 39 weeks, beginning at any point from 15 weeks prior to the expected due date up to the week following childbirth. Statutory paternity benefits are available for up to 2 weeks, at the employer's discretion.

Benefit Levels

The first 6 weeks of statutory benefits are paid at 90% of average earnings with no ceiling; remaining weeks are paid at the same rate as maternity allowances.

Maternity allowances are £108.85 ($208) per week, or 90% of weekly earnings if earnings are less than £108.85 ($208). Statutory paternity benefits are also paid at £108.85 per week (or 90% of earnings if lower than £108.85 ($208 per week)). Statutory maternity pay is subject to taxation; maternity allowances are not considered taxable income.

Other Benefits for Which Families with Infants may be Eligible

Two kinds of child benefit are available to UK residents with children under 16: (1) a universal "child benefit" paid to the primary care-giver (usually the mother); and (2) an income-tested "child tax credit". Regardless of income, the child benefit is £17 ($32) per week for the first child and £11.40 ($22) for each additional child. The value of the child tax credit falls with family income, disappearing altogether for family income above £58,000 ($110,734). The benefit is higher when family size is larger, if there is a newborn present or for families of children with disabilities. The government pays the full cost of these programs through general revenue.

2.9 United States[4]

No national program of paid maternity or child-rearing benefits is available in the US; some unpaid leave is offered.

Eligibility

At the federal level, the "Family and Medical Leave Act" of 1993 provides unpaid leave for either parent if they work in the public sector or for a private-sector employer with 50 or more employees (about 60% of workers in the private sector). Further, a worker must have been employed for at least 12 months and have worked a minimum of 1,250 hours in the previous year.

Duration

Federal law entitles each eligible parent to 12 weeks of *unpaid* "family and medical leave" until the child is 1 year old (simultaneously or sequentially). Leave is available only for the period of disability, requiring a letter from a physician. Seventeen states have extended this unpaid leave in at least one way. Fifteen have expanded coverage to employees of smaller firms; six have increased duration. Five states (California, Hawaii, New Jersey, New York, and Rhode Island) offer maternity benefits through Temporary Disability Insurance (TDI) (covering 23% of the US population). The maximum possible duration of benefits offered is 26 weeks in Hawaii, New Jersey and New York; 30 weeks in Rhode Island and 52 weeks in

---

[4] This section draws heavily upon Gornick & Meyers (2003).

California (Wisensale, 2001). However, the average duration of paid benefits actually taken is much lower (4.6 weeks in Hawaii, 4.9 weeks in New York, 9.6 weeks in New Jersey, 11.6 weeks in Rhode Island and 12.6 weeks in California). Since 2002, California also offers paid leave to new fathers (Gornick & Meyers, 2003; Wisensale, 2001).

Benefit Levels

In the 5 TDI states providing cash benefits, replacement rates vary from a low of 50% in New York to a high of 66% in Hawaii; caps on benefits mean they will never be higher than $487 a week (594 Can $); average benefits vary between $142 and $273 a week (173–333 Can $).

Other Benefits for Which Families with Infants may be Eligible

No family allowances are available to US families with children. The "earned income tax credit" provides cash transfers to many low to medium-income children, provided their parents are engaged in paid work; "food stamps" are received by 2/3 of poor US children (Rainwater & Smeeding, 2003).

3 Comparative Discussion

In order to help in understanding how program details described above "work out" in terms of weeks off and/or benefits any given individual would receive, this section carries out a set of sample calculations. The thought experiment considered is: what would a Canadian new parent with particular characteristics receive if she/he were living in one of the other countries? Calculations have been carried out for five different new parents:

i) Mother with average Canadian female full-time earnings who had worked 35 hours per week for 52 weeks prior to the birth of her child;[5]
ii) Mother with "low" wage (half the Canadian average) who had also worked 35 hours per week for 52 weeks prior to the birth of her child;[6]
iii) Mother with "high" wage (1.5 times the average), who had worked 35 hours per week for 52 weeks prior to the birth;
iv) Mother with average Canadian female earnings who was self-employed in the year preceding the birth of her child;

---

[5] "Average" earnings for full-time workers are calculated as the average for all women working more than 30 hours per week at a paid job or in self-employment in the 2000 Canadian SLID survey (the Survey of Labor and Income Dynamics). This is $38,433 (converted to 2007 dollars using the Canadian Consumer Price Index).
[6] "Low" wage is calculated as 50% of the average wage received by female full-time workers ($19,217).

v) Father with average Canadian earnings who had worked 35 hours per week for
   52 weeks prior to the birth of his child.

Results of these calculations are presented in Tables 1–5. Benefit amounts have
been converted to 2007 Canadian dollars using purchasing power parities for individual household consumption (ICP, 2008) to adjust for differences in cost-of-living
across the countries. If benefits are paid by the day or by the month, "weekly" equiv-
alents are approximated and reported in these tables. When working out maximum
benefit weeks available to a mother or father, the assumption is that the individual
takes the maximum to which she or he *could* possibly be entitled (and thus that the
spouse does not take any of his/her share of benefits). In fact, in most of the countries studied, benefits must be divided between married parents, though mothers,
on average, take a much larger share (see Marshall, 2008). For France, we present
separate calculations for benefits which would be available for a first compared to
a third child, given the large differences in entitlement for these cases. The U.S. is
excluded from these calculations.

Scenario 1: New Mother, Full-Time Paid Worker with Average Canadian Earnings

As indicated in Table 1, a Canadian woman who had worked full-time in the year
preceding the birth of her child would be entitled, following a 2-week waiting
period, to 50 weeks of paid benefits, compensated at $406 per week (55% of her
weekly earnings of $739) for a potential total of $20,300.[7] In Quebec, she would
also be eligible for 50 weeks of benefits, compensated at a higher rate during the first
25 weeks (70%). Thus, total potential benefits would be higher in Quebec ($23,075).
  In terms of total duration of paid benefits, the 50-week Canadian entitlement is
longer than what is available in the UK or Norway; fairly similar to total duration
of benefits available in Italy or in France for a first child; significantly less than the
total duration available in Germany, Sweden or, especially, Finland or France for
a third or subsequent child. An interesting difference across the countries is that
France, Germany, Italy and Norway all designate a portion of maternity benefits for
prior to the expected delivery date whereas in Canada, women can (and often do)
take almost all of their weeks following delivery. This difference could be a result
of the Canadian system emerging as part of "unemployment insurance" rather than
as a health benefit.
  For a woman working full-time with average Canadian wages, the weekly benefit
rates and, correspondingly, replacement rates are lower in Canada than in most other
countries, especially for "first stage" benefits. This is *not* true of the new Quebec
benefits, which, during the first 25 weeks have 70% replacement, and thus compare
more favorably with other countries in the study.

---

[7] In fact, the effective replacement rate over the full leave will actually be slightly lower than
55% given the two-week waiting period during which no benefits are paid (serving as a form of
"deductible").

Table 1 Mother working full-time with average Canadian earnings ($38,433 annually or $739/week)—Sample benefit calculations

	Canada	Quebec basic plan	United Kingdom	Germany	France (1st child)	France (3rd child)	Sweden	Norway	Finland	Italy
Weeks of paid benefits	50	25 (1) + 25 (2)	6 (1) + 33 (2)	14 (1) + 48 (2)	16 (1) + 26 (2)	26 (1) + 138 (2)	78 (1) + 6 (2)	38	41 (1) + 115 (2)	20 (1) + 26 (2) + 0 (3)
Total potential value of benefits	$20,300 (VII)	$23,075 (VI)	$10,854 (X)	$34,106 (II)	$12,200 (IX)	$37,060 (I)	$33,780 (III)	$28,082 (IV)	$27,590 (V)	$17,592 (VIII)
Average weekly benefits	$406	$517 (1) $406 (2)	$665 (1) $208 (2)	$739 (1) $495 (2)	$470 (1)* $180 (2)	$470 (1)* $180 (2)	$430 (1)* $40 (2)	$739	$485 (1) $67 (2)	$591 (1) $222 (2)
Effective replacement rate	55%	70% 55%	90% 28%	100% (1) 67% (2)	64% (1)* 25% (2)	64% (1)* 25% (2)	58% (1)* 5% (2)	100%	66% (1) 9% (2)	80% (1) 30% (2)
Extras								Birth grant $739	Birth grant $162	Birth grant $1385 for 2nd + children

* indicates benefit ceiling is binding.

Note: Total duration of paid benefits in any country is the sum of (1)+(2) as relevant. Entitlement is broken up in this way if benefit level changes (either because replacement rate or benefit level changes within a program or as the individual switches from maternity to child-rearing benefits, for example). See text for further details. Country rank in terms of total benefits is indicated in roman numerals in parentheses.

Table 2 Mother working full-time with $^1/_2$ average Canadian women's full-time earnings ($19,217 annually or $370 week)—Sample Benefit Calculations

	Canada	Quebec basic plan	United Kingdom	Germany	France (1st child)	France (3rd child)	Sweden	Norway	Finland	Italy
Weeks of paid benefits	50	25 (1) + 25 (2)	6 (1) + 33 (2)	14 (1) + 56 (2)	16 (1) + 26 (2)	26 (1) + 138 (2)	78 (1) + 6 (2)	38	41 (1) + 115 (2)	20 (1) + 26 (2) + 0(3)
Total potential value of benefits	$10,200 (V)	$11,575 (V)	$8,862 (VII)	$25,900 (II)	$10,600 (VI)	$34,460 (I)	$17,622 (IV)	$14,060 (V)	$18,324 (III)	$8,806 (VIII)
Average weekly benefits	$204	$259 (1) $204 (2)	$333 (1) $208 (2)	$370 (1) $370 (2)	$370 (1) $180 (2)	$370 (1) $180 (2)	$223 (1) $38 (2)	$370	$259 (1) $67 (2)	$296 (1) $111 (2)
Effective replacement rate	55%	70% (1) 55% (2)	90% (1) 56% (1)	100% (1) 100% (2)	100% (1) 49% (2)	100% (1) 49% (2)	80% (1) 13% (2)	100%	70% (1) 18% (2)	80% (1) 30% (2) 30% (3)
Extras	If eligible for maximum FS, weekly benefits = $296 (80%) total benefits = $14,800	If eligible for maximum FS, weekly benefits = $296 (80%) total benefits = $14,800		Lone mother would receive 8 weeks more than married mother	May be eligible for birth grant $1,159	May be eligible for birth grant $1,159			Birth grant $162	Birth grant $1,385 for 2nd + children

Table 3 Mother working full-time with 1.5 times average Canadian earnings ($57,650 annually or $1109/week)—Sample Benefit Calculations

	Canada	Quebec basic plan	United Kingdom	Germany	France (1st child)	France (3rd child)	Sweden	Norway	Finland	Italy
Weeks of paid benefits:	50	25 (1) + 25 (2)	6 (1) + 33 (2)	14 (1) + 48 (2)	16 (1) + 26 (2)	26 (1) + 138 (2)	78 (1) + 6 (2)	38	41 (1) + 115 (2)	20 (1) + 26 (2) + 0 (3)
Total potential value of benefits	$21,750 (VIII)	$34,250 (IV)	$12,852 (X)	$45,430 (I)	$12,200 (IX)	$37,060 (III)	$33,780 (V)	$42,142 (II)	$32,838 (VI)	$26,398 (VII)
Average weekly benefits	$435*	$767 (1)* $603 (2)*	$998 (1) $208 (2)	$1109 (1) $623 (2)	$470 (1)* $180 (2)	$470 (1)* $180 (2)	$430 (1)* $40 (2)	$1,109	$613 (1) $67 (2)	$887 (1) $333 (2)
Effective replacement rate	39%*	69% (1)* 54% (2)*	90% 19%	100% (1) 56% (2)	42% (1)* 16% (2)	42% (1)* 16% (2)	39% (1)* 4% (2)	100%	55% (1) 6% (2)	80% (1) 30% (2)
Extras									Birth grant $162	Birth grant $1385 for 2nd + children

* indicates ceiling is binding.

Note: Total duration of paid benefits in any country is the sum of (1)+(2) as relevant. Entitlement is broken up in this way if benefit level changes (either because replacement rate or benefit level changes within a program or as the individual switches from maternity to child-rearing benefits, for example). See text for further details. Country rank in terms of total benefits is indicated in roman numerals in parentheses.

Table 4 Mother, self-employed working full-time with average Canadian earnings ($38,433 or $739/week)—Sample Benefit Calculations

	Canada	Quebec basic plan	United Kingdom	Germany	France (1st child)	France (3rd child)	Sweden	Norway	Finland	Italy
Weeks of paid benefits:	0	25 (1) + 25 (2)	39	0	0	0	78 (1) + 6 (2)	38	41 (1) + 115 (2)	20 (1) + 12(2)
Total potential value of benefits	0	$23,075 (III)	$8,112 (VI)				$33,780 (I)	$18,240 (IV)	$27,590 (II)	$11,820 (V)
Average weekly benefits	0	$517 (1) $406 (2)	$208				$430 (1)* $40 (2)	$480	$485 (1) $67 (2)	$591 (1) $222 (2)
Effective replacement rate	0	70 (1) 55 92	28%				58% (1)* 5% (2)	65%	66% (1) 9% (2)	80% (1) 30% (2)
Extras									Birth grant $162	Birth grant $1.385 for 2nd + children

* indicates ceiling is binding.

Note: Total duration of paid benefits in any country is the sum of (1)+(2) as relevant. Entitlement is broken up in this way if benefit level changes (either because replacement rate or benefit level changes within a program or as the individual switches from maternity to child-rearing benefits, for example). See text for further details. Country rank in terms of total benefits is indicated in roman numerals in parentheses.

Table 5 Father working full-time with average Canadian male earnings ($54,170 annually or $1042/week)—Sample Benefit Calculations

	Canada	Quebec basic plan	United Kingdom	Germany	France (1st child)	France (3rd child)	Sweden	Norway	Finland	Italy
Weeks of paid benefits:	35	12 (1) + 25 (2)	2	0 (1) + 48 (2)	2 (1) + 26 (2)	2 (1) + 138 (2)	78 (1) + 6 (2)	35	28 (1) + 115 (2)	0 (1) + 26 (2)
Total potential value of benefits	$15,225 (VII)	$23,073 (VIII)	$416 (IX)	$29,904 (III)	$5,620 (VIII)	$25,780 (IV)	$33,780 (II)	$36,470 (I)	$24,393 (V)	$8,112 (VIII)
Average weekly benefits	$435*	$729 (1) $573 (2)	$208*	0 (1) $623(2)*	$470 (1)* $180 (2)*	$470 (1)* $180 (2)*	$430 (1)* $40 (2)	$1,042	$596 (1) $67 (2)	0 (1) $312 (2)
Effective replacement rate	42%	70% (1) 55% (2)	20%	0% (1) 60% (2)	45% (1) 17% (2)	45% (1) 17% (2)	41% (1) 4% (2)	100%	57% (1) 6% (2)	0% (1) 30% (2)
Extras										

* indicates ceiling is binding.

Note: Total duration of paid benefits in any country is the sum of (1)+(2) as relevant. Entitlement is broken up in this way if benefit level changes (either because replacement rate or benefit level changes within a program or as the individual switches from maternity to child-rearing benefits, for example). See text for further details. Country rank in terms of total benefits is indicated in roman numerals in parentheses.

As is clear from Table 1, some countries with very long total benefit durations have two stages of paid benefits with either a lower replacement rate or else flat rate, sometimes income-tested benefits (which are typically a relatively small fraction of average Canadian female full-time weekly earnings), in the second stage.

Taking into account both duration and benefit levels, total *potential* dollar compensation in Canada ranks 7th (out of the 10 cases considered—the new Quebec basic plan ranks 6th). Only Italy, France (for a first child) and the UK offer less. Of course, in countries with two stages of benefits and much lower compensation during the second stage, it may be less attractive for women with average full-time earnings to take up the full leave available (e.g., 138 weeks with only 25% replacement for a third child in France).

Another point illustrated in Table 1 is that some new mothers receive benefits paid at less than the nominal earnings replacement rate. Ceilings on benefits can be very important in determining "effective" replacement rates. In both France and Sweden, a woman with average Canadian earnings for full-time workers would encounter the ceiling on maternity benefits payable, thereby significantly reducing her effective replacement rate. For example, for the first 78 weeks, the Swedish replacement rate is nominally 80% to a maximum of $86 per day (or $430/week, assuming 5 work days per week). If average earnings per week are $739, then the effective replacement rate is actually only $430/$739 = 0.58. Similarly, in France the nominal replacement rate is 100%, but the ceiling on benefits (during the first stage) is $470 so that a woman with average Canadian earnings would, effectively have only 64% of earnings replaced ($470/$739). While benefit ceilings exist in both Canada (for both maternity and parental benefits) and Germany (for parental benefits), these ceilings are high enough that they have no impact on the benefit levels or replacement rates received by a woman with average Canadian earnings. Although there is no ceiling on benefits in Finland, replacement rates fall as earnings increase.

Scenario 2: New Mother, Full-Time Paid Worker with Low Canadian Wages (50% of Average)

In all countries studied here, a woman who had worked full-time at low wages would be entitled to the same total duration of paid benefits as a woman working full-time at average wages, assuming continuous employment prior to the child's birth in both cases (see Table 2). Benefits paid as a percentage of past earnings would, of course, be lower when earnings are lower. However, for low-wage workers, benefit ceilings do not generally bind (except for second stage UK benefits), so that the portion of earnings replaced for low wage workers is higher in some cases (e.g., France and Sweden) for low-wage new mothers than for new mothers with average wages. Also, "second stage" benefits paid at flat rates constitute a larger fraction of past earnings for low-wage workers. This means that the "opportunity cost" of lost earnings is less for low-wage than for higher-wage new mothers; they are giving up less income when they stay at home for another week with the baby. Thus, staying out longer may be a relatively more attractive option. On the other hand, affordability is likely to be more of an issue since the actual flow of funds to the household will be smaller.

Table 2 also illustrates that several countries enhance benefits for low-wage workers. In both Canada and Quebec, if net *family* income is low, replacement rates can increase from 55% to as much as 80%. A recent EI monitoring report indicates that the FS supplement is received by 22% of maternity claimants; 21% of parental claimants (CEIC, 2003). In Canada and Quebec, the entitlement to the higher replacement for a woman with low earnings would depend on her husband's income as well as her own. Of course, this family income test assumes sharing of income within the family, which may not always be the case (see Phipps, Burton, & Lethbridge, 2001). In Germany, replacement rates for parental benefits can increase from 67 to as much as 100%, depending only upon the net income of the person making the claim.

From a cross-national comparative perspective, Canadian benefits are relatively more generous for a low-wage new mother as compared to a new mother with average wages. Total potential compensation is $10,200 in Canada ($11,575 in Quebec) if family income is high enough that the family supplement to her benefits is not available. If, however, the low-wage woman had no other sources of family income (e.g., a lone mother), total potential benefits could be as high as $14,800 (in either Canada or Quebec). In either case, Canadian total compensation ranks fifth (ahead of the UK, Italy and France, in the case of a first child). With the full family supplement (and so an 80% replacement rate), Canadian total potential compensation is very similar to that available in Norway. France, for a third or higher child, stands out with very high levels of potential compensation for a low-wage new mother (very long duration of potential benefits with relatively high benefit levels); Germany is second most generous (with reasonably long duration and very high levels of compensation).

Although we do not explicitly consider the case where the new mother has recently experienced time unemployed or out of the labor market, this possibility seems increasingly likely in a time of global economic recession. In some countries, a period of unemployment (or even reduced hours without actually losing a job) could mean dis-entitlement from paid benefits, depending upon how many hours/weeks of paid work the woman had completed. Dis-entitlement in this case would be particularly likely in Canada, requiring 600 hours in the last year, France, requiring 200 hours in the past 3 months; Norway, requiring 6 months during the preceding 10 months, and the UK, requiring 26 weeks of continuous employment with the same employer. In other countries, eligibility would not be affected and, women experiencing economic hardship could also be entitled to higher replacement rates (Germany, for parental allowance) or extra weeks of benefits (6 months of income-tested benefits in Italy).

Scenario 3: New Mother, Full-Time Paid Worker with High Wages

New mothers with 1.5 times average earnings for a Canadian woman working full time will also be eligible for the same duration of benefits as women with average benefits. More affluent new mothers fare particularly well in Germany, Norway and Quebec, where weekly benefit levels are highest. However, the main point illustrated in Table 3 is that the higher the wages, the more important is the benefit ceiling level for effective replacement rates. For example, in Canada, a higher wage new mother would receive the ceiling benefit payment of $435 per week and so have past earnings re-imbursed at only 39% (rather than the nominal 55%). In Quebec, on the other hand, the ceiling would be less binding so that the same woman would receive $767 per week in the first stage (69% replacement) and $603 per week in the second stage, with 54% replacement.

As well, flat-rate child-rearing or parental benefits in some countries replace a much smaller share of a high-earner new mother's wages (e.g., 16% in France or only 6% in Finland).

It seems less likely that high-earner new mothers in France, for example, would avail themselves of the full child-rearing leave when effective replacement is very low. Professional commitment may also reinforce a tendency not to take long periods away from paid work. There is certainly a strong possibility that higher-wage women will take shorter leaves while lower-wage women will take longer leaves with a two-stage system of this type, perhaps exacerbating future differences in labor market outcomes. That is, if higher-wage women spend less time out of the labor market, they are more likely to receive promotions, for example, and thus to experience relative gains in earnings compared to lower-wage colleagues who stay home longer.

Scenario 4: New Mother Working Full-Time in Self-Employment with Average Wages

Self-employed women (or men) would not be eligible for any paid benefits in Canada outside Quebec, in France or in Germany. Benefits would be available on the same terms as for employees in Quebec, Finland and Sweden. Self-employed new mothers would be eligible for the same duration of benefits as employees in the UK and Norway, but at reduced rates of compensation. In Italy, a self-employed new mother would be entitled to fewer total weeks, but compensated at the same rate (see Table 4).

Scenario 5: New Father Working Full-Time at Average Male Wages

The final set of calculations carried out in this chapter focuses on what is available to a "typical" male full-time worker, receiving average Canadian male earnings (see Table 5).

New fathers are entitled to cash benefits in all countries studied, with three general approaches apparent. In the UK, new fathers receive only a very short, specially designated "paternity benefit". In Canada and Italy, a "parental benefit" can be shared between fathers and mothers as they choose. In Quebec, Finland,[8] Germany, Norway and Sweden, although benefits can be shared, a portion of the total is reserved for the father. "Father quotas" have been introduced to encourage

---

[8] Finland adds to the total entitlement if fathers take some of the benefit.

Table 6 Receipt of social transfers and social transfers as a fraction of DPI

	Children < 1				Children < 3				Children < 18			
	Sample size	Receives social transfers (%)	Social Transfers as a fraction of DPI		Sample size	Receives social transfers (%)	Social transfers as a fraction of DPI		Sample size	Receives social transfers (%)	Social transfers as a fraction of DPI	
			Includes zeros	Excludes zeros			Includes zeros	Excludes zeros			Includes zeros	Excludes zeros
Canada 2004	644	97.7	22.7	23.3	1804	94.9	21.6	22.7	8361	89.6	17.3	19.4
US 2004	2796	90.6	14.7	16.2	8208	91.5	14.3	15.6	32900	89.6	13.7	15.3
UK 2004	805	95.9	38.5	40.2	2246	97.5	35.3	36.2	8515	97.2	31.2	32.1
Germany 2000	66	***	***	***	635	94.6	22.3	23.6	3387	98.4	21.0	21.4
France 2000	311	95.7	27.0	28.2	882	93.9	27.0	28.7	3438	86.1	22.2	25.8
Sweden 2005	438	100.0	45.7	45.7	1154	100.0	43.1	43.1	4452	100.0	31.7	31.7
Norway 2004	434	99.6	44.2	44.4	1137	99.8	39.2	39.3	4798	99.5	28.2	28.4
Finland 2004	305	99.5	37.9	38.1	1	99.7	37.2	37.3	3735	99.4	25.7	25.8

*** sample size is too small for analysis.

fathers to take at least some benefits since evidence suggests that mothers are other-wise more likely to take the vast majority of benefits (e.g., Marshall, 2003 or 2008; OECD, 2001).

In addition to traditional gender roles, one important economic reason why men may be less likely than women to take benefits is that men earn more than women in all countries studied. With less than 100% replacement, lost earnings for the family will be higher when the father takes maternity leave rather than the mother. This is true despite the fact that men would typically receive higher weekly benefits than their wives (e.g., a father with average earnings in Quebec would receive $729 per week while his wife with average earnings would receive $517).

Notice, as well, that effective replacement rates for men are usually lower than for women (see Table 6) because with higher male earnings, ceilings on benefits are more likely to be encountered. For example, in Canada, a new mother with average female earnings would receive the full replacement rate of 55% whereas a new father with average earnings would receive a replacement rate of only 42%. Effective replacement rates can also be lower in countries with flat rate parental or child-rearing benefits since these constitute a smaller share of male earnings (e.g., the U.K. or France). Finally, men are less likely to be eligible for income-tested top-ups to replacement rates (e.g., Germany).

In the Canadian case, the decision in 2001 to waive a second waiting period for fathers sharing parental benefits with mothers has been important for encourag-ing more fathers to take parental benefits (Perusse, 2003). Particularly for fathers considering taking a short leave, the 2-week waiting period previously in place had a large impact on effective replacement rates. In Quebec, the 5 weeks of parental benefits now only available to fathers has had a dramatic impact on take-up (Marshall, 2008).

Like higher-wage new mothers, new fathers are likely to receive high weekly benefits when ceilings are high (e.g., Quebec) or non-existent (e.g., Norway). Although potential total benefits are high when the total duration of paid leave is high (e.g., France or Finland), the very low replacement rate during this period make it unlikely that many fathers would in fact exercise their full entitlement.

4 The Over-All Financial Well-Being of Families with Infants in 9 Affluent Countries

Over-all financial well-being of households will depend upon the family (e.g., marital status, number of children), the market (e.g., number of earners, hours of paid work and rates of compensation) and the state (e.g., social transfers available for families of young children). This section of the chapter uses the most recent microdata available from the Luxembourg Income Study (LIS)[9] to compare the

---

[9] The Luxembourg Income Study is a set of cross-sectional microdata files, housed in Luxembourg by accessible via the internet. Member countries contribute microdata sets with a focus on income information (e.g., the Canadian data are the Survey of Consumer Finances and then the Survey of

over-all financial well-being of families with very young children. In general, this means outcomes are being compared in the early years of the new century. The U.S. is included in this section of the chapter.

4.1 Social Transfers

Although the focus of the chapter is on maternity and parental benefits, at the end of the day, it is important to keep in mind that different countries package support for families with infants and young children in different ways. Thus, country A may offer less generous maternity/parental benefits than country B but a very generous child allowance, for example. It would then be inappropriate to conclude that country A is less generous to families with newborns. This section of the chapter attempts to present a broader picture of the over-all package on offer in each country.

Since maternity or parental benefits might be reported, variously, as "unemployment insurance" (Canada), as sickness benefits or as family benefits (and in several countries, maternity benefits would be considered "sickness" benefits while parental benefits would be considered "family" benefits), Table 6 begins by simply reporting on receipt of *any* social transfers. As noted above, this further has the advantage of taking account of all forms of cash support received by families with young children. Throughout this section of the paper outcomes are reported separately for families with a youngest child aged less than 1 year[10] (which would be most relevant for countries with a fairly short total duration of benefits), for families with a youngest child under 3 (most appropriate for countries with a longer duration of benefits) and for all families with children aged 0–17 (for comparative purposes).

As Table 6 indicates, families with children typically receive social transfers. This is least likely in the U.S., where nonetheless about 90% of families with infants report receiving a social transfer.[11] While nearly all families with young children receive social transfers in Canada and France, benefit receipt falls after children reach the age of 3 in these countries (from 97.7 to 89.6% in Canada and from 95.7 to 86.1% in France). In the Scandinavian countries, families with children are almost certain to receive social transfers, regardless of the age of the child.

Table 6 also reports social transfers as a percent of disposable personal income[12] received by families with children. It is quite clear that social transfers comprise

---

Labor and Income Dynamics, cross sections). Great attention has been paid by LIS staff to re-codes which ensure maximum comparability of variables across the countries.

[10] The German sample is too small to allow separate reporting for families with children aged less than one year. In the Italian data, maternity benefits and child allowances are reported as part of "net income" rather than as part of "social transfers," so we are unable to include Italy in Table 6.

[11] In the US case, food stamps are included as "cash transfers." There has been a dramatic increase in the proportion of U.S. families with children receiving social transfers from only about half in 2000.

[12] As noted in the policy summaries, a number of the European countries guarantee child support payments to lone mother households. Thus, child support can be a social transfer whereas in North America, this would be a private transfer. Social transfers as reported here do not include child support, but these are added in to compute total disposable income.

the largest share of income for families with very young children in Norway and Sweden. Social transfers as a fraction of disposable income are next highest for Finland and the UK.[13] In these four countries, families with older children receive considerably less than those with newborns; however, even families with older children still receive higher transfers than elsewhere. Social transfers as a fraction of family disposable income are next highest in France; they are lowest in Canada and the U.S. In the U.S., since there are no specially designated maternity/parental or young child benefits, there is no noticeable falling off in terms of what is available for older children.

4.2 Labor Market Participation of Mothers with Young Children

Table 7 contrasts labor market behavior of new mothers across the 9 countries.[14] Women with a youngest child aged 0–3 years are least likely to report earnings in Italy (40.6%), the UK (45.3%) and Germany (49.5%). At the other end of the spectrum, women with a youngest child aged 0–3 years are most likely to report earnings in Norway (82.3%) and Sweden (79.4%). Thus, the countries with the most generous maternity/parental benefits programs also have the highest labor-force participation rates for young mothers—whether as a cause or as an effect of policy is not, of course, entirely clear. High rates of labor force participation by young parents may focus attention on the issue and encourage policy development; generous maternity/parental benefits programs may encourage labor-market participation of young parents.

Table 7 Percentage of Mothers with Positive Wages/Salaries

	Children < 1		Children < 3		Children < 18	
	Sample size	%	Sample size	%	Sample size	%
Canada 2004	638	72.3	1768	69.6	7939	73.8
US 2004	2757	63.9	8041	61.6	31461	69.3
UK 2004	804	40.7	2235	45.3	8301	59.9
Germany 2000	66	***	633	49.5	3350	64.1
France 2000	309	61.1	876	56.2	3378	67.8
Sweden 2005	437	79.1	1149	79.4	4331	85.1
Norway 2004	429	84.3	1120	82.3	4663	86.2
Finland 2004	302	69.9	799	68.2	3633	81.7
Italy 2000	154	43.0	443	40.6	2396	39.8

*** sample size is too small for analysis.

---

[13] Note that transfers will be high when labor market earnings are low and vice versa. This may help in understanding why UK average social transfers appear high by comparison with Norwegian average transfers. While Norway offers very generous programs, labor market participation and market earnings are very high. The UK offers less generous benefits, but more families need to rely upon them.

[14] In all countries except the UK, fathers are almost certain to report earnings.

It is also interesting to note that 52% of women in the UK agree that "a pre-school child is likely to suffer if his/her mother works" compared to 48% of women in Canada and to 36% of women in Norway (Phipps, 1999, p. 35). Different attitudes across countries about what is the "best" way to care for infants presumably influence the shape of maternity/parental benefits programs as well as choices about labor market behavior by parents of newborns.

Finally, recall that although these Scandinavian countries offer very long and relatively generously compensated leaves, women also have the option of extending their leaves by returning to work part-time while continuing to collect benefits part-time (e.g., a woman would be allowed to stretch 6 months of benefits over a full year by working half time for pay). "Keeping one's oar in the labor market" in this way could help to mitigate documented negative consequences of staying out of paid work for long periods of time (i.e., the "mommy gap"—see Phipps et al., 2001).

4.3 The Incidence and Depth of Poverty

Table 8 compares the incidence and depth of poverty for families with very young children before and after taxes/transfers in each of the 9 countries studied. "Depth of poverty" indicates, for each poor family, how *far* below the poverty line family income actually falls. (For example, if the poverty line is $10,000 and income is $8,000, then "depth" of poverty is $2,000. To facilitate comparisons across countries, we express the average depth of poverty, calculated for all poor families in each country, as a proportion of the poverty line.)

If they were to rely only upon market earnings, 21.4% of Canadian families with a youngest child aged 0–3 years would have income below the poverty line[15] and the average depth of poverty, for those poor, would be 54.3% of the poverty line. After taxes and transfers, 13.3% remained poor, with an approximate halving in the average depth of poverty (to 28.6%).

This important reduction in the depth of young child poverty notwithstanding, Canada's record on poverty for families with very young children is only better than that of Italy and the US. Poverty rates are lower in all other countries studied, generally as a result of more generous social transfers. For example, for families with children aged 0–3, French transfers reduce the incidence of poverty from 31.8 to 9.2%; Swedish transfers reduce the incidence of poverty from 21.2 to 5.8%; Norwegian transfers reduce poverty from 22.8 to 7.0%; Finnish transfers reduce poverty from 22.0 to 7.6%.

A final important point to take from Table 8, however, is that the Scandinavian countries also *start* with relatively low levels of market poverty, perhaps because in addition to the generous social transfers they provide, they also have other policies which are supportive of labor market participation of parents with young children (e.g., childcare—see Rainwater & Smeeding, 2003).

---

[15] Poverty lines are constructed in relative terms for each country as 50% of median equivalent income for that country.

Table 8 Rate and depth of poverty—with and without taxes and transfers

	Children < 1				Children < 3				Children < 18			
	Pre taxes/transfers		Post taxes/transfers		Pre taxes/transfers		Post taxes/transfers		Pre taxes/transfers		Post taxes/transfers	
	Rate (%)	Relative depth (%)	Rate (%)	Relative depth (%)	Incidence (%)	Relative depth (%)	Rate (%)	Relative depth (%)	Incidence (%)	Relative depth (%)	Rate (%)	Relative depth (%)
Canada 2004	21.6	48.1	11.6	24.5	21.4	54.3	13.3	28.6	21.1	54.5	13.3	26.5
US 2004	27.6	53.8	23.6	40.8	26.6	52.5	22.4	39.4	22.8	53.3	17.4	38.6
UK 2004	28.7	87.8	11.9	27.2	25.9	85.7	11.7	25.0	22.9	80.1	8.9	23.7
Germany 2000	11.0	40.5	15.5	28.3	15.4	68.0	8.8	29.8	15.4	66.0	8.3	27.0
France 2000	27.9	49.7	9.7	15.1	31.8	46.3	9.2	15.9	26.3	49.1	8.4	17.9
Sweden 2005	24.0	63.3	8.2	26.7	21.2	65.9	5.8	26.0	18.4	64.1	4.3	26.3
Norway 2004	24.4	58.8	6.6	28.2	22.8	65.4	7.0	24.8	17.0	61.6	4.9	24.2
Finland 2004	21.3	69.5	7.5	13.2	22.0	67.2	7.6	14.2	15.9	63.9	4.6	19.6
Italy 2000	NA	NA	12.7	32.9	NA	NA	15.8	38.8	NA	NA	14.7	37.2

5 Conclusions

This comparison of Canadian maternity and parental benefits with those available in 9 other affluent countries suggests the following key points:

- Since 2001, the total duration of Canadian benefits compares relatively favorably by international standards. Most countries with a longer duration eventually move to a flat-rate benefit or a lower replacement rate towards the end of the extended period.
- However, the level of benefits offered in Canada is rather low, particularly by comparison with first-stage maternity benefits available elsewhere.
- Ceilings on maximum benefits payable (e.g., in Canada, France, Sweden) or flat-rate benefits for some part of the covered period (e.g., Germany, France) mean that the effective replacement rate for men is usually lower than for women (because men generally have higher earnings). This may discourage men from taking a larger share of benefits. A tension is that with a higher replacement rate, men receive higher weekly benefits than women.
- Some countries have implemented inducements for men to take parental leaves (e.g., by allocating a portion of the leave for men only in Sweden, Norway or Quebec); by adding to the total entitlement if men take part of the leave in Finland).
- Scandinavian countries are particularly flexible about allowing parents to choose whether to take full-time leave or to receive the same total payment, but spread out over a longer time by returning to work part-time. In Canada, new parents receiving parental leave are now able to earn up to 25% of their weekly benefit or $50 without any deduction in that benefit, though they are not able to *extend* their benefit period in this way. Allowing mothers the flexibility to return to work part-time when they are ready may help to minimize some of the adverse earnings consequences of long periods of time spent outside the paid labor market. This may also encourage more men to take leave, if they are reluctant to stay away from their paid jobs full-time.
- Although Canadian social transfers play a vital role in reducing the depth of poverty experienced by very young children, the full social transfer package leaves more very young children in poverty than is the case in any of the other countries studied here except Italy and the US.

Acknowledgments I would like to thank Sarah MacPhee for excellent research assistance and both the Canadian Institute for Advanced Research and the Social Sciences and Humanities Research Council of Canada for funding

References

Canada Employment Insurance Commission. (2003). *Employment insurance 2002 monitoring and assessment Report.* Canada Employment Insurance Commission.
Esping-Andersen, G. (1990). Three worlds of welfare capitalism. Cambridge: Polity Press.

Gornick, J., & Meyers, M. K. (2003). *Families that work: Policies for reconciling parenthood and employment*. New York: Russell Sage Foundation.

Marshall, K. (2003). Benefiting from extended parental leave. *Perspectives on Labor and Income, 4*(3), 5–11.

Marshall, K. (2008). Fathers' use of paid leave. *Perspectives on Labor and Income, 9*(6), 5–14.

Missoc (serial). *Social protection in the member states of the community*. Brussels: EC. On-line version: http://europa.eu.int/comm/employment_social/missoc/missoc2004_en.pdf. Accessed 25 October 2004.

OECD. (2001). *Balancing work and family life: Helping parents into paid employment*. OECD Employment Outlook, Ch. 4, Paris.

Perusse, D. (2003). New maternity and parental benefits. *Perspectives on Labor and Income, 4*(3), 1–4.

Phipps, S. (1994, December). *Maternity and parental leaves and allowances: An international comparison*. Report to Human Resources Development Canada, Department of economics, Dalhuosie University.

Phipps, S. (1998, May). *Maternity and parental benefits: An international comparison*. Update, mimeo. Department of economics, Dalhousie University.

Phipps, S. (1999). *An international comparison of policies and outcomes for young children*. Canadian Policy Research Networks Study No. F/05.

Phipps, S. (2006). Working for working parents: The evolution of maternity and parental benefits in Canada. *Choices, 1*(2). Available at: www.irpp.org

Phipps, S., Burton, P., & Lethbridge, L. (2001). In and out of the labor market: Long-term income consequences of interruptions in paid work. *The Canadian Journal of Economics, 34*(2), 411–429.

Phipps, S., MacDonald, M., & MacPhail, F. (2001). Gender equity within families versus better targeting: An assessment of the family income supplement to employment insurance benefits. *Canadian Public Policy, 27*(4), 423–446.

Rainwater, L., & Smeeding, T. M. (2003). *Poor kids in a rich country: America's children in comparative perspective*. New York: Russell Sage Foundation.

Social Security Programs Throughout the World. (2004, September). Washington, DC: U.S. Dept. of Health, Education and Welfare, Social Security Administration, Division of Program Research.

The world Bank (2008). International comparison program. Availabe at www.worldbank.org/data/icp

Wisensale, S. K. (2001). *Family leave policy: The political economy of work and family in America*. Armonk, New York: M.E. Sharpe.

Child Poverty in Upper-Income Countries: Lessons from the Luxembourg Income Study

Janet C. Gornick and Markus Jäntti

1 Introduction and Background

Few social and economic problems are more compelling than child poverty. While poverty is evident throughout the life cycle—affecting children, prime-age adults and the elderly—poverty among children has particular resonance. Child poverty captures our attention for several reasons: it is widely held that children need and deserve protection from hardship; most children have no control over their economic circumstances; deprivation during childhood can have lifelong consequences; and some of the effects of child poverty have spillover effects. Child poverty in rich countries is especially compelling, because it is rooted not so much in scarce aggregate resources but mainly in distributional arrangements, both private and public.

It is well-established that, within most industrialized countries, children's likelihood of being poor is shaped, in part, by their family demography and by their parents' attachment to the labor market. It has also been established that child poverty varies widely across countries, and a substantial share of that variation is due to cross-national diversity in core institutions, including labor market structures and tax and transfer policies. A growing body of research, much of it drawing on the Luxembourg Income Study (LIS), demonstrates that upper-income countries with relatively similar demographic characteristics report remarkably different poverty outcomes. Stark variation is evident in child poverty rates based on both market-income and post-tax-and-transfer income.

As we report in this chapter, for example, after accounting for taxes and transfers, fewer than 5% of children in Denmark, Finland, Norway and Sweden live in poor

J.C. Gornick (✉)
Luxembourg Income Study; Political Science and Sociology, The Graduate center, City University of New York, USA
e-mail: jgornick@gc.cuny.edu

For readers' ease, throughout this chapter, when we cite studies based on LIS, we cite the versions that appear in the LIS Working Paper series. Several of these LIS Working Papers have been subsequently published; the publication information appears on-line.

S.B. Kamerman et al. (eds.), *From Child Welfare to Child Well-Being*, Children's Well-Being: Indicators and Research 1, DOI 10.1007/978-90-481-3377-2_19, © Springer Science+Business Media B.V. 2010

households. In comparison, 6–9% of children are poor in Germany, the Netherlands and Switzerland; 11–20% in Australia, Canada, the United Kingdom (UK), Israel and Poland; and fully 22% in the United States (US). Two countries with much in common, the UK and the US, provide a telling illustration of the powerful role played by both labor market patterns and public policy. In the UK, before accounting for taxes and transfers, 34% of children are poor; after taxes and transfers, 19% (about half as many) are poor. In the US, before taxes and transfers, 25% are poor (a lower rate than in the UK) and, after taxes and transfers, still 22% (higher than in the UK).[1] While market outcomes clearly matter, for many children, their risk of living in poverty is strongly shaped by the design of their countries' instruments of redistribution.

In this chapter, we draw on the resources of the Luxembourg Income Study, a cross-national data archive and research institute, to sketch a portrait of children's poverty across a large number of upper-income countries. In Section 2, we present highlights from over two decades of LIS-based research on child poverty. We first draw on a set of country-level indicators that LIS makes available (known as the LIS *Key Figures*) to sketch a broad-brush portrait of child poverty across 30 countries over time. We then survey the large LIS-based literature on child poverty that has been reported in scores of articles and books. We focus on research that seeks to explain cross-national variation in child poverty levels and synthesize in detail findings from three especially comprehensive studies of child poverty.

In Section 3, we present an original snapshot of contemporary child poverty, in which we focus on 13 upper-income[2] countries as of approximately 2000. After describing our data and methods, we present our findings. We begin by offering a descriptive overview of poverty among all households and among households with children. In these comparisons, we present multiple poverty measures—both relative and absolute, both pre- and post-taxes and transfers—and we report the magnitude of poverty reduction due to taxes and transfers. Drawing on substantive lessons from the LIS-based literature on the determinants of child poverty (including our own earlier work), we assess, within countries, the association between child poverty and three consequential characteristics: the type of family in which a child resides, parents' level of educational attainment, and parents' engagement in paid work. Throughout this section, we report child poverty outcomes—poverty levels and intra-country disparities in children's risk of poverty—across countries. We emphasize variation across established models of social welfare provision. In Section 4, we offer conclusions.

---

[1] The poverty outcomes reported in the paragraph are taken from Table 2, presented later.

[2] The World Bank classifies countries into four income categories—high, upper-middle, lower-middle, and low-based on per capita GDP. As of the early 2000s, 12 of our 13 study countries were classified as "high income". One, Poland, was classified as "upper-middle income". Throughout this chapter, we use the term "upper income" to refer to the top two groups: high and upper-middle.

2 Quarter Century of LIS Research: What Have We Learned?

2.1 The Luxembourg Income Study as a Resource

Since its founding in 1983, LIS has been a valuable, and widely used, resource for studying children's economic wellbeing across countries and over time. LIS is a public-access data archive, now containing microdata (i.e., data at the household- and person-level), from over 30 countries, for up to six time points (or more in a few cases). The LIS staff acquires datasets, mostly based on national household income surveys, harmonizes these datasets *ex post* into a common template, and makes the harmonized data available to researchers around the world.[3] Thus far, LIS primarily contains datasets from high-income countries—the majority of which are in Europe—with a relatively small number from upper-middle income countries. Over the next 3–5 years, datasets will be added from 15 to 20 middle-income countries; that expansion will enable researchers to study children's economic wellbeing in a more globalized context.

The LIS data are made available through two main channels. First, LIS produces a set of national-level statistics, known at the LIS *Key Figures*. These include a series of poverty and inequality measures, over time, disaggregated across various demographic groups, one of which is children. These standardized indicators are available for public use, with no restrictions, on the LIS website. Second, LIS makes the harmonized microdata available to registered users, via a remote-access system, enabling researchers to use the LIS microdata to tackle highly tailored questions and to use a range of statistical tools. In the next section, we summarize the main patterns and recent trends in child poverty, as evident in the LIS *Key Figures*. After that, we review core findings from the large body of LIS research on child poverty; most of that research has been conducted using the LIS microdata directly.

2.2 The LIS Key Figures: Variation Across Countries and Over Time

Across the 30 countries included in the LIS *Key Figures*, the likelihood that children live in poverty varies dramatically. Child poverty rates—defined as the percentage of children living in households with post-tax-and-transfer income less than 50% of the country's household-size-adjusted median—are available for all 30 countries, at some point during the years bounded by the middle 1990s and approximately 2000. During that time period, child poverty varied from 5% or less in four countries (Denmark, Finland, Norway, Sweden), 6–10% in 13 countries (Netherlands, Czech Republic, Slovenia, Taiwan, Belgium, Austria, France,

---

[3] The LIS datasets include income, labor market, and demographic indicators. Detailed information on the original surveys and on the harmonized datasets is available at http://www.lisproject. org/techdoc

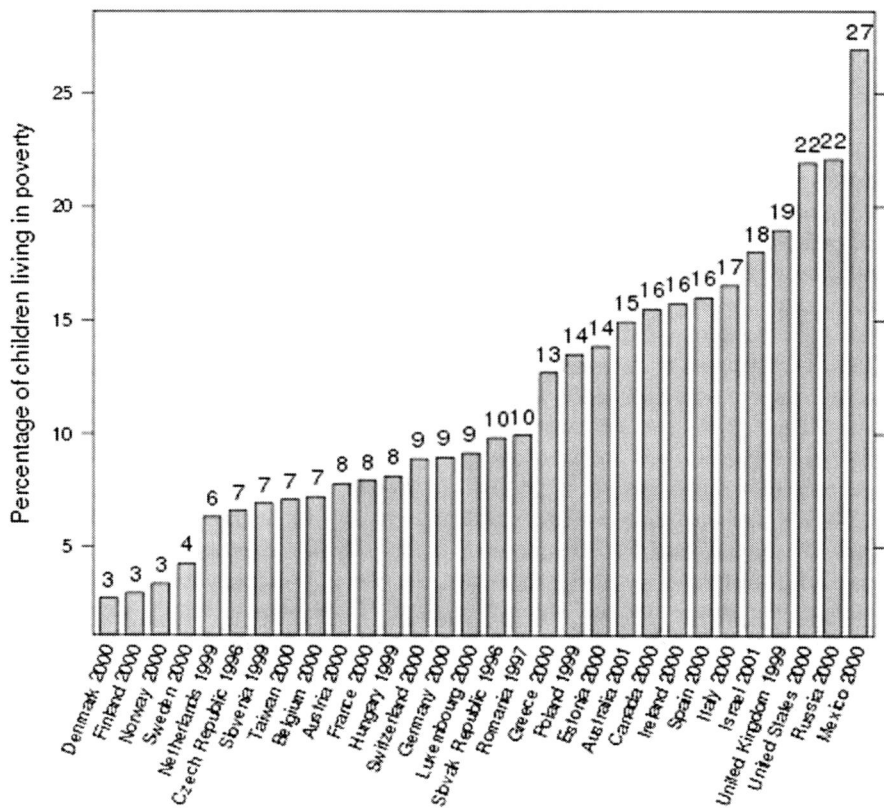

Fig. 1 Child poverty rates (disposable household income of less than 50% median household income).
Source: LIS datasets, late 1990s to early 2000s

Hungary, Switzerland, Germany, Luxembourg, Slovak Republic, Romania), 11–20% in 10 countries (Greece, Poland, Estonia, Australia, Canada, Ireland, Spain, Italy, Israel, UK), and more than 20% in 3 (Mexico, Russia, and the US). These child poverty rates are depicted in Fig. 1:

Moreover, the LIS *Key Figures* reveal that children's *relative* economic wellbeing within their own countries also varies sharply. Using the same poverty measure as in Fig. 1, the *Key Figures* indicate that in nine countries (Belgium, Denmark, Finland, Greece, Norway, Slovenia, Sweden, Taiwan, and the UK) children are substantially *less* likely to be poor than the population at large, while in two countries (Austria and Ireland) they are about equally likely to be poor as all persons. In the other nineteen countries, remarkably, children are substantially *more* likely to be poor than is the larger population. In fully nine countries, children are more than 20% more likely to be poor than is the overall population. This result—disproportionately high child poverty—is found in countries with otherwise diverse child poverty outcomes: Canada, Czech Republic, Hungary, Italy, Luxembourg, Mexico, Netherlands, Slovak Republic, and the US.[4]

Finally, the LIS *Key Figures* enable an assessment of child poverty rates over time. For most (but not all) of the countries included in LIS, we can assess child poverty trends during the decade of the 1990s. The *Key Figures* reveal an overall worsening of the economic wellbeing of children during the 1990s, as captured in relative poverty rates (using the 50% of median standard). In most of the LIS countries, child poverty rates increased during these years—in some cases, by a small increment, in others by a substantial amount. For example, in Israel, child poverty rose from 12% in 1992 to 18% in 2001; in Luxembourg, from 5% in 1991 to 9% in 2000, in Poland, from 8% in 1992 to 18% in 1999; and in Spain from 12% in 1990 to 16% in 2000. While governments across the upper-income countries often cite reducing child poverty as a policy priority, in more cases than not, its prevalence has risen in recent years. At the same, in a few countries, child poverty rates declined during the 1990s. That was the case in 2 high-poverty countries, the UK and the US. In the UK, the poverty rate among children fell from 18% in 1991 to 10% in 1999; in the US, child poverty dropped from nearly 26% in 1991 to 22% in 2000. In neither case was a similar decline seen in the overall national poverty rate.

2.3 The LIS Literature: The Search for Explanations

The issue of child poverty has attracted considerable attention among scholars using the LIS microdata. Over the last 25 years, nearly fifty LIS Working Papers have included child poverty outcomes; in many of these, child poverty is the *central* concern of the paper.[5] These studies are diverse with respect to conceptual approaches, poverty measures, countries included, years covered, and substantive focus. Several focus on cross-national variation in within-country poverty determinants; many aim to identify and decompose the determinants of cross-national variation.

Several LIS-based studies have assessed child poverty outcomes in general, often with a focus on measurement standards and methods (see, e.g., Brady, 2004; Corak, 2005; Findlay & Wright, 1992; Marx & van den Bosch, 1996; Smeeding & Rainwater, 1995). Many studies have focused on the effects of household composition on children's likelihood of being poor (see, e.g., Bane & Zenteno, 2005; Beaujot & Liu, 2002; Gornick & Pavetti, 1990; Redmond, 2000; Weinshenker & Heuveline, 2006); throughout these studies, single motherhood has received the most sustained attention. Other studies have focused on the effects of parents', especially mothers' employment and earnings (see, e.g., Bradbury & Jäntti, 1999; Misra, Budig, & Moller, 2006; Moller & Misra, 2005; Munzi & Smeeding, 2006;

---

[4] It should be noted that whether children have higher or lower poverty rates, compared to the overall population, may depend on the specific equivalences scale that is used.

[5] All LIS Working Papers are available on-line; see http://www.lisproject.org/publications/wpapers.htm

Smeeding, Christopher, Phillips, McLanahan, & England, 1999; Solera, 1998). Not surprisingly, a central theme cutting across LIS studies on child poverty is the impact of country-level institutions, primarily income tax and transfers policies (see, e.g., Bäckman, 2005; Bradshaw & Chen, 1996; Brady, 2005; Brady, Fullerton, & Cross, 2008; Cantillon & van den Bosch, 2002; D'Ambrosio & Gradin, 2000; Jäntti & Danziger, 1992; Jeandidier & Albiser, 2001; Kuivalainen, 2005; Makines, 1998; Orsini, 2001; Scott, 2008; Skinner, Bradshaw, & Davidson, 2008; Smeeding, 2005; Smeeding & Torrey, 1988; Smeeding, Rainwater, & Danziger, 1995; Waddoups, 2004).

In the remainder of this section, we synthesize the primary findings from three especially comprehensive studies of child poverty, all using the LIS data: a 1999 UNICEF report by Bruce Bradbury and Markus Jäntti, a 2003 book by Lee Rainwater and Timothy Smeeding, and a 2008 journal article by Wen-Hao Chen and Miles Corak. In each of these three studies, the core questions concern explanations for cross-country variation in child poverty outcomes.

Bradbury & Jäntti (1999) studied child poverty across 25 LIS countries as of the early and middle-1990s. One of their central goals was to analyze the sources of cross-national variation, using both relative and absolute measures of poverty. First, Bradbury and Jäntti found that the Nordic and Western European countries usually have low rates of child poverty, whereas Southern European and English-speaking countries typically report high rates. They noted that, while the country rankings differ somewhat between results using relative versus absolute poverty measures, this broad grouping of countries was robust across these two approaches. In contrast, the rankings of most of the transition countries (mainly the former Eastern bloc countries) with respect to child poverty rates depended on which poverty measure was used—a result that is not especially surprising, given that average real incomes in the transition countries are markedly lower than in most of the other study countries. They also found that, across the upper-income countries studied, those with higher levels of national income tended to have lower real poverty rates—although the US emerged as a marked exception, with a substantially higher level of child poverty than its national income would predict.

Bradbury and Jäntti reported that, while much literature appropriately focuses on variation in welfare state institutions when accounting for the diversity of child poverty outcomes across countries, variation in the market incomes received by the families of disadvantaged children was an even more powerful explanatory factor. With regard to market income, they found that the English-speaking countries in particular stood out. Even though these countries are usually categorized as "welfare laggards" due to their low aggregate levels of social expenditures, the tight targeting of these expenditures means that, in most cases, governments actually provide substantial income transfers to their most needy children (the US being an exception). The living standards of disadvantaged children in these countries, however, remain relatively low because of their families' limited labor market incomes. They reported that the higher living standards of the most disadvantaged children in the "welfare leaders" (particularly the Nordic countries) is due largely to the higher market incomes in these families.

In the end, Bradbury and Jäntti conclude that it is not clear whether diverse labor market outcomes are driven by varied employment and social policies (such as child care subsidies), by the different incentive structures imposed by different targeting patterns, or by other factors. However, their results do suggest that an understanding of child poverty variation requires that serious attention be paid to labor market environments and outcomes. They close with this observation: "It appears to us, in conclusion, that policy-makers who are seriously concerned about the economic well-being of their countries' children, need to closely and critically examine the answer to this question: 'Which features of labor markets best protect the living standards of children?' (Bradbury & Jäntti, 1999, p. 72)."

Rainwater and Smeeding consolidated much of their earlier LIS-based research on child poverty, and expanded it, in their 2003 book *Poor Kids in a Rich Country: America's Children in Comparative Perspective.* The book is organized around several lines of inquiry, among them: cross-national variation in child poverty rates; the effects of inequality and population characteristics on child poverty; and the role of different forms of income in alleviating child poverty in both one-parent families and two-parent families.

Focused on the middle-1990s, Rainwater and Smeeding assessed child poverty variation across 15 countries: Australia, Canada, the US, and twelve diverse European countries. Overall, they found the same country clusters reported by Bradbury and Jantti. Using the 50%-of-median standard, Rainwater and Smeeding report the highest child poverty rate in the US (20%), followed by Italy, the UK, Canada, Australia, and Spain (12–20%). Moderate child poverty rates (5–10%) were reported across five Western European countries (Germany, France, Netherlands, Switzerland, Belgium) and the lowest poverty rates (2–4%) were found in the four Nordic countries (Denmark, Norway, Finland, and Sweden).

To understand the inequality context of this observed variation in child poverty, Rainwater and Smeeding ranked their study countries by the size of their middle class and arrived at nearly the same findings (as their poverty results). They found, at one inequality pole, several countries in northern Europe (with large middle-classes and low poverty) and, at the other inequality pole, they placed the US along with Italy and the UK. They conclude this analysis with a finding about the US that is at odds with the traditional "American story"—which tells us that the high level of income inequality in the US generates favorable levels of economic growth, which in turn raises the standard of living of the worst-off Americans, relative to their European counterparts. In fact, Rainwater and Smeeding find that the real income level of America's poorest children is actually *lower* than that of their counterparts in many other LIS countries. Specifically, in half of their comparison countries, the poorest third of children are better off in real terms than are their American peers. In most of the remaining comparison countries, children in the lowest fifth of the income distribution are as well off, or better off, than are similarly positioned American children.

Rainwater and Smeeding assessed the role that demography plays in explaining variability in child poverty rates, where demography includes the household's age composition, gender composition, and size, as well as the earning status (yes/no) of the head, spouse and other household adults. With their eye on explaining the exceptionally high US child poverty rates, they concluded that demography is by no means destiny: the demographic composition of the US contributes to its higher child poverty with respect to only half of their study countries and, in most of those cases, its contribution is modest. Rainwater and Smeeding summarize their conclusion: "Compared with institutional factors, demographic differences play only a minor role in the differences among countries. It is primarily the US income packaging that produces high child poverty rates, not exceptional US demography (Rainwater & Smeeding, 2003)." Keeping their focus on the US, Rainwater and Smeeding further conclude that variation across countries in the number of household earners explains little of the child poverty variation: "Whatever the differences between the United States and other countries in the proportion of children who live in families with no earners, one earner, or two earners, we observe that American child poverty rates are considerably higher for each earner type" (Rainwater & Smeeding, 2003, p. 56).

At the heart of Rainwater and Smeeding's book is an analysis of cross-country variation in income packaging. Noting that the vast majority of children in all of their study countries live in two-parent families, they first focus on these families. Here, their bottom-line finding is largely consistent with that of Bradbury and Jäntti: earnings received by the families of children in the lowest income quintile are slightly less strongly related to poverty rates than is transfer income—but both are important explanatory factors. In other words, among two-parent families, in addition to the structure and generosity of income supports, earnings matter a great deal in explaining cross-country variation in child poverty rates.[6]

Rainwater and Smeeding then analyze single-parent families, among whom child poverty rates are higher in all countries. As with two-parent families, they conclude that the demographic and labor-supply variations in single-mother families in these fifteen countries do not have much effect on child poverty rates. On the other hand, Rainwater and Smeeding conclude, again as with two-parent families, levels of earnings matter: "if we think of the poverty rate for children in single-mother families as a function of mothers' earnings and social transfers, we find that across these fifteen countries market income (principally earnings) seems to play a larger role than transfers, although both are important (Rainwater & Smeeding, 2003, p. 122)".

Finally, we turn our attention to Chen and Corak, whose 2008 *Demography* article, "Child Poverty and Changes in Child Poverty", assessed child poverty trends during the 1990s in the US and eleven European countries. Chen and Corak take a somewhat novel approach to studying change over time. To adopt what they describe as "the least challenging standard by which to judge progress (Chen & Corak, 2008, p. 538)", they use a poverty line fixed in the early 1990s (using the

---

[6] Rainwater and Smeeding address the somewhat puzzling contradiction between their finding (above), that the number of earners explains little (across countries), yet the level of earnings is important: "the reason that some countries have high two-parent child poverty rates and others have low rates has more to do with the mix of earnings and transfers and the level of earnings than with whether families include an earner per se (Rainwater & Smeeding, 2003, p. 95)."

50%-of-median standard) and adjust it over time only by applying country-specific consumer price indices. Using their fixed-line standard, they found that, during the 1990s, child poverty rates rose in three countries (West Germany, Italy and Hungary); remained essentially unchanged in six (Canada, Sweden, Luxembourg, Belgium, the Netherlands, and Finland); and fell in three—one low-poverty country (Norway) and two high-poverty countries (the UK and the US).

Based on a complex analysis of the factors underlying the trends that they report, Chen and Corak draw three lessons. First, family and demographic shifts played a relative minor role in explaining child poverty trends throughout the 1990s (partly because these factors evolve slowly). That said, in eleven of the twelve study countries, to the extent that changes in parental characteristics had an effect, they lowered child poverty rates. Second, changes in employment and earnings mattered much more. In nine of the twelve countries in their study, the increased labor market engagement of mothers consistently mattered—in the direction of lowering child poverty rates. Chen and Corak also found that, in several countries, decreases in the employment rates and earnings of fathers also mattered, contributing to increased child poverty rates. Third, income transfer policy reforms aimed at raising labor supply may or may not increase families' post-tax-and-transfer income. Social policy reforms interact in complex ways with other factors, such as the overall level of child poverty, the extent and functioning of the service and other sectors, and the overall hospitability of the labor market to low-skilled and other disadvantaged workers. Chen and Corak sum up with a cautionary note to policy-makers: "there is no single road to lower child poverty rates. The conduct of social policy needs to be thought through in conjunction with the nature of labor markets (Chen & Corak, 2008, p. 552)." Thus, like both Bradbury & Jäntti (1999), and Rainwater & Smeeding (2003), Corak and Chen find that, in explaining cross-national variation in child poverty, demographic variation matters modestly, while national labor market patterns and social policy factors both matter a great deal—and they matter via complex and interacting mechanisms.

3 Snapshot of Contemporary Child Poverty: A Comparison of 13 Countries

3.1 Data and Methods

For our own empirical analyses, we use datasets from LIS's Wave V (Release 2), which is centered on the year 2000.[7] We selected thirteen diverse countries for comparison: Australia, Canada, Denmark, Finland, Germany, Israel, the Netherlands, Norway, Poland, Sweden, Switzerland, the UK and the US. The main criterion for

---

[7] There is some variation within this wave. The datasets from the Netherlands, Poland and the UK pertain to 1999. The datasets from Australia and Israel report income in 2001. The rest are from the year 2000.

inclusion was the availability of pre-tax ("gross") income, so that we could meaning-fully assess, across all of our study countries, the extent to which taxes and transfers reduce market-generated poverty. While all LIS datasets provide data on pre-transfer income, only a subset provides data on pre-tax income.

Income indicators. As is common in research using the LIS data, we use two main income variables, market income and disposable income; both are summary income variables, constructed and provided by LIS. Market income (referred to by LIS as MI) includes earnings, cash property income, and income from occu-pational pensions. Household disposable income (known in the LIS literature as DPI) is the sum of market income plus private transfers, public social insurance, and public social assistance—net of income taxes and mandatory payroll taxes.[8] Throughout this chapter, we adjust household income for household size (to "equiv-alize" wellbeing across households of different sizes), using a common equivalence scale transformation, in which adjusted income equals unadjusted income divided by the square root of household size; that represents the mid-point between the two extreme assumptions of no economies of scale and perfect economies of scale.

Poverty measures. We report poverty rates, using multiple measures. In each case, we capture person-level poverty rates, although they are based on household incomes. In other words, our unit of analysis is the individual; we report the prob-ability that individuals—primarily children—live in poor households. Specifically, we assign the equivalized household income to each household member and esti-mate all results at the person level. In the first three tables, we report relative poverty rates, based on both market income and disposable income, in each case using three poverty lines: 40, 50, and 60% of median (size-adjusted) household disposable income. Each of these three poverty lines captures a different depth of poverty. The 50% standard is most often used in the LIS literature on poverty; the 40% line captures what is sometimes referred to as "severe poverty" while the 60% line, commonly employed by the European Union, is often labeled "near poverty".

In these first three tables, we also report poverty rates, using the United States' poverty line (marked "US line") as the threshold. The US line, usually described as an *absolute* poverty line, is based on a longstanding US government measure derived from the estimated cost of a basket of food for a given family size, and annually adjusted for inflation. We convert the US line for a family of four to a single-person poverty line using our equivalence scale—the square root of family size—and apply that to all cases. We use the OECD's purchasing power parity (PPP) exchange rates to convert those amounts to international dollars.

Finally, we calculate and report poverty reduction across countries, which is cap-tured as the poverty rate based on market income minus the poverty rate based on disposable income. This difference is an indicator, albeit a somewhat crude one, of the extent to which states lift poor populations out of poverty, using the main instruments of income redistribution. It is important to note that this indicator of

---

[8] Imputed rents, and irregular incomes, such as lump sums and capital gains and losses are not included in LIS DPI.

poverty reduction reflects an accounting exercise; it does not account for the possibility that market income (and thus poverty patterns based on market income) might be quite different if tax-and-transfer programs did not exist. The final four tables—which disaggregate poverty rates by (household) demographic and labor market characteristics—report poverty based on disposable income only, using the 50%-of-median relative poverty measure.

Demographic and labor market variables. To assess the influence of factors that affect the risk of poverty among children, we construct indicators of family structure, educational attainment, and labor market status. We first classify children as living with their *single parent* (mother or father), with *two parents*, or in *other* families (i.e., families in which children reside with persons other than their own parents). We also classify children according to their parents' educational attainment, more precisely the educational attainment of the head of the household in which they live. Attainment is measured as *low*, *medium* or *high*, using the standardized recodes provided by LIS.[9] Low educational attainment includes those who have not completed upper secondary education; medium refers to those who have completed upper secondary education and non-specialized vocational education, and high includes those who have completed specialized vocational education, post-secondary education and beyond. Where LIS did not provide recodes, we constructed them, adhering to these educational cutoffs as closely as possible.

In addition, we construct a measure of labor market attachment, categorizing parents as having either *low* or *medium/high* labor market status. We code persons as having low labor market status if their earnings are in the lowest fifth of the earnings distribution, including those with no earnings; women's and men's distributions are constructed separately. Persons not in the bottom fifth are coded as having medium/high labor market status.

3.2 Social Policy Regimes

To place the variation across our thirteen countries into institutional context, when we present our results, we group the countries into four country clusters. In the text and tables, we refer to these groupings by their geographic/regional or linguistic characteristics. We classify Germany, the Netherlands and Switzerland as *Continental* countries; Denmark, Finland, Norway and Sweden as *Nordic* countries; and Australia, Canada, the UK and US as *Anglophone* countries.[10] We also include but do not categorize, two other countries, Israel and Poland. Of course, ultimately it is not geography, region or language that makes these groupings

---

[9] LIS education recodes are available at http://www.lisproject.org/techdoc/education-level/education-level.htm

[10] Following the convention in cross-national research, we refer to Canada as Anglophone, although it is officially bilingual, part Anglophone and part Francophone.

meaningful for our analyses of child poverty across countries. These clusters are meaningful for our study because of their well-established institutional commonalties. Substantial within-cluster variability is evident in all of these groups, but overall they are characterized by important common features. In this section, we offer a brief synopsis of these institutional features—with a focus on policy configurations as they shape both redistribution overall and women's employment patterns.

The clusters that we employ here draw heavily on the work of Danish sociologist Gøsta Esping-Andersen (1990)—and on the many extensions to his work contributed by feminist scholars (for a review, see Gornick & Meyers, 2003). Esping-Andersen and other scholars have classified the major welfare states of the industrialized west into three clusters, each characterized by shared principles of social welfare entitlement and relatively homogeneous outcomes. The Continental countries are characterized as typically tying transfers to earnings and occupation, with public provisions tending to replicate market-generated distributional outcomes. In the Continental countries, social policy is also shaped by the principle of subsidiarity, which stresses the primacy of the family and community for providing dependent care and other social supports. In contrast, social policy in the Nordic countries is characterized as organized along social democratic lines, with entitlements linked to social rights. The Nordic policy framework has also historically emphasized gender equality, especially with respect to rates of labor force participation. In yet another contrast, social benefits in the Anglophone countries are typically residual in design, reflecting and preserving consumer and employer markets, with most entitlements derived from need based on limited resources. The Anglophone countries, especially the US and Canada, also have labor market and social policy features associated with relatively high women's employment rates.[11]

Many scholars, across disciplines, have criticized this regime-type framework. Some have argued that it poorly captures women's rights and needs, especially in relation to unpaid work. Others are concerned by intra-cluster heterogeneity, with some critics breaking out new clusters. While we agree with these arguments, we make use of these country clusters—however imperfect—because they provide a helpful organizing framework for assessing cross-national variation among upper-income countries. They help us to identify empirical patterns across our comparison countries and they bring into relief the importance of policy configurations for poverty reduction. Working with these well-known groupings will also allow comparative scholars to situate our findings into the larger literature on the nature and consequences of social policy variation across upper-income countries.

---

[11] While few welfare state typologies include either Israel or Poland, Israel's social policy is often described as a mix of Continental European and developing-country features, and Poland's as still transitioning from state socialist to a model that mixes liberal features (included a reliance on means-tested benefits) with elements that reduce women's labor market attachment from typically high pre-transition levels.

4 Findings

We begin with a presentation of overall poverty rates across our thirteen countries, imposing no age cut. (See Table 1, which indicates the percentage of all persons who live in poor households). We first report poverty rates based on market-income—relative to 40, 50, and 60% of median household disposable income. Considering simple (unweighted) country-group averages, at all three relative thresholds, poverty rates are ranked similarly: highest in the Israel-Poland pair, followed by the Anglophone and Nordic countries (which are nearly tied), and finally by the Continental cluster. Using the US poverty threshold, we see a similar pattern, but the magnitudes shift markedly. When poverty is captured using this real income standard, poverty rates in the Israel-Poland pair are dramatically higher. That is mainly due to the extremely high poverty rate, using this measure, reported in Poland (82.7%), the one country in our study that is not classified as high income.

Next we turn to poverty rates based on post-tax-and-transfer (or "disposable") household income (see the second vertical panel of Table 1). Three clear findings emerge. First, in every case, disposable-income poverty rates are lower than the market-based rates. This result is not surprising, but it confirms that, on average, at this part of the income distribution, the tax-and-transfer systems in these countries consistently augment household income—in other words, the incoming transfers exceed the outgoing taxes. Second, considering relative poverty rates, the disposable-income results are somewhat different than the market-income results. The ranking of the countries shifts, such that the lowest poverty cluster is now the Nordic cluster—indicating that the Nordic countries have more redistributive tax/benefit systems. Third, when the US poverty line is applied across countries, the clusters shift again, with the Continental countries now reporting lower poverty than the Nordic countries. That result is driven by the relatively high Finnish and Swedish poverty rates, in real terms, although the difference between these two country groups is small.

The magnitude of poverty reduction, calculated as the market-income poverty rate minus the disposable-income poverty rate, is also reported here (see the third vertical panel of Table 1). This indicator captures the "amount" of poverty "removed" when taxes and transfers are considered. Focusing on the 50% relative poverty standard, we see that the Israel-Poland pair (21.0 percentage points) and the Nordic countries (20.9 percentage points) report the most poverty reduction, followed by the Continental and Anglophone clusters (16.6 and 12.8 percentage points, respectively). One especially remarkable finding in this panel is the US result, where we see the least poverty reduction (7.5 percentage points) across all thirteen countries. When we consider poverty reduction based on the US real-income standard, one strong finding emerges. The amount of poverty reduced in the Nordic, Continental and Anglophone clusters remains about the same, but now the lower-income Israel-Poland pair reduces the least poverty (10.2 points in Israel and only 3.5 points in Poland). In Poland, the tax-and-transfer system clearly raises household income; however, except in a small number of cases, it does not raise Polish incomes to the

Table 1 Percentage of all persons living in poor households

	market income				disposable income				poverty reduction [MI less DPI]			
	40% DPI	50% DPI	60% DPI	US line	40% DPI	50% DPI	60% DPI	US line	40% DPI	50% DPI	60% DPI	US line
Continental												
Germany	27.6	30.0	32.6	29.1	4.6	8.4	13.4	6.7	23.0	21.6	19.1	22.4
Netherlands	17.4	20.0	22.2	18.5	2.6	5.0	11.1	3.4	14.9	15.0	11.1	15.1
Switzerland	18.0	20.7	23.2	18.0	3.9	7.7	13.5	3.9	14.1	13.1	9.6	14.1
average	*21.0*	*23.6*	*26.0*	*21.9*	*3.7*	*7.0*	*12.7*	*4.7*	*17.3*	*16.6*	*13.3*	*17.2*
Nordic												
Denmark	22.4	24.8	27.3	23.9	2.0	5.4	13.1	3.9	20.4	19.4	14.2	20.0
Finland	27.1	30.1	33.1	32.7	2.2	5.4	12.4	11.7	24.9	24.7	20.7	21.0
Norway	20.4	23.4	26.4	21.1	3.0	6.5	12.3	3.4	17.3	16.9	14.1	17.6
Sweden	26.5	29.1	31.9	30.5	3.8	6.6	12.3	9.0	22.7	22.5	19.6	21.5
average	*24.1*	*26.9*	*29.7*	*27.0*	*2.8*	*6.0*	*12.5*	*7.0*	*21.4*	*20.9*	*17.1*	*20.0*
Other												
Israel	24.7	29.9	34.6	37.4	7.5	15.6	23.4	27.1	17.1	14.3	11.1	10.2
Poland	36.1	41.7	47.0	82.7	9.5	14.1	20.0	79.2	26.6	27.6	27.0	3.5
average	*30.4*	*35.8*	*40.8*	*60.0*	*8.5*	*14.8*	*21.7*	*53.2*	*21.9*	*21.0*	*19.0*	*6.9*
Anglophone												
Australia	24.2	26.9	30.3	27.3	5.6	12.2	20.5	13.8	18.6	14.7	9.8	13.4
Canada	20.1	23.7	27.6	21.1	7.2	12.4	18.9	8.2	12.9	11.3	8.7	12.9
United Kingdom	28.6	31.6	34.2	32.3	6.2	13.7	22.0	16.6	22.4	17.9	12.2	15.8
United States	20.4	24.8	29.2	18.8	11.1	17.3	24.0	9.1	9.2	7.5	5.2	9.8
average	*23.3*	*26.7*	*30.3*	*24.9*	*7.5*	*13.9*	*21.3*	*11.9*	*15.8*	*12.8*	*9.0*	*13.0*

notes: Includes persons of all ages; in the first four columns, cells report poverty rates based on market income, with poverty lines drawn at 40, 50, and 60 percent of median disposable income, and at the US poverty line; in the second four columns, the cells report poverty rates based on disposable income, with poverty lines drawn at 40, 50, and 60 percent of median disposable income, and at the US poverty line; in the last four columns, cells report the difference between market-income poverty and disposable-income poverty (always relative to the same poverty line).

level of the US poverty threshold. That is not surprising, given that the US line falls within Poland's top quintile group, that is, at a place in the income distribution that, in Poland, would not be considered poor.

Next, we turn to child poverty rates with respect to children under age eighteen (see Table 2). The first finding in Table 2 is that the cross-country pattern with respect to market-income relative poverty is broadly similar to that of persons of all ages—with an important difference: poverty rates in the Nordic countries are now substantially lower than in the Anglophone countries. The relative poverty portrait based on disposable income is also similar (to all persons); the lowest poverty cluster is again the Nordic cluster.[12]

Second, we find that using multiple poverty thresholds increases our understanding of child poverty patterns. The cross-country rankings are quite robust with respect to which threshold is used. At all three poverty levels—40, 50, and 60% of the median—the ranking of the country cluster averages is the same. But the prevalence of poverty varies markedly across the three thresholds. For example, with respect to market income, in the Anglophone countries, while 26.4% of children, on average, are poor (at 50%), 30.7%—nearly one third—are poor when we apply the "near poor" line (at 60%). Even more remarkably, fully 22.5% are poor using the "severe poverty" line (at 40%); in other words, with respect to market income, fully 85% of poor children are severely poor. Similar results are seen elsewhere; in the other three country clusters, 80–83% of poor children are severely poor. When we turn from market- to disposable-income poverty, the story shifts. In each country group, the percentage of poor children that is severely poor is much lower—46% in the Nordic countries, 52–54% in the Anglophone and Continental countries, and 55% in the Israel-Poland pairing. This pattern indicates that, overall, taxes and transfers play an especially crucial role in preventing poverty among families with the most limited market incomes.

Third, the child poverty reduction results are somewhat similar to the all-person results with respect to mitigating relative poverty. Using the 50% relative poverty standard, we see that the Israel-Poland pair reports the most poverty reduction (16.3 percentage points), followed by the Nordic countries (12.6 percentage points), then the Anglophone (9.1 percentage points) and Continental (4.4 percentage points) countries. Again we see exceptionally little poverty reduction in the US case (3.0 percentage points), but here the US is no longer the least poverty-reducing country; Switzerland reduces even less child poverty (1.9 percentage points). In fact, Switzerland's tax-and-transfer system is so unfavorable towards families with children that—at the 60%-of-median standard—Swiss families report a modestly *higher* poverty rate after taxes and transfers (15%) than they do before (13.4%).

---

[12] There are some small discrepancies between the child poverty rates presented in Fig. 1 (based on the LIS Key Figures) and in Table 2 (based on our own calculations). Those are due to minor differences in the treatment of extreme values.

Table 2 Percentage of all children (<18 years old) living in poor households

	market income				disposable income				poverty reduction [MI less DPI]				ratio of all children to all persons *Table 2 compared to Table 1*		
	40% DPI	50% DPI	60% DPI	US line	40% DPI	50% DPI	60% DPI	US line	40% DPI	50% DPI	60% DPI	US line	market income poverty, 50% DPI	disposable income poverty, 50% DPI	poverty reduction, 50% DPI
Continental															
Germany	14.0	16.4	20.1	15.5	5.5	9.0	14.3	7.5	8.5	7.4	5.8	8.0	0.55	1.07	0.34
Netherlands	8.4	10.3	12.2	9.4	3.0	6.5	12.0	4.3	5.4	3.9	0.2	5.1	0.52	1.29	0.26
Switzerland	7.5	10.8	13.4	7.5	4.6	8.9	15.0	4.6	2.9	1.9	-1.7	2.9	0.52	1.16	0.14
average	*10.0*	*12.5*	*15.2*	*10.8*	*4.4*	*8.1*	*13.8*	*5.5*	*5.6*	*4.4*	*1.4*	*5.3*	*0.53*	*1.18*	*0.25*
Nordic															
Denmark	12.5	14.5	17.3	13.7	1.2	2.7	8.9	2.0	11.3	11.7	8.4	11.8	0.58	0.51	0.61
Finland	14.1	17.8	21.9	21.2	1.5	3.1	8.4	7.9	12.5	14.7	13.5	13.3	0.59	0.57	0.60
Norway	10.6	13.5	17.2	11.0	1.9	3.7	7.8	2.2	8.6	9.8	9.4	8.7	0.58	0.57	0.58
Sweden	16.0	18.5	22.5	20.1	1.8	4.3	9.2	5.9	14.2	14.2	13.3	14.2	0.63	0.64	0.63
average	*13.3*	*16.1*	*19.7*	*16.5*	*1.6*	*3.4*	*8.6*	*4.5*	*11.7*	*12.6*	*11.2*	*12.0*	*0.60*	*0.57*	*0.60*
Other															
Israel	28.3	34.2	39.3	42.4	7.3	18.0	28.3	33.0	21.0	16.1	11.0	9.4	1.14	1.16	1.13
Poland	29.1	36.2	42.8	83.9	13.3	19.6	27.5	84.9	15.8	16.6	15.3	-1.0	0.87	1.39	0.60
average	*28.7*	*35.2*	*41.1*	*63.2*	*10.3*	*18.8*	*27.9*	*58.9*	*18.4*	*16.3*	*13.1*	*4.2*	*1.01*	*1.27*	*0.86*
Anglophone															
Australia	20.0	23.1	27.8	23.4	5.8	11.9	19.4	13.9	14.2	11.2	8.4	9.5	0.86	0.98	0.76
Canada	19.1	22.8	27.2	20.3	8.2	15.6	23.9	9.5	10.9	7.2	3.3	10.8	0.96	1.26	0.64
United Kingdom	31.0	34.2	37.0	34.9	7.2	19.1	28.9	22.9	23.9	15.1	8.1	12.0	1.08	1.39	0.84
United States	19.7	25.2	30.8	17.7	14.4	22.2	30.4	11.7	5.3	3.0	0.5	6.0	1.02	1.28	0.41
average	*22.5*	*26.4*	*30.7*	*24.1*	*8.9*	*17.2*	*25.7*	*14.5*	*13.6*	*9.1*	*5.1*	*9.6*	*0.98*	*1.23*	*0.66*

notes: In the first four columns, cells report poverty rates based on market income, with poverty lines drawn at 40, 50, and 60 percent of median disposable income, and at the US poverty line; in the second four columns, the cells report poverty rates based on disposable income, with poverty lines drawn at 40, 50, and 60 percent of median disposable income, and at the US poverty line; in the last four columns, cells report the difference between market-income poverty and disposable-income poverty (always relative to the same poverty line).

Fourth, we calculate three key outcomes among children, compared to the same outcomes for all persons, to gauge the extent to which children are under- or over-represented among the poor and the degree to which poverty reduction is greater or lesser for children (see the far-right vertical panel of Table 2). Considering market-income poverty rates (at the 50% standard), we find that in all of the Nordic and Continental countries, children are much less likely to be poor than are all persons. In two Anglophone countries—Canada and the US—children are about equally likely to be poor as are all persons; in the UK, and especially in Israel, they are more likely to be poor than are all persons. After accounting for taxes and transfers, children are more likely to be poor in all of our study countries—except in the four Nordic countries, where child poverty rates (based on disposable income) are 51–64% of the overall poverty rate. We also see a general pattern of less poverty reduction among children than among all persons. That result is especially notable in the Continental countries, where child poverty reduction is, on average, about one-quarter of poverty reduction overall. The meager amount of child poverty amelioration in the Continental countries explains the wide discrepancy between market-income poverty (where children are much less poor than the general population) and disposable-income poverty (where children are substantially more likely to be poor).

We also assess child poverty outcomes for the youngest children—that is, children younger than age six (see Table 3). The most salient findings here concern the differences between outcomes among these young children compared to all children (see the far-right vertical panel). Here we see a widespread pattern in which poverty rates among these young children—with respect to both market-income and disposable-income poverty—are modestly higher than among all children. That finding holds even in the (generally "child friendly") Nordic countries; the Netherlands and (for market-income poverty) Switzerland are exceptions. That the youngest children are usually more likely to live in households with market income below the poverty threshold indicates that, on average, their parents bring in less income from earnings. These parents' more limited earnings are likely traced to several overlapping factors. The parents of the youngest children (especially mothers) are less likely to be in the labor force, partly because younger children need more care at home. These parents are also younger than the parents of older children, which raises both their risk of unemployment and the probability that they will hold low-paid jobs. That the youngest children, in most countries, are also more likely to be disposable-income poor (compared to all children) suggests that their parents' lower labor market income is not offset by the effects of tax-and-transfer features targeted on families with the youngest children. Also, the (younger) parents of these younger children are probably less likely than their older counterparts to receive some categories of social income, such as unemployment, disability, and retirement pensions.

As noted in the child poverty research literature, family structure explains substantial (within-country) variation in child poverty rates—and our results confirm that overwhelmingly (see Table 4). In nearly every country in this study, children who live with single mothers are more likely to be poor than are children who live

Table 3 Percentage of young children (< 6 years old) living in poor households

	market income				disposable income				poverty reduction [MI less DPI]				ratio of young children to all children *Table 3 compared to Table 2*		
	40% DPI	50% DPI	60% DPI	US line	40% DPI	50% DPI	60% DPI	US line	40% DPI	50% DPI	60% DPI	US line	market income poverty, 50% DPI	disposable income poverty, 50% DPI	poverty reduction, 50% DPI
Continental															
Germany	16.3	18.2	22.0	17.6	7.3	11.3	16.5	9.3	9.0	6.9	5.6	8.3	1.11	1.25	0.94
Netherlands	6.9	8.2	9.6	7.5	2.7	5.7	12.4	4.0	4.2	2.6	-2.8	3.5	0.80	0.88	0.66
Switzerland	6.4	8.7	12.4	6.4	4.0	9.2	17.1	4.0	2.5	-0.5	-4.7	2.5	0.81	1.03	-0.26
average	*9.9*	*11.7*	*14.7*	*10.5*	*4.7*	*8.7*	*15.3*	*5.7*	*5.2*	*3.0*	*-0.6*	*4.8*	*0.91*	*1.05*	*0.45*
Nordic															
Denmark	14.3	16.7	19.6	15.8	1.5	3.4	10.6	2.4	12.9	13.3	9.0	13.5	1.15	1.23	1.13
Finland	15.9	20.2	26.5	25.3	2.2	4.3	11.5	10.8	13.7	15.8	15.0	14.6	1.13	1.39	1.08
Norway	12.1	14.7	18.9	12.4	2.3	4.4	8.2	2.6	9.7	10.3	10.7	9.8	1.09	1.18	1.06
Sweden	18.3	20.6	24.5	22.5	3.1	7.1	12.9	9.4	15.2	13.5	11.6	13.0	1.11	1.66	0.95
average	*15.1*	*18.0*	*22.4*	*19.0*	*2.3*	*4.8*	*10.8*	*6.3*	*12.9*	*13.2*	*11.6*	*12.7*	*1.12*	*1.37*	*1.05*
Other															
Israel	29.2	35.1	40.6	43.9	8.3	20.3	31.5	36.4	20.9	14.7	9.1	7.4	1.03	1.13	0.91
Poland	29.6	37.0	44.5	86.6	13.4	20.3	28.8	86.0	16.2	16.7	15.6	0.6	1.02	1.03	1.01
average	*29.4*	*36.0*	*42.5*	*65.2*	*10.8*	*20.3*	*30.2*	*61.2*	*18.6*	*15.7*	*12.4*	*4.0*	*1.02*	*1.08*	*0.96*
Anglophone															
Australia	--	--	--	--	--	--	--	--	--	--	--	--	--	--	--
Canada	20.7	24.1	28.7	21.7	9.3	17.8	26.2	10.7	11.4	6.3	2.5	11.1	1.06	1.14	0.88
United Kingdom	33.3	36.5	39.7	37.2	9.0	23.8	33.9	28.0	24.3	12.7	5.9	9.3	1.07	1.25	0.84
United States	20.4	26.1	32.1	18.3	15.5	23.9	32.6	12.6	4.9	2.3	-0.5	5.7	1.04	1.07	0.76
average	*24.8*	*28.9*	*33.5*	*25.7*	*11.2*	*21.8*	*30.9*	*17.1*	*13.5*	*7.1*	*2.6*	*8.7*	*1.05*	*1.15*	*0.82*

notes: In the first four columns, cells report poverty rates based on market income, with poverty lines drawn at 40, 50, and 60 percent of median disposable income, and at the US poverty line; in the second four columns, the cells report poverty rates based on disposable income, with poverty lines drawn at 40, 50, and 60 percent of median disposable income, and at the US poverty line; in the last four columns, cells report the difference between market-income poverty and disposable-income poverty (always relative to the same poverty line).

Australia could not be included due to incomplete information on children's ages.

Table 4 Percentage of children (<18 years old) living in poor households, by family type

	single-mother family		single-father family		two-parent family		ratio of single-mother to two-parent families	
	MI 50% DPI	DPI 50% DPI	MI 50% DPI	DPI 50% DPI	MI 50% DPI	DPI 50% DPI	MI 50% DPI	DPI 50% DPI
Continental								
Germany	61.7	38.3	34.1	16.1	9.3	4.7	6.7	8.2
Netherlands	57.8	38.4	NA	NA	5.4	3.2	10.7	11.9
Switzerland	58.0	22.3	8.2	7.8	7.4	8.1	7.9	2.7
average	*59.2*	*33.0*	*21.2*	*12.0*	*7.4*	*5.3*	*8.4*	*7.6*
Nordic								
Denmark	45.3	6.4	29.5	11.5	9.1	1.9	5.0	3.3
Finland	52.1	8.2	29.9	2.8	12.1	2.2	4.3	3.7
Norway	53.8	10.9	23.9	5.0	5.7	2.0	9.4	5.5
Sweden	54.2	12.9	18.7	4.2	10.4	2.3	5.2	5.6
average	*51.3*	*9.6*	*25.5*	*5.9*	*9.3*	*2.1*	*6.0*	*4.5*
Other								
Israel	69.7	36.3	NA	NA	31.0	16.7	2.3	2.2
Poland	58.7	21.0	47.6	17.4	31.8	20.0	1.8	1.0
average	*64.2*	*28.6*	*47.6*	*17.4*	*31.4*	*18.3*	*2.0*	*1.6*
Anglophone								
Australia	68.9	32.7	46.1	34.4	17.1	8.9	4.0	3.7
Canada	62.7	43.6	27.4	18.6	16.1	11.2	3.9	3.9
United Kingdom	82.4	45.4	57.3	37.6	20.0	11.3	4.1	4.0
United States	61.2	51.5	29.6	26.3	15.6	14.6	3.9	3.5
average	*68.8*	*43.3*	*40.1*	*29.2*	*17.2*	*11.5*	*4.0*	*3.8*

notes   NA means results cannot be reported due to small cell sizes (N<30).

with single fathers[13] *and* children who live with single fathers are more likely to be poor than are those who live with two parents. Children in single-mother families have extremely high market-income poverty rates—in all countries and in all country clusters. The market-income child poverty rate varies from 68.8% age, on average, in the Anglophone countries (with a stunningly high rate of nearly 82.4% in the UK), to 64.2 in the Israel-Poland pair, to 59.2% in the Continental countries, to a low of 51.3 in the Nordic countries—where the most favorable rate across the thirteen countries, still 45%, is reported in Denmark.

Market-income poverty is consistently lowest among children in two-parent families. Among these children, the risk of market-based poverty is highest (31.4%) in the Israel-Poland pair, more moderate, on average, in the Anglophone (17.2%) and Nordic countries (9.3%), and lowest (7.4%) in the Continental cluster. Using the market-income standard, the *greater* poverty risk associated with living with a single mother is especially marked in the Continental countries—where, on average, children in single-mother families are over eight times as likely to be poor as are children in two-parent families. Remarkably, in the Netherlands, the market-income poverty rate among the children of single mothers is ten times the poverty rate among children who live with two parents.

Taxes and transfers, of course, reduce child poverty across all family types. However, with post-tax-and-transfer income, family structure still matters a great deal. Considering the ratio of single-mother to two-parent poverty rates, we see that the greater risk associated with living with a single mother is approximately the same with disposable-income poverty as with market-income poverty. With post-tax-and-transfer poverty, the children of single mothers, compared to the children of two parents, are (on average) 7.6 times as likely to be poor in the Continental cluster, 4.5 times as likely in the Nordic countries, and 3.8 times as likely in the Anglophone countries.[14]

Our review of the child poverty literature underscored that labor market income is an enormously influential factor in shaping the likelihood that any given household is poor. Clearly, a household's earnings are shaped by another important demographic factor—the educational attainment of the household head. In Table 5, we report market- and disposable-income poverty rates for children living in households headed by adults with low, medium, and high educational attainment. The

---

[13] We do not report poverty rates for children in single-father families in the Netherlands and Israel, as the sample sizes in the raw data are too small.

[14] The results reported here indicate that the likelihood that children in any given family type are poor varies widely across our study countries. This variation in group-specific poverty rates is compounded by variation, across countries, in the prevalence of these various family types. The percentage of children, for example, that live with single-mothers ranges from 6 to 9% in Switzerland, Israel, Poland, and the Netherlands; to 11–14% in Australia, Finland, Germany, Canada, Denmark, and Norway; to 16–21% in the US, Sweden, and the UK. Across these countries, variation in the probability of living with a single father is much less; it never exceeds 3% of children. Furthermore, one family type was excluded from Table 4—children living exclusively with adults *other than their parents*. That category includes in most cases 1–4% of children across these countries—with the exception of Poland (7%) and the US (where it reaches 10%).

Table 5 Percentage of children (< 18 years old) living in poor households, by educational level of household head

	low education		medium education		high education		ratio of low to high education	
	MI 50% DPI	DPI 50% DPI	MI 50% DPI	DPI 50% DPI	MI 50% DPI	DPI 50% DPI	MI 50% DPI	DPI 50% DPI
Continental								
Germany	35.0	23.9	17.5	8.6	4.7	3.0	7.5	8.1
Netherlands	27.6	20.8	8.7	4.2	2.4	1.5	11.6	13.6
Switzerland	21.2	13.4	10.6	8.7	7.1	7.7	3.0	1.8
average	*27.9*	*19.4*	*12.3*	*7.2*	*4.7*	*4.0*	*7.4*	*7.8*
Nordic								
Denmark	27.4	3.8	10.5	2.5	6.8	1.5	4.0	2.6
Finland	32.8	6.0	20.1	2.7	4.7	1.6	6.9	3.9
Norway	20.1	6.0	14.9	3.2	4.9	1.0	4.1	5.9
Sweden	30.6	5.9	17.5	3.9	10.1	3.3	3.0	1.8
average	*27.7*	*5.4*	*15.7*	*3.1*	*6.6*	*1.8*	*4.5*	*3.5*
Other								
Israel	52.4	32.6	30.9	14.8	20.4	8.7	2.6	3.7
Poland	61.7	38.4	31.2	17.9	4.7	1.8	13.2	21.5
average	*57.1*	*35.5*	*31.0*	*16.3*	*12.5*	*5.2*	*7.9*	*12.6*
Anglophone								
Australia	–	–	–	–	–	–		
Canada	39.1	28.9	25.5	17.8	16.0	10.6	2.4	2.7
United Kingdom	53.9	29.5	28.9	16.3	10.0	6.9	5.4	4.3
United States	54.6	51.4	26.1	22.6	7.9	6.7	6.9	7.6
average	*49.2*	*36.6*	*26.8*	*18.9*	*11.3*	*8.1*	*4.9*	*4.9*
notes	Australia could not be included due to incomparable data on educational attainment.							

results clearly show that heads' educational attainment is highly (negatively) correlated with child poverty. Within all thirteen countries, poverty rates—based on both
market and disposable income—are highest in the least educated group, lower in
the medium-education group, and lower yet in the most highly educated group. The
greater risk of poverty, for children, associated with living in a house headed by an
adult with low educational attainment varies markedly across countries (see the far
right panel of Table 5), but no clear cluster pattern emerges. For example, considering market-income poverty, low educational attainment (of the head), compared to
high educational attainment, approximately triples the probability of being poor in
Israel—while it raises the likelihood of poverty more than thirteen-fold in Poland.

In our final empirical analyses, we consider the role played by parents' labor market status combined with family structure and gender. We first consider four types
of two-parent households: both parents have low labor market status (as defined
in the methods section); the mother's status is medium/high status and the father's
is low; the father's is medium/high and the mother's is low; and they both have
medium/high labor market status (see Table 6). As with educational attainment,
the results clearly show that parents' labor market status is highly correlated with
child poverty. In nearly of our study countries, poverty rates—based on both market
and disposable income—fall systematically as we move (left to right) across the
subgroups in Table 6; Israel is an exception.

Market-income poverty is most prevalent when both parents have low labor market engagement; in most cases, the child poverty rate in these households is 50%
or higher, with the highest poverty rate—somewhat surprisingly—seen in Sweden,
where it is nearly 80%. On the other end of the spectrum, when both parents have
medium/high labor market status, poverty rates are dramatically lower—in fact, less
than 4% in all countries. In between those extremes, we see a consistent pattern in
which gender clearly matters. Among children who have only one of their parents
strongly attached to the labor market, those for whom that parent is their father are
better off—and often by a substantial margin; again, Israel is an exception.

In these two-parent families, overall, the results with respect to disposable-
income poverty are similar: in nearly all countries, disposable-income poverty
rates fall systematically as we move (left to right) across the subgroups. Also,
some country cluster patterns emerge. In the third subgroup, for example—father
medium/high, mother low—poverty rates are consistently low (4% or less) in the
Continental and Nordic countries, while they are much higher (10% or more)
in the Anglophone countries (except Australia) and in Israel. Finally, in these
results we see the importance of maternal employment in two-parent families with
substantially employed fathers. Nearly everywhere, the fourth subgroup reports considerably less poverty than the third group[15]—with the sharpest differences seen in
three Anglophone countries and in Israel. In Canada, the UK, and the US, even
after taxes and transfers, poverty rates range from 10 to 15% among households
headed by a couple in which the father is strongly attached to paid work and the

---

[15] The one exception is in Finland, where poverty rates are very low in both groups.

Table 6 Percentage of children (< 18 years old) living in poor households, by labor market status of parents, two-parent families

	both low		father low, mother medium/high		father medium/high, mother low		both medium/high	
	MI 50% DPI	DPI 50% DPI	MI 50% DPI	DPI 50% DPI	MI 50% DPI	DPI 50% DPI	MI 50% DPI	DPI 50% DPI
Continental								
Germany	42.7	24.4	20.3	7.8	7.9	4.0	1.6	0.8
Netherlands	47.7	33.8	13.7	3.5	0.5	0.9	0.0	0.0
Switzerland	--	--	--	--	--	--	--	--
average	*45.2*	*29.1*	*17.0*	*5.7*	*4.2*	*2.4*	*0.8*	*0.4*
Nordic								
Denmark	72.4	12.8	16.7	5.1	7.5	1.3	0.1	0.1
Finland	59.8	12.9	23.8	5.2	17.1	0.9	2.9	0.6
Norway	54.2	20.9	14.8	3.9	2.6	1.0	0.0	0.0
Sweden	78.7	16.1	28.1	6.1	6.3	1.8	0.4	0.2
average	*66.3*	*15.7*	*20.9*	*5.1*	*8.4*	*1.3*	*0.9*	*0.2*
Other								
Israel	72.7	42.8	30.8	10.0	30.1	17.0	2.7	1.0
Poland	--	--	--	--	--	--	--	--
average	*72.7*	*42.8*	*30.8*	*10.0*	*30.1*	*17.0*	*2.7*	*1.0*
Anglophone								
Australia	64.0	38.1	18.9	10.1	10.9	3.1	0.8	0.2
Canada	69.3	59.7	33.3	22.8	17.8	10.3	3.8	1.7
United Kingdom	67.8	36.6	25.8	16.6	19.1	10.8	1.6	1.2
United States	67.7	63.4	41.2	36.6	15.1	15.0	2.8	2.7
average	*67.2*	*49.4*	*29.8*	*21.5*	*15.7*	*9.8*	*2.3*	*1.4*

notes   Switzerland and Poland could not be included due to incomplete data on person-level earnings.

Table 7 Percentage of children (< 18 years old) living in poor households, by labor market status of parents, single-parent families

	single mother, low		single father, low		single mother, medium/high		single father, medium/high	
	MI 50% DPI	DPI 50% DPI	MI 50% DPI	DPI 50% DPI	MI 50% DPI	DPI 50% DPI	MI 50% DPI	DPI 50% DPI
Continental								
Germany	91.8	55.4	NA	NA	44.4	28.4	18.4	0.0
Netherlands	97.7	73.5	NA	NA	33.9	17.3	NA	NA
Switzerland	-	-	-	-	-	-	-	-
average	*94.7*	*64.5*	*NA*	*NA*	*39.1*	*22.9*	*18.4*	*0.0*
Nordic								
Denmark	92.7	15.3	82.9	32.2	22.2	2.1	1.1	0.4
Finland	97.8	20.6	71.9	11.3	38.3	4.5	15.7	0.0
Norway	97.1	24.9	73.9	15.7	36.8	5.4	0.8	0.0
Sweden	95.8	31.9	NA	NA	34.9	4.1	0.0	0.0
average	*95.9*	*23.2*	*76.2*	*19.8*	*33.0*	*4.0*	*4.4*	*0.1*
Other								
Israel	96.0	61.1	NA	NA	40.4	8.6	NA	NA
Poland	-	-	-	-	-	-	-	-
average	*96.0*	*61.1*	*NA*	*NA*	*40.4*	*8.6*	*NA*	*NA*
Anglophone								
Australia	91.3	51.1	74.4	59.5	35.1	4.9	7.3	0.0
Canada	96.2	82.7	81.9	62.1	50.0	28.8	13.1	7.2
United Kingdom	97.5	64.8	89.4	61.5	56.0	11.6	20.4	10.1
United States	93.1	84.6	75.3	68.7	53.6	43.6	9.5	7.7
average	*94.5*	*70.8*	*80.3*	*62.9*	*48.6*	*22.2*	*12.6*	*6.3*

notes   Switzerland and Poland could not be included due to incomplete data on person-level earnings.
NA means results cannot be reported due to small cell sizes (N<30).

mother is not. In these three countries, among households in which both parents are strongly attached, the poverty rates are much lower, approximately 1–3%. In these Anglophone countries, maternal employment clearly matters—and it matters a lot.

Last, we consider the association, among the children of single parents, between child poverty, parents' labor market attachment, and parents' gender (see Table 7). We assess households headed by four subgroups: a single mother with low labor market status; a single father with low status; a single mother with medium/high labor market status; and a single father with medium/high status. Again, in nearly every study country, poverty rates—based on both market and disposable income— fall systematically as we move (left to right) across these subgroups. When we consider market-income poverty, households headed by single mothers with low labor market status are almost all poor—poverty rates are 90% or higher in all countries. Likewise, among single fathers with low labor market engagement (in the seven countries where we have data and sufficient sample sizes), market-income poverty is less prevalent but still widespread (72–89%). In the third subgroup (children whose single mothers have medium/high status), market-income poverty ranges from 22.2% in Denmark to 44.4% in Germany, and is 50% or higher in three Anglophone countries, Canada, the UK, and the US. Among single-parent households, market-income poverty is lowest everywhere in those households headed by single fathers with medium/high labor market attachment—although it remains 15–20% in three diverse countries, Germany, Finland and the UK.

Finally, in these single-parent families, the results with respect to disposable-income poverty are again quite similar: in all countries, disposable-income poverty rates fall systematically as we move (left to right) across the subgroups. Perhaps the most salient finding here is the consistently large difference in the risk of being poor—even after taxes and transfers—when we compare single mothers with low labor market engagement to single mothers with high labor market status. It is interesting that the two most extreme examples are two markedly different countries. In Sweden, households headed by a single mother with low employment attachment are over eight times more likely to be poor than are households headed by a single mother with stronger engagement (32% compared to 4%). In Australia, households headed by a single mother with low employment status are over ten times more likely to be poor than are households headed by her counterpart with stronger labor market engagement (51.1% compared to 4.9%). Across all of these countries—before as well as after taxes and transfers—in single-mother households, employment matters, and it matters a great deal.

5 Conclusions

For more than two decades, diverse researchers have drawn on the resources of the Luxembourg Income Study to study poverty among children. In this brief conclusion, we revisit the descriptive information provided in the LIS *Key Figures*, the rich analytical literature produced by dozens of scholars, and our own contemporary snapshot of child poverty in thirteen countries, to draw some general conclusions.

First, it is clear that child poverty rates vary markedly across the mostly high-income countries included in the LIS data archive. The variation in child poverty takes many forms; it is evident with both market- and disposable-income poverty, at multiple relative poverty thresholds, using a real-income threshold, and within nearly every demographic and labor market status subgroup. As we learned from the LIS *Key Figures* (and reported in Fig. 1), in the middle-1990s/early 2000s, child poverty rates—based on disposable income and the 50%-of-median standard—vary dramatically. The lowest rates (5% or less) are reported in four Nordic countries (Denmark, Finland, Norway, Sweden) and the highest rates (more than 20%) are seen in three diverse countries, Mexico, Russia, and the US.

Second, child poverty rates shift over time, and in complex ways. Our review of the LIS *Key Figures* highlights diverse patterns of change during the 1990s. These figures reveal an overall worsening of the economic wellbeing of children during the 1990s. In most of the LIS countries, child poverty rates increased during the 1990s—in some cases, by a small increment, in others by a substantial amount—although in some countries (including the US) the prevalence of child poverty declined in recent years. Chen & Corak (2008), in their comprehensive review of children's poverty trends during the 1990s, also found a varied picture with both rising and falling levels of poverty. Of course, findings about trends are highly sensitive to the time period chosen. Rainwater & Smeeding (2003), for example, considered a longer period of time and concluded that child poverty in the US had, in general, risen in recent decades—a result clearly confirmed in the LIS *Key Figures*. Using the 50% standard, the *Key Figures* reveal that US child poverty rose from 19% in 1974, to 20% in 1979, to 25% in 1986, and 26% in 1991—before the period of decline seen in the 1990s.

Third, within countries, family demography and parents' labor market engagement matter enormously with respect to children's likelihood of living in a poor household. Our own empirical work demonstrates, for example, that, in nearly all of our study countries, younger children are more at risk than older children; children who live with single parents are more likely to be poor than are children who live with two parents; and children who live with less educated parents are more likely to be poor than are their peers whose parents are more highly educated. Furthermore, among both one- and two-parent families, the risk of child poverty (before and after taxes and transfers) consistently falls as parents' labor market attachment rises. And, not surprisingly, parents' gender matters too. The children of single mothers are more likely to be poor than are the children of single fathers nearly everywhere; among children with one of their two parents strongly attached to the labor market, those for whom that parent is their father are less likely to be poor.

Fourth, as many LIS studies have demonstrated, taxes and transfers powerfully shape the economic wellbeing of children in all countries. Our own results (reported in Table 2) indicate that taxes and transfers reduce child poverty everywhere, although the amount of poverty reduction varies sharply across countries. Using the 50% relative poverty standard—and relying on the simple difference between market-income and disposable-income poverty rates—we see that the Israel-Poland pair reports the most poverty reduction, followed by the Nordic and Anglophone countries, followed by the Continental cluster. Our results turned up especially little reduction of child poverty in the US case (about 3 percentage points) and in Switzerland (about 2 percentage points). Of course, as we noted earlier, this indicator captures only the mechanical relationship between pre- and post-tax-and-transfer poverty rates. It does not account for the ways in which these public programs shape the market-based outcomes; nonetheless, it is an illuminating indicator of the reach of public policy and clearly demonstrates that policy responses to poverty vary markedly across these upper-income countries.

Fifth, several studies have concluded that the explanatory factors that matter within countries are not necessarily the same as those that matter across countries. In short, because demographic composition across the 30 LIS countries varies relatively modestly, and because demography changes slowly, several studies—including the three that we reviewed in detail in this chapter—find that demography is not an especially powerful factor for explaining variation in child poverty rates, or trends, across the LIS countries. Instead, the most important explanatory factors are institutional, and they concern both labor market structures (and outcomes) and policy configurations. Bradbury & Jäntti (1999) concluded that, while variation in welfare state institutions is important when accounting for the diversity of children's poverty outcomes across countries, variation in the market incomes received by their families is a more powerful explanatory factor. Rainwater & Smeeding (2003) largely concur, concluding that, at the bottom of the household income distribution, both earnings received and transfer income are important factors underlying cross-national child poverty variation. Chen & Corak (2008) also found that, in explaining cross-national variation in child poverty trends, demographic variation matters modestly, while national labor market patterns and social policy factors both matter a great deal—and they matter via complex and interacting mechanisms.

Sixth, over-arching institutional models—as captured in the country clusters that we employ in this chapter—also seem to matter. Presenting poverty outcomes by country clusters is an admittedly crude way of assessing the role of institutions; it is an approach that aggregates a large number of national features into a single institutional designation. However, as our own results indicate, the clusters do correspond to child poverty outcomes—in a number of ways. Child poverty based on market income, for example, is consistently highest in the Anglophone countries, followed by the Nordic, then the Continental, countries. In contrast, disposable-income poverty is systematically lower in the Nordic than in the Continental cluster, indicating a pattern of more extensive income redistribution (among households with children) in the Nordic countries. We also find patterns with respect to children's over- (or under-) representation among the poor. Based on market income, children throughout the Nordic and Continental clusters are less likely to be poor than the general population; after taxes and transfers, children in all of the Continental countries are more likely to be poor—a result found in none of the Nordic countries. Clearly, institutional designs in the Nordic countries include elements that are particularly favorable towards children and that are not universally operating across Europe.

Furthermore, these welfare state models, and the country clusters that correspond to them, are correlated with more than patterns of taxing and transferring; they are also associated with patterns of female (especially maternal) employment. While a full assessment of mothers' employment is outside the scope of this chapter, cross-country variation in employment outcomes also shapes the child poverty results that we have reported. For example, when we consider the prevalence of the four subgroups in Table 6 (the various combinations of two-parent employment statuses), we find that the fourth subgroup (both parents medium/highly engaged) is most prevalent in the Nordic countries (results not shown). In the four Nordic countries, between 63 and 69% of children (in two-parent families) have two parents with medium/high labor market attachment. In none of the other countries in our study does that figure exceed 60%. The Nordic institutional design is both strongly redistributive and most highly associated with structural features that encourage and enable maternal employment; both elements shape the prevalence of child poverty.

The Luxembourg Income Study will remain a rich resource in the years to come, allowing researchers in many countries to track families' economic wellbeing across countries, through economic upturns and downturns. The current recession, which is affecting all industrialized countries—and diverse government responses to it—will shed light on how the interaction between labor market characteristics and public policies either protect or fail to protect children from shocks to the market system. After LIS adds more middle-income countries to its archive, a process now in the early stages, researchers will be able to study child poverty in a much more globalized context. The integration of microdata from an increasingly diverse set of countries will enable researchers, across disciplines, to tackle entirely new questions about the determinants and nature of child poverty.

References

Bäckman, O. (2005). *Welfare states, social structure and the dynamics of poverty rates: A comparative study of 16 countries, 1980–2000.* Luxembourg: Luxembourg Income Study Working Paper No. 408.

Bane, M. J., & Zenteno R. (2005). *Poverty and place in North America.* Luxembourg: Luxembourg Income Study Working Paper No. 418.

Beaujot, R., & Liu, J. (2002). *Children, social assistance and outcomes: Cross national comparisons.* Luxembourg: Luxembourg Income Study Working Paper No. 304.

Bradbury, B., & Jäntti, M. (1999). *Child poverty across industrialized nations.* Innocenti Occasional Papers, Economic and Social Policy Series, no. 71. Florence, Italy: UNICEF. (originally Luxembourg Income Study Working Paper No. 205)

Bradshaw, J., & Chen, J. R. 1996. *Poverty in the U.K.: A comparison with nineteen other countries.* Luxembourg: Luxembourg Income Study Working Paper No. 147.

Brady, D., Fullerton A., & Cross J. M. (2008). *Putting poverty in political context: A multi-level analysis of working-aged poverty across 18 affluent democracies.* Luxembourg: Luxembourg Income Study Working Paper No. 487.

Brady, D. (2004). *Reconsidering the divergence between elderly, child and overall poverty.* Luxembourg: Luxembourg Income Study Working Paper No. 371.

Brady, D. (2005). *Structural theory and relative poverty in rich western democracies, 1969–2000.* Luxembourg: Luxembourg Income Study Working Paper No. 407.

Cantillon, B., & Van den Bosch, K. (2002). *Social policy strategies to combat income poverty of children and families in Europe*. Luxembourg: Luxembourg Income Study Working Paper No. 336.

Chen, W. H., & Corak, M. (2008). Child poverty and changes in child poverty. *Demography, 45*(3), 537–553. (originally Luxembourg Income Study Working Paper No. 405)

Corak, M. (2005). *Principles and practicalities for measuring child poverty in rich countries*. Luxembourg: Luxembourg Income Study Working Paper No. 406.

D'Ambrosio, C., & Gradin, C. (2000). *Are children in growing danger of social exclusion? Evidence from Italy and Spain*. Luxembourg: Luxembourg Income Study Working Paper No. 262.

Esping-Andersen, G. (1990). *The three worlds of welfare capitalism*. Cambridge: Polity Press.

Findlay, J., & Wright, R. (1992). *Gender, poverty and intra-household distribution of resources*. Luxembourg: Luxembourg Income Study Working Paper No. 83.

Gornick, J. C., & Meyers, M. K. (2003). *Families that work: Policies for reconciling parenthood and employment*. New York: Russell Sage Foundation.

Gornick, J.C., & Pavetti, L. (1990). *A demographic model of poverty among families with children: A comparative analysis of five industrialized countries based on microdata from the Luxembourg income study*. Luxembourg: Luxembourg Income Study Working Paper No. 65.

Jäntti, M., & Danziger, S. (1992). *Does the welfare state work? Evidence on antipoverty effects from the Luxembourg income study*. Luxembourg: Luxembourg Income Study Working Paper No. 74.

Jeandidier, B., & Albiser, E. (2001). To *what extent do family policy and social assistance transfers equitably reduce the intensity of child poverty? A comparison between the US, France, Great Britain and Luxembourg*. Luxembourg: Luxembourg Income Study Working Paper No. 255.

Kuivalainen, S. (2005). *Families at the margins of the welfare state: A comparative study on the prevalence of poverty among families receiving social assistance*. Luxembourg: Luxembourg Income Study Working Paper No. 403.

Makines, T. (1998). *Contradictory findings? The connection between structural factors, income transfers and poverty in OECD countries*. Luxembourg: Luxembourg Income Study Working Paper No. 179.

1996 Marx, I., & Van den Bosch, K. (1996). *Trends in financial poverty in OECD countries*. Luxembourg: Luxembourg Income Study Working Paper No. 148.

2006 Misra, J. Budig, M., & Moller, S. (2006). *Reconciliation policies and the effects of motherhood on employment, earnings, and poverty*. Luxembourg: Luxembourg Income Study Working Paper No. 429.

Moller, S., & Misra, J. (2005). *Familialism and welfare regimes: Poverty, employment and family policies*. Luxembourg: Luxembourg Income Study Working Paper No. 399.

2006 Munzi, T., & Smeeding, T. (2006). *Conditions of social vulnerability, work and low income, evidence for Spain in comparative perspective*. Luxembourg: Luxembourg Income Study Working Paper No. 448.

Orsini, K. (2001). *Yet the poorest, relatively speaking: Italian poverty rates in international perspective*. Luxembourg: Luxembourg Income Study Working Paper No. 261.

Rainwater, L., & Smeeding, T. M. (2003). *Poor kids in a rich country: America's children in comparative perspective*. New York: Russell Sage Foundation.

Redmond, G. (2000). *Children in large families: Disadvantaged or just different?* Luxembourg: Luxembourg Income Study Working Paper No. 225.

Scott, K. (2008). *Growing up in North America: The economic well-being of children in North America*. Luxembourg: Luxembourg Income Study Working Paper No. 482.

Skinner, C., Bradshaw, J., & Davidson, J. (2008). *Child support policy: An international perspective*. Luxembourg: Luxembourg Income Study Working Paper No. 478.

Smeeding, T. (2005). *Government programs and social outcomes: The United States in comparative perspective*. Luxembourg: Luxembourg Income Study Working Paper No. 426.

Smeeding, T., & Torrey, B. (1988). *Poor children in rich countries.* Luxembourg: Luxembourg Income Study Working Paper No. 16.

Smeeding, T., Christopher, K., Phillips, K. R., McLanahan, S., & England, P. (1999). *Poverty and parenthood across modern nations: Findings from the Luxembourg income study.* Luxembourg: Luxembourg Income Study Working Paper No. 194.

Smeeding, T., Rainwater, L., & Danziger, S. (1995). *The Western welfare state in the 1990s: Toward a new model of antipoverty policy for families with children.* Luxembourg: Luxembourg Income Study Working Paper No. 128.

Smeeding, T., & Rainwater, L. (1995). *Doing poorly: The real income of American children in a comparative perspective.* Luxembourg: Luxembourg Income Study Working Paper No. 127.

Solera, C. (1998). *Income transfers and support for mothers' employment: The link to family poverty risks.* A Comparison between Italy, Sweden and the UK. Luxembourg: Luxembourg Income Study Working Paper No. 192.

Waddoups, C. (2004). *Welfare state expenditures and the distribution of child opportunities.* Luxembourg: Luxembourg Income Study Working Paper No. 379.

Weinshenker, M., & Heuveline, P. (2006). *The international child poverty gap: Does demography matter?* Luxembourg: Luxembourg Income Study Working Paper No. 441.

Part V
Issues in Child Well-Being

Early Childhood Education and Care

Peter Moss

1 Introduction

Since the 1970s, there has been a growing interest in the comparative study of what today is most often referred to as "early childhood education and care" (ECEC), services providing non-parental care and education for children under compulsory school age; these services include nurseries, nursery schools, kindergartens, various types of "age-integrated" centres for children under and over 3 years, and family day care provided by home-based workers. Some of this work has been initiated by academics, interested in better understanding political, social and cultural differences in policy, provision and practice; it is here that Al Kahn and Sheila Kamerman have played a leading role (I first met them in the 1970s, as a junior researcher knowing nothing of ECEC beyond my own shores, when they called on me in London during one of their regular swings through Europe to keep themselves informed about policies).

But much of this work has been initiated by international organisations. My own induction into comparative work came about through coordinating a group of experts set up by the European Commission (EC) to do work on ECEC services and other measures to support (in Eurospeak) "the reconciliation of employment and family responsibilities". The EC Childcare Network undertook a wide range of comparative work between 1986 and 1996 including three reviews of ECEC services in EU member states. Non-governmental international organisations that have become increasingly interested and active include the World Bank, the Council of Europe, UNESCO, UNICEF and the Organisation for Economic Cooperation and Development (OECD).

OECD's role in this field is long-standing and of particular interest. As far back as 1976 they published a comparative study on "child care programs" prepared for a working party on the role of women in the economy—and authored by Alfred Kahn and Sheila Kamerman (Kahn & Kamerman, 1976). Their continuing interest

P. Moss (✉)
Thomas Coram Research Unit, Institute of Education University of London, London, UK
e-mail: Peter.moss@ioe.ac.uk

S.B. Kamerman et al. (eds.), *From Child Welfare to Child Well-Being*, Children's
Well-Being: Indicators and Research 1, DOI 10.1007/978-90-481-3377-2_20,
© Springer Science+Business Media B.V. 2010

in this field has culminated in what many would consider the most important and comprehensive comparative study of ECEC, at least amongst rich countries: the thematic review of early childhood education and care (note, no longer just "child-care") in 20 countries, widely referred to as *Starting Strong*, and producing two major reports (OECD, 2001, 2006). (Interestingly, *Staring Strong* was paralleled by a second OECD thematic review, launched in 2001, of "family friendly" policies in 13 member states, and commonly known as *Babies and Bosses* (2007). This review included "child care arrangements", involving overlap with *Starting Strong*. The two reviews, however, came out of different parts of OECD—the Directorate for Education and the Directorate for Employment, Labour and Social Affairs—adopted different perspectives and arrived at rather different conclusions. For a unique analysis of OECD's work in this field, revealing the workings of an international organisation undertaking comparative studies into ECEC see Mahon, (2009).

This growth in comparative research in ECEC services has paralleled a growth of policy interest, both by national governments (and, in the case of the European Union, by a regional government) and international organisations. Both have seen in ECEC an important means for pursuing a range of key policy objectives, including employment growth, gender equality, family support, poverty reduction, and educational enhancement. What is less clear, because the subject is unresearched, is how cross-national studies by the latter have influenced policy-making by the former.

2 Comparative Work on ECEC: What We Know Today

By the end of the first decade of the 21st century, we have a good knowledge of the ECEC systems in place in a range of richer countries, broadly speaking OECD member states, which are the countries where ECEC services have been most widely developed; most children living in OECD countries now spend at least 2 years in ECEC settings before beginning primary school (OECD, 2001). However, growing interest in and provision of ECEC is a global trend: global estimates suggest enrolment in pre-primary programmes increased by 11% during the 5 years up to 2004, by which time 124 million young children were attending some form of ECEC before starting school. Increases were most pronounced in the regions that were also witnessing the strongest growth in primary education, notably sub-Saharan Africa (43.5% increase), Caribbean (43% increase) and South and West Asia (40.5%) (Woodhead, 2007, p. 8).

Focusing on the richer, OECD world, we can divide countries into three groups.

1. A group of countries that have integrated government responsibility for ECEC, mostly into education though sometimes into welfare, and have further integrated key policy dimensions—such as funding, workforce and regulation. In some cases, but not all, ECEC provision is based around a single age-integrated type of provision, variously termed (e.g. "preschool" in Sweden, "kindergarten" in

Norway, "playschool" in Iceland). These countries have high levels of provision, a well-developed workforce with a high or rising proportion of graduate workers, and have accepted ECEC services, across the age range, as primarily a public good and responsibility, requiring high levels of public funding, mostly applied through directly financing services themselves (i.e. supply funding). Main examples include the five Nordic countries, New Zealand and Slovenia; the five Nordic countries are in the top six of 25 OECD countries included in the recent UNICEF "league table of early childhood education and care in economically advanced countries" (UNICEF, 2008).

2. A group of countries whose ECEC provision is split between "childcare" and "education", with divided government responsibility, and separate funding, workforce and regulation for each part. Typically "childcare" services, mainly intended for employed parents and their children, are seen as primarily a private responsibility, albeit it with lower income parents able to access some form of financial subsidy, and are provided through a market of mainly private provision, often with a substantial for-profit element; the "childcare" workforce in these services has lower qualifications and far lower pay than teachers in the "education" workforce. The "education" part is relatively under-developed, usually consisting of 1 or 2 years of often part-time provision, immediately before school entry. Such countries also have programmes targeted at disadvantaged families, based on the premise that early intervention will help reduce their high levels of poverty and inequality. Levels of public expenditure on ECEC are lower, less than half that in the first group of countries, and for "childcare" mainly takes the form of "demand subsidy", that is parents rather than services are subsidised. Main examples include English-speaking countries such as Australia, Canada (excluding Quebec), Ireland and the United States, which come bottom in the UNICEF league table.

3. A group of countries whose ECEC provision is also split between "childcare" and "education", again with divided government responsibility. But unlike the second group, "childcare" services are seen as primarily a public responsibility, often provided by local government or else by non-profit private organisations, with direct public funding through parents are also expected to contribute financially. The main feature, however, of these countries is a well-developed "education" sector with the universal provision of at least 3 years of free and often full-time education, for children from 3 years of age upwards. If "care" and "education" are integrated in the first group of countries and "care" dominates ECEC in the second, in this third group education is the dominant player. Main examples include Belgium, France, Italy, and much of Central and Eastern Europe; these countries occupy the middle part of the UNICEF league table.

Of course, like all attempts to categorise, some countries do not fit comfortably. England and Scotland, in the United Kingdom, have integrated responsibility for all ECEC services into education, and England has developed an integrated system of regulation across all ECEC services. But other key structural aspects of services—notably access, funding and workforce—remain divided, reflecting a strong and continuing tendency to see "childcare" and "education" as separate; both countries straddle groups 1 and 2. Spain similarly has integrated responsibility for ECEC into education, and has also developed an integrated approach to workforce, built around a new profession of a specialised early years teacher. Yet it has not followed through to develop a fully integrated 0-6 system, building up education for over 3s while leaving provision for under 3s largely to a market of separate, often private for-profit services; it is left straddling groups 1 and 3.

A schema such as this offers a broad brush picture of ECEC policy and provision. It reflects the emphasis of much comparative work, which has been on the quantitative and structural. We can get some idea, too, of how countries think about the purposes of services and who has responsibility for what aspects of them. But this is only the tip of the iceberg, a large tip certainly, but still only a part of a much larger whole, the easily visible part of policy. Comparative work has paid far less attention to such large areas as history, traditions and politics; understandings (social constructions) of the child or of key concepts, such as "care" and "education"; and actual practice—how and why early childhood workers and children do what they do and how they understand their practice.

There are some important exceptions. The work of Joseph Tobin and his colleagues, comparing understandings of practice in ECEC services in China, Japan and the United States, has been ground-breaking in demonstrating how this important area can be studied cross-nationally and that there are substantial cultural differences in how early childhood work is understood and practiced (Tobin, Wu, & Davidson, 1989). Their work required the development of innovative video-based methods, and Tobin and new partners have taken these methods further in a recent comparative study—*Children crossing borders*—of children of immigrants in ECEC services in five countries (for more information, see http://www.childrencrossingborders.org/uk.html).

The *Starting Strong* reports for OECD have also attempted to go deeper under the policy surface, to reveal the complex infrastructure of purpose, orientation and content. For example, John Bennett, the main coordinator of the whole project, has drawn attention to important differences between countries with what he terms a "social pedagogic" approach to ECEC (including the Nordic states) and those with a "pre-primary" approach (including many of those with strong systems of nursery education for children over 3 years).

In the former,

> The focus was traditionally on the social development of the child and family outreach. Pedagogues work with the whole child, and broad developmental goals as well as learning and language development are pursued. Programmes are child centred—interactivity with peers and educators encouraged and the quality of life in the institution is given high importance ... a balance is struck between culturally-valued *topics of learning* (such as, music, song, dance, environmental themes ...) on the one hand, and on supporting the child's meaning-making acquired through relationships and experience of the world. This requires reasonable child: Staff ratios so that staff can attend to each child, and organise interesting group or project work.

By contrast, in the pre-primary approach:

> The focus is increasingly on learning and skills in areas useful for school. Class groups are mainly teacher directed ... Teacher-child relationship may be *instrumentalised* because of large numbers of children per teacher, and the need to achieve detailed curriculum goals ... clear learning goals are established, generally in the cognitive domain, and especially as children approach school age. Phonic and syllabic recognition, and exercises in counting and calculation are often formally practised. Readiness for school is well assured in the teaching subjects that are privileged in the curriculum (Bennett, 2006).

Another interesting and telling example of more qualitative national differences, also highlighted in *Starting Strong*, is the importance attached in some countries, notably the Nordic states, to democracy as a basic value of ECEC services, a pedagogic approach going hand-in-hand in these countries with a democratic approach. Wagner (2006) argues that democracy is central to the Nordic concept of the good childhood and notes, in support of this contention, that "official policy documents and curriculum guidelines in the Nordic countries acknowledge a central expectation that preschools and schools will exemplify democratic principles and that children will be active participants in these democratic environments" (p. 292). The Swedish pre-school curriculum, for instance, states that: "democracy forms the foundation of the pre-school. For this reason, all pre-school activity should be carried out in accordance with fundamental democratic values" (Swedish Ministry of Education and Science, 1998, p. 6). For a fuller discussion of democracy and ECEC, see Moss (2007).

So a lot has been achieved over 30 or more years. We have a clear if partial picture of cross-national similarities and differences. But we also can see, more clearly, some of the issues yet to be fully addressed in the conduct of comparative studies.

3 Some Issues in the Comparative Study of ECEC Services

3.1 Methods

Anyone who has attempted to undertake a cross-national comparison of ECEC data quickly comes up against two fundamental issues: getting comparable and reliable data and the equivalence of concepts and terms. Countries do not collect the same information in the same way, in some cases because they have differently structured systems and policy agendas, in other cases because some have more centralised and effective data collection systems than others. Even the most basic of information (or information that the researcher may consider to be "most basic", a view not necessarily shared) can be frequently missing or else is collected using particular and unique methods and definitions; the end result can be tables full of gaps or numbers that do not compare like with like. In urging countries to pay "systematic attention to data collection and monitoring", the second *Starting Strong* report suggests that one problem may by the newness of the field: "the large-scale information systems on population, households, social policy and education that are routinely managed by national statistical bureaus were not initially set up to deliver the kinds of data needed to advance ECEC policy and provision" (OECD, 2006, p. 15).

But things get more difficult when it comes to concepts and terms, and indeed more generally trying to get below the numerical surface to a deeper understanding of what underlies and shapes ECEC systems. Researchers from another country, often bringing their own national baggage with them, can fail to see, hear or understand important features of the countries they are studying. This can be partly a matter of language and partly a matter of tradition and culture. A good example is provided by the example of "pedagogy", an holistic approach to working with children practiced by the profession of "pedagogue", which is long-established and widespread throughout most of Continental Europe; indeed it is difficult to understand services and practices in many countries without understanding the key role of "pedagogy" (which, confusingly to the English ear, appears as "éducation" in French-speaking countries, the pedagogue as "éducateur"). Yet "pedagogy" and "pedagogue" have been rendered almost invisible in English-speaking countries, often lost in translation ("pedagogy" typically appearing as "the science of education", "pedagogues" as "teachers") and not part of the mainstream tradition of these countries (perhaps the best translation into English, if translation should be made, is "pedagogy" as "education in its broadest sense") (for a fuller discussion of pedagogy, see Moss & Petrie, 2002; Petrie, Boddy, Cameron, Wigfall, & Simon, 2006).

One reason for the high standing achieved by the OECD *Starting Strong* review was the methodology it applied, in part to address some of these issues (described in detail in OECD, 2006, Annex B). This was "both quantitative, based on statistical data, and phenomenological, that is, based on actual visits to countries to experience their early childhood systems in a personal and experiential manner" (OECD, 2006, p. 234). Each country reviewed prepared a Background Report, providing "core quantitative and descriptive information for the review" (OECD, 2006, p. 233). A review team, consisting of 3 or 4 external experts with a member of the OECD review staff, then spent time in the country to visit services and speak to a wide range of stakeholders. After their visit, the review team produced an evaluative report, or Country Note, which was discussed and agreed with the country's government. Through this process of exchange and dialogue, the opportunities for deepening understanding were improved and the risks of deep misunderstandings (for example, from inadequate textual translation) or serious omissions were reduced, while the OECD staff accompanying each visit provided both continuity and consistency and accumulated experience and knowledge reflected in the final reports of the overall review.

The case of "pedagogy", just referred to, illustrates another methodological problem, one that is, I believe, of profound importance yet relatively little discussed: the dominance of English as a language of research and knowledge transfer. Most (I hesitate to say all) cross-national work on ECEC is conducted and reported on in English, reflecting the dominance of this language in academia (including journals and other forms of dissemination) and international organisations. This has two immediate consequences. Countries whose first language is not English are studied in English, their concepts, terms and practices translated from their own language into another language, in the process of which much may be lost—perfect translation, providing exact understanding, is an impossibility. Second, participation in such research is increasingly limited to those with a good command of English, and is in fact dominated by native English speakers, who see the world in a particular way, not only because English is their language (and the importance of language for constructing meaning is now widely appreciated) but also because they come from English-speaking societies where certain assumptions, values, practices and policies are widespread; researchers may not necessarily subscribe to these dominant discourses, yet cannot stand entirely outside of them.

Most non-English speakers involved in cross-national work are reluctant to raise the matter of language, either through politeness or perhaps a sense of the futility of doing so. The following comment by a German participant in a European training project is, therefore, unusual to see in print, but may well reflect the views of many others and could apply more generally to cross-national research:

> (The difficulties in acquiring a foreign language) has led to a pragmatism of settling for more commonly-spoken languages and of course among them for the English language predominantly with all the associated exclusionary consequences.... There is always the need to get results, to be pragmatic, to overcome language differences as barriers, and not enough time and space to explore the subtleties of discovering meaning through non-comprehension, through the pain not only of working through interpreters but of clarifying terminology so that it can be used reliably by interpreters and shared among all participants. This seems to hold up the works, those representing lesser spoken languages come to regard this as a personal problem.... Despite decades of exchanges and collaboration it is still almost impossible to make English-speaking colleagues and students in social work understand the nature of social pedagogy (Lorenz, 1999, p. 20).

A central problem, it seems to me, is that native English-speakers, surrounded by a world that seems ready to speak English, have not been aware of or taken moral responsibility for the consequences of the dominance of their language. Not having to work in other languages, they can be unaware of the demands posed by having to do so, of the complexities of translation and of the difficulty for native English-speakers to understand non-English speaking societies. They too readily take English for granted and apply, unquestioningly, an English (or perhaps I should say an Anglo-American) frame to the interpretation of a non-English experience.

Yet an awareness of linguistic diversity and a willingness to work with it can be a valuable tool in cross-national research, a means of digging down to deeper understanding of difference as well as similarity. The German researcher just quoted goes on to make an important observation, that should inform methodology on cross-national work by emphasising the potential importance of identifying and struggling with areas of incomprehension: "And yet, it would be precisely the non-understanding which could give us the most valuable clues to differences in meaning, to the need for further clarification of familiar terms and concepts, to the transformation of taken-for-granted perspectives into creative, shared knowledge"

(Lorenz, 1999, p. 21). This reflection raises a key question—why do cross-national research? I will return to this later on.

3.2 Interpretation

The question of language is of course central to making sense of cross-national data, as well as deciding what data to seek out. More generally, interpretation requires a deep knowledge of history, culture and contemporary context, as well as of related policies, such as parental leave or the compulsory school system. But even at a more superficial and quantitative level, interpretation of comparisons is rarely simple, and usually requires careful attention to detail. Producing international league tables is a case in point.

Such tables are both beguiling and dangerous, if sometimes useful. Beguiling because they appear to offer a clear comparison between disparate countries, dangerous because the appearance of comparability usually masks substantial and important differences, leading to the possibility of misleading conclusions. Any meaningful, and useful, comparative table is almost certain to include a plethora of footnotes, careful reading of which is essential to adequate interpretation. Yet footnotes go often unread, even by the most rigorous academic. So the devil is in the detail, but the detail can be readily overlooked.

A recent example of the problem with interpreting league tables is provided by the European Commission. The member states of the European Union committed themselves in 2002 to achieving "childcare" places for 33% of children under 3 and 90% of children between 3 and school age, by 2010—the so-called "Barcelona targets" (the use of "childcare" reflects how the EC, like many member states, has a split approach to ECEC services, with one Directorate-General— Employment, Social Affairs and Equal Opportunities—focusing on "childcare", a second—Education and Culture—on "early education", and a third—Justice, Freedom and Security—on children's rights). In October 2008, the European Commission published a note entitled "Childcare services in the EU", in which it assesses member states' progress towards achieving the targets (European Commission, 2008). Graph 1 provides a league table of "the proportion of children up to 3 years cared for by formal arrangements", based on the European Survey of Income and Living Conditions for 2006.

The graph shows five countries have surpassed the 33% target: Denmark, Netherlands, Sweden, Belgium and Spain. Denmark and Sweden may not be a surprise, although the substantially lower level of coverage for Sweden than Denmark needs to be read in the context of Sweden's stronger leave provision, meaning fewer children under 3 years in services (leave policy is a typical contextual issue that needs to be factored in to interpretations of ECEC data for children under 3 years, just as varying compulsory school ages need to be factored in to the other end of the ECEC spectrum, when comparing data for children over 3 years). Belgium benefits, in part, from admitting 2 year olds to nursery school. But the inclusion of Netherlands and Spain are harder to understand, as they are not known for having high levels of provision for younger children.

More careful scrutiny of the graph reveals part of the reason; the Netherlands has an attendance rate of about 45%, but on closer inspection it can be seen that nearly all of this group are attending less than 30 hours a week, in sharp contrast to the other four countries where half or more attend 30 hours a week or more. This is accounted for by the very high level of part-time employment among Dutch mothers (the highest, by far, in Europe) and also by high numbers of under 3s attending playgroups, a form of provision open for short hours and often attended by children whose mothers are not employed. In other words, if a comparison had been made of volume of attendance—the number of hours attended per week—rather than numbers of children attending, the Netherlands would not only be far outstripped by the other four countries, but would drop far down the league table. As for Spain, it is impossible to understand the high level of children in "formal arrangements", not least because there is no further detail apart from hours of attendance, for example no explanation of what arrangements are in use in each country.

3.3 Consequences

Having worked in this field for many years, I am a great enthusiast for cross-national work and believe it can make a major contribution to policy and practice. The key question is why? My answer is because such work is invaluable for stimulating critical thinking: "a matter of introducing a critical attitude towards those things that are given to our present experience as if they were timeless, natural, unquestionable... [it is a matter] of interrupting the fluency of the narratives that encode that experience and making them stutter" (Rose, 1999, p. 20). At its best, cross-national work makes us question our taken-for-granted assumptions, makes the implicit explicit, makes the familiar strange. It raises awareness of otherness and alternatives, so helping us break free from what Unger (2005) calls "the dictatorship of no alternative" (p. 1). If we believe that policy making should be, first and foremost, a democratic political and ethical process, supported by but not led by technical practice, then we need critical thinking and awareness of alternatives.

Cross-national study can also deepen our awareness of the processes and forces by which policies come to be made and maintained and discourses attain dominance. It is, therefore, a necessary condition for understanding the politics of ECEC policy and, by definition, understanding how change has come about in the past and might be brought about in the future.

But we should remember Foucault's comment that "not everything is bad but that everything is dangerous". Cross-national comparisons can, I believe, be dangerous, especially if they are used as part of a managerial exercise in benchmarking, best practice or whatever other term is used to describe processes of standardisation and normalisation based on a belief in and search for universal, objective and stable standards and norms—processes that give primacy to technical practice. This is not to deny the importance of coherence, the case for certain democratically-agreed common principles and values; but it is to recognise the importance also of diversity—of perspectives, values, purposes—and of the inevitable and necessary tension in the relationship between coherence and stability, a relationship that has been with us for millennia and can never be reduced to a final position.

I have been involved and continue to be involved in a search for a common set of European goals and principles for ECEC services, and this search has been and continues to be informed by cross-national comparison. In 1996, the EC Childcare Network that I coordinated produced a ground-breaking document, *Quality Targets in Services for Young Children*, which set out 40 targets whose achievement would implement the political principles and objectives agreed by EU member state governments in a 1992 Council Recommendation on Child Care. While in 2008, *Children in Europe*, a multi-lingual European magazine published by a network of national magazines, produced a Policy Paper outlining the rationale for and components of a European approach to ECEC policy, including a common image of the child and 10 principles (Children in Europe, 2008). Both of these exercises have convinced me that, informed by cross-national knowledge of different perspectives and systems, it is possible to arrive through democratic negotiation at substantial agreement on shared goals and principles, albeit always subject to review and revision.

In this search I have drawn particular inspiration and knowledge from particular places, both countries and communities. These places have shown me that there are alternatives, that other ways of thinking and practicing ECEC are possible, and have provoked me to think about my own understandings, values and theories about ECEC. This experience of the importance of "islands of dissensus" has led me to believe that as well as needing a framework of democratically-negotiated common goals and principles, there is a need not just for diversity but for the welfare state to actively espouse and support local and democratic experimentation (Unger, 2005), whether it be in the delivery of services or in pedagogical theories and practices—or, in the words of the director of an Italian city's ECEC services, the need to stimulate and nurture "local cultural projects of childhood".

In short, we need more discussion about the potential uses and abuses of comparative work. And we need to recognise that comparative work can involve the study of both mainstream policies, service systems and discourses, but also of local knowledge and minority experiences. If it is to avoid the trap of furthering standardisation and normalisation, it needs to keep a critical stance and an openness to alterity.

4 What Next?

Looking forward I would like to suggest three strands in the future direction for comparative work on ECEC.

1. **Continuing strong**: the *Starting Strong* review has left the ECEC world with an invaluable resource of information. What is needed now, I believe, is to ensure that this resource is maintained and improved to provide an accessible

data base—combining quantitative and qualitative material—for researchers, students, policy makers and others wanting information on ECEC in different countries. Annex E of the 2006 report is titled "Country Profiles", and contains an extensive and detailed account of the ECEC systems in all 20 participating countries. These profiles should be extended to include other countries and some additional items (for example, more material on concepts and pedagogical practice and more information on complementary policies such as parental leaves), regularly updated by an agency working with an advisory group of leading experts, and made generally available for research, study, policy making and other purposes.

The data base of country profiles might also be used to conduct a regular (5 yearly) international overview of the current situation and recent developments in ECEC; and to develop and regularly produce a set of comparable, meaningful and useful ECEC indicators.

2. **Focused comparative studies**: Such a regular overview should preclude the need for further general one-off studies. Instead, cross-national work should now focus on the study of more specific topics and developments, for example:

- *Evaluations*: examples might include market approaches to ECEC; education-based integrated systems (a pilot project on this subject is, at the time of writing, underway with the support of UNESCO); and the relationship between ECEC and the school system (the *Starting Strong* reports propose a "strong and equal partnership", which might provide one frame of reference for such a study).
- *Politics and history* of ECEC policies and discourses. A recent study of the politics of leave policies (Kamerman & Moss, 2009) reveals the importance of such work for analysis and understanding of current policies, as well as the role of path dependency and the possibilities for "paradigm" change. Another related area meriting more study is the role of governance, for example the particular issues arising in federal states, and the relationship between national and local government in unitary states.
- *ECEC practice and understandings of practice* among children, parents and ECEC workers. The work of Joseph Tobin and others provides a good basis for further comparative studies to explore not only if and how practice itself differs between countries but also how stakeholders understand practice.
- *Understandings (or images)* of the child, services themselves and early childhood workers. The world famous pedagogical practice in Reggio Emilia is famously based on the question "what is your image of the child?", which captures the notion, now deeply embedded in the sociology of childhood, that childhood is a social construction. The same holds true for all other aspects of ECEC. The significance is that understandings (or images or social constructions) are arguably highly productive of policy, provision and practice. Once again, deep knowledge requires digging deep below the surface, to explore the extent and nature of fundamental differences of perception.

3. **Comparative local studies of innovative communities and services** that share similar values, ways of working and/or purposes, to better understand the conditions under which, for example, democratic experimentation ("local cultural projects of childhood") may develop and thrive. One approach would be to look at local experiences in different countries which share a common source of inspiration, for example centres working with inspiration from Reggio Emilia in Northern Italy. This city, whose pedagogical theories and practices have developed over more than 40 years, has influenced practitioners and services in many countries, from Korea to Sweden, generating many questions about how local knowledge can be distributed and adapted, as well as providing a fascinating example of what has been termed glocalisation (for further discussion of the pedagogical theories and practices of Reggio Emilia, see Dahlberg, Moss, & Pence, 2007; Rinaldi, 2005).

Another potential example would be to compare examples of centres which have developed as social movements, moving in Manual Castell's terms from a "resistance identity" to a "project identity". Project identities emerge from local demands struggling to change perceived conditions of exclusion and existing power relationships. In extraordinary circumstances, groups such as Sheffield Children's Centre not only resist their conditions but also are able to propose alternatives to mainstream views by attempting to reconcile and overcome such contradictions. The story of the centre is, by and large, a history of the construction of alternative ways to engage with the children and families with whom the centre is connected, and with communities within which it has come to be embedded (Broadhead, Meleady, & Delgado, 2008).

This excerpt comes from a book which is a case study of an extraordinary and important local experience, the Sheffield Children's Centre, a community-based centre that has developed a wide range of services for children and families, as a result of deep engagement with its local community and its democratic ethos. The book exemplifies Lather's call for "qualitative policy analysis", involving "a form of applied social science that can cope with the multiplicity of the social world". In this work, Lather argues, "Case studies assume prime importance as critical cases, strategically chosen, providing far better access for policy intervention than the present social science of variables. . . Simultaneously 'sociological, political and philosophical' (Flyvbjerg, 2001, p. 64), this is a kind of science that does not divest experience of its rich ambiguity because it stays close to the complexities and contradictions of existence". (Lather, 2006, p. 785).

The book on the Sheffield Children's Centre is co-authored by a Mexican undertaking doctoral studies in England, and who is able to make some connections between the Sheffield centre and the "example of a community-based preschool scheme that began in 1981 in one of the rapidly growing shanty towns of Mexico City" (Broadhead et al., 2008, p. 21). This comparison is not, however, developed at length, but hints at the potential for more comparative work at the level of local ECEC projects, cross-national studies of critical cases that engage with complexity and diversity.

5 Conclusion

I have spent half my working life struggling to understand policy systems and structures in a range of richer countries, and I still find this interesting and important. But over the years I have become increasingly drawn to the idea that systems and structures, not just in ECEC but more generally across the welfare state, are produced by deeply embedded political and cultural values and understandings. This can lead down the reductionist road of path dependency, which may lead to the (mistaken) conclusion that no change is possible, that there is no alternative. But it can also open up the prospect of thinking and doing differently, that there are alternatives directions and, therefore, democratic choices to be made between different pathways.

Two understandings of early childhood services that are widespread, especially in the English-speaking world, are as businesses, supplying a marketised commodity for sale to parents; and as factories, applying technologies to children to produce predetermined outcomes. Through my cross-national work, especially in Italy and Sweden, my own understandings have been challenged, provoked and stimulated, until today I find myself drawn down another path, towards another understanding of early childhood services: as "public forums in civil society in which children and adults participate together in projects of social, cultural, political and economic significance" (Dahlberg et al., 2007, p. 73). As such they can also be seen as laboratories or workshops (Rinaldi, 2005), where citizens, younger and older, collaborate to enhance individual and public well-being by producing many outcomes, only some of which are predetermined.

I realise, of course, that such an understanding is neither universal nor inevitable. It is a choice and one at odds with understandings of services as businesses and factories. But it is a possibility, it is an alternative, it opens up for a democratic politics of early childhood—and it owes everything, in my case, to cross-national work and to the inspiration of leaders in this field such as Al Kahn.

References

Bennett, J. (2006, 10 May). 'Schoolifying' early childhood education and care: Accompanying preschool into education. Public lecture given at the Institute of Education University of London.

Broadhead, P., Meleady, C., & Delgado, M. A. (2008). *Children, families and communities: Creating and sustaining integrated services.* Maidenhead: Open University Press.

Children in Europe. (2008). *Young children and their services: Developing a European approach.* Children in Europe Policy Paper. http://www.childrenineurope.org/docs/PolicyDocument_001.pdf. Accessed 5 December 2008.

Dahlberg, G., Moss, P., & Pence, A. (2007). *Beyond quality in early childhood education and care: Languages of evaluation* (2nd ed.). London: Routledge.

European Commission. (2008). *Childcare services in the EU* (Memo/08/592, Brussels, 3 October 2008). http://europa.eu/rapid/pressReleasesAction.do?reference=MEMO/08/592&type=HTML. Accessed 5 December 2008.

Flyvbjerg, B. (2001). *Making social science matter: Why social inquiry fails and how it can succeed again.* Cambridge: Cambridge University Press.

Kahn, A. J., & Kamerman, S. B. (1976). *Child care programs in nine countries: A report prepared for the OECD working party on the role of women in the economy.* Paris: Organisation for Economic Cooperation and Development.

Kamerman, S., & Moss, P. (forthcoming, 2009). *The politics of parental leave policies: Children, parenting, gender and the labour market.* Bristol: Policy Press.

Lather, P. (2006). Foucauldian scientificity: Rethinking the nexus of qualitative research and educational policy analysis. *International Journal of Qualitative Studies in Education, 19*(6), 783–791.

Lorenz, W. (1999). The ECSPRESS approach – Guiding the social professions between national and global perspectives. In O. Chytil & F. W. Seibel (Eds.), *European dimensions in training and practice of social professions* (pp. 13–28). Boskovice: Verlag Albert.

Mahon, R. (2009). *The OECD's discourse on the reconciliation of work and family life.* Global Social Policy, *9*(2): 183–204 .

Moss, P. (2007). Bringing politics into the nursery: Early childhood education as a democratic practice. *European Early Childhood Education Research Journal, 15*(1), 5–20.

Moss, P., & Petrie, P. (2002). *From children's services to children's spaces: Public policy, children and childhood.* London: Routledge.

OECD (Organisation for Economic Cooperation and Development). (2001). *Starting strong I: Early childhood education and care.* Paris: Organisation for Economic Cooperation and Development.

OECD (Organisation for Economic Cooperation and Development). (2006). *Starting strong II: Early childhood education and care.* Paris: Organisation for Economic Cooperation and Development.

OECD (Organisation for Economic Cooperation and Development). (2007). *Babies and bosses: reconciling work and family life.* Paris: Organisation for Economic Cooperation and Development.

Petrie, P., Boddy, J., Cameron, C., Wigfall, V., & Simon, A. (2006). *Working with children in care: European perspectives.* Maidenhead: Open University Press.

Rinaldi, C. (2005). *In dialogue with Reggio Emilia: Listening, researching and learning.* London: Routledge.

Rose, N. (1999). *Powers of freedom: Reframing political thought.* Cambridge: Cambridge University Press.

Swedish Ministry of Education and Science. (1998). *Curriculum for preschool* (English translation). Stockholm: Swedish Ministry of Education and Science.

Tobin, J., Wu, D., & Davidson, D. (1989). *Preschool in three cultures: Japan, China and the United States.* New Haven, CT: Yale University Press.

Unger, R. (2005). *What should the left propose?* London: Verso.

UNICEF. (2008). *The child care transition: A league table of early childhood education and care in economically advanced countries* (Innocenti Report Card 8). Florence: UNICEF Innocenti Research Centre.

Wagner, J. T. (2006). An outsider's perspective: Childhoods and early education in the Nordic countries. In J. Einarsdottir & J. T. Wagner (Eds.), *Nordic childhoods and early education: Philosophy, research, policy and practice in Denmark, Finland, Iceland, Norway, and Sweden* (pp. 289–306). Greenwich, CT: Information Age Publishing.

Woodhead, M. (2007). Early childhood and primary education. In M. Woodhead & P. Moss (Eds.), *Early childhood and primary education: Transitions in the lives of young children* (Early childhood in focus 2, p. 8). Milton Keynes: Open University.

Childcare Policies in France: The Influence of Organizational Changes in the Workplace

Jeanne Fagnani

Along with the Nordic countries, France leads the European Union in public child-care provision and benefits aimed at reducing child care costs for families (Adema & Thévenon, 2008; Fagnani & Math, 2008) (see Chapter 17 in this book). In a recent cross-national study, OECD[1] has also shown that family spending has the greatest focus on childcare services in France and the Nordic countries. As a matter of fact, the progressive arrival of mothers on the labour market since the 1970s has, through an interactive process, prompted French family policy decision makers to introduce a whole range of services for parents in paid employment, which has in turn enabled a growing number of mothers to gain access to jobs. This has helped to place the question of the work/family life balance firmly onto the policy agenda.

However, since the nineties, significant organizational changes entering the workplace have marched hand in hand with a trend toward the development of atypical, irregular and/or unforeseeable working time schedules. Against this background, how do decision makers involved in family policies tackle the issue of children' s well-being—in particular as far as their everyday life is concerned—when both parents are in paid work? By focusing specifically on preschool children (aged under 6 years) I will attempt to demonstrate that the real driver for current childcare policies, while couched in terms of the "best interest" of the child, is in fact the combined forces of labour market pressure and demands for a mother's right to paid work.

The first part of my paper will offer an historical overview of childcare policies since the seventies by placing emphasis on continuities and changes and highlighting the ways in which the boundaries between the state, families, and the market

J. Fagnani (✉)
Centre d'Economie de la Sorbonne-Team Matisse, University of Paris, France

Source: Report of the "Cour des Comptes", Les aides à la garde des jeunes enfants, July 2008, http://www.ccomptes.fr/CC/documents/RELFSS/Chap10-aides-garde-jeunes-enfants.pdf

Note: A child can attend the nursery school in the morning and be cared for by a childminder in the afternoon or looked after by a nanny after having spent the day in a crèche.

[1] Family spending in services represents 1.6 percentage of GDP compared to 0.77 in Germany for instance. http://www.oecd.org/dataoecd/15/47/39680843.xls

S.B. Kamerman et al. (eds.), *From Child Welfare to Child Well-Being*, Children's Well-Being: Indicators and Research 1, DOI 10.1007/978-90-481-3377-2_21, © Springer Science+Business Media B.V. 2010

have been redrawn where childcare responsibilities are concerned. Additionally, rationales which underpinned the successive policy changes at various stages as they were introduced will be explored. In the second part, I will provide an analysis of the reforms introduced since the nineties and shed light on what was at stake from the perspective of the children' s well-being and public support to mothers' employment. To conclude, I will point out some of the tensions and dilemmas policy makers currently face in regard to childcare policies.

1 Problematic and Theoretical Background: What is at Stake?

In France, during the week, around a third (36%) of children aged three years or under receive care solely from their parents, in most cases the mother (Ruault & Audrey, 2003). Indeed, a significant proportion of mothers of young children are in fact on parental leave and therefore don't work at all (and are eligible for a flat-rate benefit)—or only on a part-time basis—until the child is able to attend nursery school. The decision made by many to become full-time parents comes down to a number of factors: harsh working conditions, in particular working schedules that don't match the opening hours of public childcare facilities; long commute times; and the numerous difficulties they often have to cope with to reconcile work with family responsibilities. The remaining two-thirds of children have mothers who resume their job after maternity leave and rely on publicly subsidized child care arrangements.[2] In reality, families with young children often need two earners in order to afford housing and to achieve a certain level of lifestyle, in particular in families whose mother's potential wage is high enough to make employment worthwhile and who can choose to "outsource" care as the opportunity (Bloemen & Stancanelli, 2008) cost of using their own time to provide care rose.

Many of these mothers and especially the ambitious or career-oriented are forced to devote large chunks of time to their job, in spite of the implementation of the 35-hour laws on working time (Fagnani & Letablier, 2004). It is in fact important to mention that the 35 working hours are calculated on an average annual basis, which means that employees may sometimes work 42 hours or more a week for a few months and much less at other periods. A wide range of options may be developed within the same company, which reinforces the general movement towards the individualisation and fragmentation of working schedules. As far as management is concerned, the units of reference are working days, which imply that employees may, for example, have a day off every two weeks (or have a longer holiday period). But, at the same time, they may continue to work for long hours everyday day, which does not help them to devote more time to family obligations.

---

[2] 80.6% of mothers with only one child, under three years of age, were economically active in 2007. Among them, 57.0% were working full-time (Employment survey, INSEE, 2008).

The legislation on working hours is very complex and diversity has been the rule in introducing new forms of work organisation. Against the background of unbalanced power relationships between employers and employees (taking into account a high unemployment rate and a low level of trade union representation), employees have sometimes been obliged to accept flexible working schedules and practices to which they traditionally objected. Therefore a wide range of patterns of reduction in working time was observed. Moreover from 2007, employees are encouraged to work additional hours which are paid 25% more per hour (50% more on Sundays).

Indeed, in France as in other countries, firms are compelled to operate within an intensely competitive global market, which in turn shapes their internal working patterns and practices (Perrons, Fagan, McDowell, Ray, & Ward, 2006). With the development of flexible and not always family friendly work schedules and an increase in workload, dual-earner parents are frequently facing enormous difficulties in managing their everyday life (Bressé, le Bihan, & Martin, 2007). Therefore, they are often obliged to rely on multiple—both formal and informal—child care arrangements (Fagnani & Letablier, 2005) and their children are likely to spend large amounts of time outside of the home.

Within this context the need to investigate what effects changing working conditions, and consequently the daily patterns of parents lives, are having on the well being of children is clear. Should there in fact be any guarantees on what constitutes adequate time for children to spend with their parents? Where and how are young children cared for when both parents are in full time employment? Have decision makers properly taken into account France's long standing tradition of focusing on the quality of care and the benevolent effects it provides on the early socialisation of young children? Our aim will be to partially answer these questions.

In analysing changes in child care policies since the seventies, borrowing from Peter Hall (1993), I will distinguish at each stage:

- A process of first order change: the process whereby instrument settings are changed (i.e., the level at which child care benefits and related tax deductions are set), while the overall goals and instruments of policy remain the same.
- A process of second order change: when the instruments of policy as well as their settings (i.e., successive governments decided in the eighties and nineties to create new child care allowances and to increase regularly their respective levels), are altered even though the overall goals of policy remain the same which, in the case of France, means supporting mothers' employment and creating jobs in the caring sector.
- A process of third order change or paradigm shift: when a radical shift (i.e., when French family policy shifted from the *male-breadwinner model* to the *dual-earner model*), entails simultaneous changes in all three components of policy, the instruments settings, the instruments themselves, and the hierarchy of goals behind policy.

These three types of policy change (or variables) are used by Peter Hall to disaggregate the concept of "social learning" which is defined "as a deliberate attempt to adjust goals or techniques in response to past experience and new information. Learning is indicated when policy changes as the result of such a process". We can draw upon French family policy to provide a salient illustration of the appropriateness of these concepts. In the eighties policy makers at the governmental level learned from research reports that West German fertility rates were significantly lower than those found in France but—no doubt to their surprise—so was the rate of female employment. A decision was thus made to increase caring services and extend support for mothers' employment (Fagnani, 2007). Despite the reluctance of some organized social interests (i.e., the most conservative family associations), boundaries between the state, families, and the market were redrawn. This evidence is consistent with the progressive entry of women into the workforce. Therefore this theoretical approach provides a useful framework to analyze the course of French child care policymaking since the paradigmatic shift which took place from the 1970s onwards.

The theory of *path dependency* (according to which all reforms are framed by past commitments and specific institutional arrangements) (Pierson, 2001), would also seem relevant to any investigation into how the policies and their underlying logic have been moving in these areas. Moreover, it should be noted that child care provision and the public delivery of services provided to working parents are nested within a set of broader institutional arrangements; France has an "explicit" family policy that is overseen by government institutions and the subject of official reports produced annually. The "family" as such is legally recognized as an institution that plays an important role in the maintenance of social cohesion. The appointment of a minister responsible for family issues further demonstrates the importance given to this issue.

The principal institution in charge of family policy is the *National Family Allowance Fund* (CNAF), with its large network of 123 *Local Allowance Funds* (CAFs). Theoretically, the social partners as well as family organisations represented on the Executive Board of the CNAF meet periodically to determine the orientations for intervention in family policy. In actual practice, decisions are made by the government, whether approved or not by the Executive Board. It is solely at the local level that the Executive Boards of the CAFs have any real decision-making power, and in particular, a margin for manoeuvre in the provision and development of childcare services.

Focusing on child care policies in isolation will provide few compelling insights and our aim will be to look at their overall organisation and then place it in its institutional, historical and cultural context.

1.1 The Development of an Extensive System of Public Day Care Since the Seventies: a Paradigmatic Shift

In order to understand the foundations of the current child care policy we need to realize that in France children have been historically considered as not only a private but a public resource as well. They represent a "common good" and indeed the "wealth of the Nation" which in turn bears certain obligations towards them. This long-standing tradition stretching back to the 19th Century (Morgan, 2002) also helps to explain why *crèches* and nursery schools enjoy such widespread popular support. Indeed, since the end of World War II, *Protection Maternelle et Infantile* (PMI) services, a national public system of preventive health care and health promotion for all mothers and children from birth through age 6, has played an important role and is responsible for the quality of public childcare provision. They license and monitor all care services falling outside the public school system which include: the monitoring of compliance with health (including preventive health exams and vaccinations); safety; nutrition; and staffing standards. They are additionally occupied with the supervision of the training and licensing of childminders. Additionally, an office of the child ombudsmen (*défenseur des enfants*) was created in 2000 and is charged with protecting the "interests of the child". Nevertheless, it lacks funding and because of limited means its missions are largely focused on high profile subjects which have provoked some sort of public outcry such as the abuse of children or juvenile delinquency.

1.1.1 Public Childcare Provision: An Historical Legacy

The history of public childcare in France is intimately bound up with the notion that the state has an obligation to protect maternity, childhood, and the capacity of women to work outside the home (in particular during the first World war when the economy needed the women on the labor market) (Luc, 1999). This conception, deeply embedded in Republican ideals, manifested itself in the latter stages of the 19th century, when demographic trends suggested to the state that motherhood needed more attention, and was closely bound up with the prevailing views of how to define the idea of citizenship.

Later, from the post-war years to the seventies, legislators focused their attentions on reducing the high infant mortality rate. They assumed that the most efficient way to achieve this goal was to encourage mothers to stay at home. This was at odds with a longstanding tradition of labour force participation of women in France (Pedersen, 1993). Protecting the physical health of children and of pregnant women moved to the forefront of the policy agenda and it was within this context that PMI services were reinforced and developed. In accordance with these measures, and in order to encourage mothers to stay at home, couples with at least two children were offered financial incentives in the form of the "*Allocation de Salaire Unique*" (Single Salary Allowance). Additionally, until the 1960s, France promoted the "male breadwinner" model by providing generous assistance to families where only the male was in paid employment (Fagnani, 2006). Accordingly, the labour force participation rate of mothers remained very low until the mid 1960s.

However from the seventies onwards, the hierarchy of goals and set of instruments employed to guide childcare policy shifted progressively and radically. This was accompanied by substantial changes in the type discourse employed by policy makers. The level of the "Single Salary Allowance" was progressively reduced, then restricted only to low-income families, and eventually abolished in 1978. Against the background of an acute labour shortage, and a growing demand for qualified women to occupy jobs in the tertiary sector (education, health, social services, administration and banking), the French government began to set up community-funded day care centres (*crèches*) in an attempt to attract women into the work force. At the same time, as the result of an interactive process, the increase in the participation of married women in the labour force stimulated demand by couples for the expansion of public day care facilities and other social services. The primary source of this demand came directly from the urban middle classes and was actively supported by the women's movement, a movement which placed strong emphasis on equality issues in the labour market. All of these factors provided a strong impetus for childcare policy change and French family policy took steps to incorporate the model of the "working mother". A growing proportion of unpaid private care-giving responsibility was progressively transferred into the domain of paid public provision.

Against this background, political actors were inclined to win women's votes on the basis of their support for child care provision. Policy makers became increasingly receptive to the arguments of early childhood specialists in favour of *crèches*: local Family Allowance Funds (*Caisse d'Allocations Familiales*, CAFs) obtained additional funding to take partial responsibility for the running costs of public childcare services, including *crèches*, and to improve the quality of care for infants and young children. At the same time, legislators took a further decisive step with the creation of a childcare allowance for families where the mother worked outside the home. This decision was particularly symbolic in that it also decreed that the Single Salary Allowance would henceforth only be granted to low-income families. Within this context, recreational centres, and holiday camps for employees' children were also organized by several companies at the instigation of their respective Works Committees.

In the second half of the 1970s the rise in the number of *crèche* slots and the increasing attendance of young children in nursery schools (*écoles maternelles*) finally gave decisive impetus to childcare policies which placed emphasis on the "quality" aspect of child care provision. A 1977 law allowed registered "child minders" access to proper employee status and its associated rights which had up to that point been restricted by the vagueness and ambiguity of their positions. This law also marked the first steps toward social recognition of the importance of the quality of childcare. Militant action and information campaigns organized by the National Association of Nursery Nurses, doctors in the PMI services and psychologists were beginning to bear fruit. The early socialization of young children was promoted by stressing that *crèches* provided an "ideal" preparation for the transition to nursery school.

When the left came to power at the beginning of the 1980s, trade unionists and political decision makers spoke increasingly of the need to develop a childcare policy "to assist mothers" to combine paid work and family responsibilities. As a result funding allocated by both local authorities and the CNAF for the construction of *crèches* was substantially increased. The progressive construction of policy oriented towards working mothers interacted with the change in women's attitudes vis-à-vis paid work in a snowball effect that resulted in a rise in women's employment rates.

The existence of the "*école maternelle*" (nursery school), an institution created in the late nineteenth century under the Third Republic (Morgan, 2002), added to the growing movement in favour of shared public responsibility for young children. Around 8% of children aged between two and three and 99% of those aged 3–6 now attend (either on a full-time or part-time basis) these free *école maternelle*. On site cafeterias and out of school hours care centres have enabled more mothers to work full-time. Furthermore, local authorities have considerably developed recreational infrastructure to keep schoolchildren occupied on lesson free Wednesday afternoons, or after school, using financial assistance from the local CAFs.

It has therefore become quite socially acceptable for a child less than three years of age to be taken care of in public day care facilities for the whole day while his or her parents are at work. The early socialization this provides is additionally held in high esteem, particularly by the educated middle classes and the probability that a child will attend a *crèche* increases significantly when his or her mother has reached a high level of educational attainment. In France, 12% of those children whose parents are in senior or middle management or occupying supervisory roles are enrolled (despite the fact that this childcare arrangement is more costly for them than for low-income families), compared with only 7% of children from working-class families (Ruault & Audrey, 2003). Among children aged under three with a mother working full-time, 30% of those living in well off families (top fifth quintile of income) are cared for in a *crèche* compared to only 22% of those living in the poorest families (first and second quintiles) (Bressé & Galtier, 2006) because for them it is still cheaper to rely on family members (most often grand parents).

Therefore, developments of public infrastructure and the resulting benefits linked to childcare have gone hand in hand with changes in childrearing norms. It is undeniable that France's historical legacy has created a favourable context for these changes to occur.

1.2 The Development of Individualized Formal Childcare Arrangements: Promoting "Freedom of Choice" or Fighting Unemployment?

France is well known for having pursued demographic objectives in its social policy, until the 1970s. However given the country's relatively high fertility rates[3] (2.0 compared to 1.3 in Germany by 2007), from the 1990s onwards socio-economic constraints and public concern about the dramatic rise in unemployment rates have

---

[3] This high fertility rate partly explains why the pronatalist lobby is no more so influential as before.

been the main drivers for second order change in childcare policies. Against a background of rising unemployment the right-wing government decided, in 1994, to exploit the job creating potential of the childcare sector by dramatically increasing child care allowances and introducing special tax breaks in order to help families better meet the costs of "individualized" child care arrangements (registered child minders and home helps like "nannies"). The government hoped to encourage families with young children to create employment and at the same time bring more domestic workers into the formal economy. Adopting the rhetoric of "free choice for parents", and "diversification of childcare arrangements" to draw popular support, successive governments began to use family policy as a tool to fight unemployment without challenging the overall terms of *the working mother* model. Concomitantly, increasing internal flexibility (often employer driven and not always family friendly), in the workplace—in particular development of irregular or atypical working hours—has led to a rising demand for more "flexible" forms of child care arrangements.[4]

Against this background, the issue of the child's interest from the point of view of the time spent with both parents and of the protection of their biological rhythms, seems to have been relegated to the background of the policy agenda. Policy makers (the ministry in charge of family policies, local authorities, and the CNAF) refocused their energies and began to place more emphasis on the following issues: how to increase the number of available slots in *crèches* and the number of licensed child minders; finding new funding structures for childcare facilities; and making regulation more flexible in regard to the skills of the staff in *crèches*.

1.2.1 Outsourcing of Care Work and the Promotion of Individualized Formal Child Care Arrangements

Successive governments, regardless of their political stripes, began to favour the development of individualized childcare arrangements with the underlying aim being to reduce the cost of hiring someone in the sector which cared for young children. The CNAF and the State agreed to pay a portion of the social security contributions and salaries of registered child minders and "nannies". From 2004, these childcare allowances are income-related. To be eligible both parents with at least one child aged under 6 have to be employed or registered as unemployed or attending a training course.

---

[4] Over the last decade, there has been an increase in the number of "Multi-accueil" services, sometimes also called "Maisons de la petite enfance". They currently account for nearly three quarters of childcare facilities (Bailleau, 2007). The rationale is to group together in one place, multiple and flexible childcare arrangements: crèches, halte-garderies (half-time), emergency care for children at risk, meeting rooms for childminders who look after children in their own home but who regularly attend "Multi-accueil" facilities to provide the children with opportunities to play together. The objective was to meet parents' needs by providing them with opportunities to modify their childcare arrangement along with their professional constraints and to get in the same place another one more fitted to their current obligations (from part-time to full-time for instance, on a regular basis or from time to time, etc.). The use of some slots in "Multi-accueil" is therefore not defined in advance.

Parallel to the reduction in the cost of this type of childcare was an accompanying increase in the professionalism of child minders, who are now required to receive two years of additional training in the 5 years following their initial registration. These measures have achieved considerable success, with the number of families receiving the child-care allowance associated with a registered child minder[5] rising from 110,000 in 1991 to 685,000 in 2005 (Caisse Nationale des Allocations Familiales, CNAF). As a result, the most common type of care arrangement for children of working parents, with the exceptions of the actual parent on parental leave, is now the registered child minder (Table 1).

Table 1 Childcare arrangements for children aged under 3 (2006)

	Number of children under 3
Collective childcare facilities	327,600
	30.1%
Kindergarten and nursery schools	184,600*
	17.0%
Registered childminders	535,000
	49.3%
Nanny at home (publicly subsidized)	37,300*
	3.4%
Total	1,085,100
	100%
	46.4%
Looked after by parents (with paid parental leave or not) or other people (relatives, friends . . .)	1,253,900
	53.9%
Total number of children 0–3 years	2,339,000
	100%

* Estimations
Source: Report of the *'Cour des Comptes', Les aides à la garde des jeunes enfants, July 2008*
Note: A child can attend the nursery school in the morning and be cared for by a childminder in the afternoon or looked after by a nanny after having spent the day in a crèche.

A second childcare allowance covers a part of the social security contributions which must be paid by families who employ a person in their home (a "nanny") to care for their child(ren) aged under 6 years. In addition, these families are entitled to a deduction of 50% of the real costs from their income tax up to a limit of 6,000 Euros per year.

Despite vociferous criticism emanating from women's associations, the government also decided in 1994 to provide encouragement to active parents who, upon giving birth to a second child, opt for "staying-at-home" after the maternity (or paternity) leave. A new flat rate childrearing benefit (not income-related) is now provided on the condition that they stop working or work only on a part-time basis until the child reaches the age of three (Fagnani & Math, 2009). To be eligible

---

[5] This child-care allowance covers the social security contributions to be paid by the employer of the registered childminder. An additional and income-related financial contribution is also given to the family.

for this benefit, parents are required to have worked or have been registered as unemployed before the birth. Despite a gender-neutral discourse, 98% of beneficiaries are currently women. This reinforces therefore the widely held view that caring remains the primary responsibility of the mother. In this context, under the Socialist government, a serious attempt was made to encourage a less unequal division of unpaid work within couples; official rhetoric on family issues emphasized the right of *both parents* to be present with a newborn baby. This resulted in a decision to extend paternity leave (paid at full rate under a certain ceiling) from three to eleven days from January 2002.

In total, in dual-earner families, approximately seven out of ten children under three years of age attend either a *crèche* (the fees are income-related) or nursery school (which is free but fees for lunch are income-related) or are the subject of subsidized childcare whether this be a registered child minder; help in their own home; or one of the two parents receiving the Child Rearing Benefit. All these figures are already beyond the targets for 2010 that were set at the European Summit of Barcelona held in 2002.

1.2.2 Changes in Instrument Settings: The Reform Introduced in 2004

In 2004 a process of first order change took place under the right-wing government (headed by Prime Minister de Villepin) and a reform of the child care allowances system was introduced. In fact, the two former child care allowances were replaced by a single one, namely the *"Complément de libre choix du mode de garde"* (Supplement for the freedom of choice of the child care arrangement). This allowance is income related and its amount also varies according to the type of child care arrangement and the age of the child. Thanks to the significant increase in its amount, it has become cheaper for low-income families to rely on a registered childminder than before.

In reality, the only change of real consequence contained in the reforms consisted of providing parents with a single child aged under three, with an allowance[6] (*Complément de libre choix d'activité*, Supplement for the freedom of choice to work or not), which is an equivalent of the former child rearing benefit. Eligibility criteria is strict and requires that the mother or father has been continuously working for at least two years before the child's birth which has meant that parents holding precarious or undeclared jobs are all but disqualified from qualifying for this allowance.

In 2006 the government introduced further measures which benefited only larger families, defined as having at least three children. Following the birth of a third child or more one of the two parents can take advantage of an allowance of 766 Euros per month (in 2008) for a total of 12 months on condition that one parent stops working completely. The aim of this measure is to encourage fathers who earn modest salaries to consider taking parental leave.

---

[6] Its amount is 552 Euros per month in 2009 if the parent does not work and this amount decreases if the parent works part-time.

2 The Predicament of Childcare Policy: What is at Stake?

In spite of its many successes, in particular a spectacular decline in the infant mortality rate since the end of World War II,[7] French family policy is facing new challenges linked to the numerous and dramatic changes which have occurred both on the labour market and in the family sphere. This has forced policy makers and social partners (Executive Boards of CAFs, local authorities, and trade-unions), to confront the resulting tensions which have arisen because of conflicting interests within the family.

2.1 Dilemmas for Policy Makers: Coping with Conflicting Interests Within the Family

Between 1998 and 2000, average working time was reduced by the 35-hour legislation (Fagnani & Letablier, 2004). As a result, significant organizational changes in the workplace and intensification of work have gone hand in hand with a development of atypical, irregular and/or unforeseeable working time schedules. For instance, the results of a survey conducted among a representative sample of recipients of child benefits, and having a child aged less than three years, demonstrate that 19% of parents (father or mother) have irregular and unforeseeable work schedules (CREDOC, 2006). Parents are feeling the strain and often declare that their professional constraints make it difficult to organize child care. This complaint is most pronounced among mothers and fathers in senior or middle management or occupying supervisory roles as they are the ones most likely to be confronted with long working hours. Thirty three percent of parents having a child aged under three declare that their work schedules make it "sometimes" or "often" difficult to organise child care. This is the case for 67% of parents—most of them being upper-middle income families—relying on a home helper to look after their child(ren) (CREDOC, 2006).

Although there is a dearth of reliable data in this area, it is likely that the time parents are able to devote to their children is being squeezed and has become limited during the working week and in some cases the weekend. The institutions charged with upholding childcare policies which provide parents with the ability to cope with their professional constraints can provide some useful indicators here. For instance, according to regulations children can by right attend a *crèche* as well as an *école maternelle* up to10 hours a working day: over the last decade, there has been an increase in the number of childcare services (run by private organisations but publicly funded) and *crèches* which operate 24 hours a day and 7 days a week in order to allow working parents to meet the demands of their employer. Therefore, we can

---

[7] Infant mortality rate declined from 52 per thousand in 1950 to 7.3 in 1990 and 4.1 in 2002 (INSEE).

infer that a significant proportion of children under three are spending large amounts of their time in outside care.

A survey carried out on a representative sample of families having at least one child aged under seven has shown that among children aged under three and cared for in *crèches*, 25% spend more than 42 hours and a half per week in *crèches*. For those being cared for by registered childminders, 25% spend more than 44 hours in care and for those being cared for by a nanny at home 25% spend more than 46 hours with the nanny (Ruault & Audrey, 2003). Concomitantly, in 2005, nearly 60% of full-time registered childminders declared that they work more than 45 hours a week (Blanpain & Momic, 2007). Moreover, parents are often obliged to rely on multiple child care arrangements during the same day and/or during the week, in particular when they have work schedules which overlap. Consequently, staff in the child care sector have begun to voice criticisms and often mention that parents are frequently neglecting their child's daily and biological rhythms in favour of their own work schedules and in the process neglecting their child's well being (Renaudat, 2006).

In this context, childcare facilities and child minders have been placed under increasing pressure to accept and adapt their own working hours to the needs of the increasing number of parents confronted with flexible or unsocial working hours. Taking into account their personal family obligations, individuals employed in the childcare sector are all striving to protect their own interests and are very reluctant to accept ever more flexible working schedules. Registered child minders, if they can afford to,[8] will often refuse to look after a child outside of standard working hours. The result is that young children are often cared for by a rotating cast of characters and institutions within the same day. This is particularly so when both parents have non-standard work schedules; when the parent is living alone; or, when there is an only child (Bressé et al., 2007).

A report ordered, in 2003, by the *"Haut Conseil de la Population et de la Famille"* (established in 1985, this committee with only advisory powers provides advice to the government on family issues and demography), placed emphasis once again on both the advantages and drawbacks of the prevailing child care arrangements from the point of view of the child. It underlined the importance of language learning on cognitive and psychomotor development of children while at the same time warning of the risks of infectious diseases in *crèches*. It recommended, on one hand, an increase in places in *crèches* and, on the other hand, the further development of training programs to improve the skills of childminders and nannies at home.

The current situation is indeed far from adequate. Research on child minders has provided alarming evidence that 49% have no qualification whatsoever and 35% have very low qualifications (Blanpain & Momic, 2007). The problem becomes all the more glaring if we take into account the lack of professional training for carers engaged as home helps: they are exempt from all training/education requirements and receive no supervision from PMI services despite the fact that the state (through

---

[8] For instance, if it is difficult for parents to find out another child care arrangement or if she is highly valued by the family.

tax concessions and child care related allowance), heavily subsidizes this form of child care arrangement. What the report did not mention were the other aspects and components related to children's well-being (i.e., the potential impact of widespread changes in working conditions which could force parents to risk further disrupting the child's daily rhythms by decreasing time spent together).

In reality, it is difficult to force these issues onto the policy agenda or achieve increased media visibility. The reasons for this are numerous:

Firstly, these issues are relatively new and still not well documented. Surveys on parental time invested in children are scarce and lack the adequate data to investigate the impact of working conditions on the time spent with children and its effects on their daily rhythms. The most recent one, drawn on data from the "Time Use" survey conducted in 1998–1999 by the National Institute for Economic Studies (INSEE), made an assessment of the time invested in family life but neglected any consideration of child care arrangements (Lesnard & Chenu, 2003). Moreover this study was prior to the implementation of the 35-hour laws.

A second reason is that fighting unemployment and promoting gender equality on the labour market has been given greater priority on the policy agenda. Successive governments and advisory boards of family allowance funds have placed strong emphasis on the promotion of opening hours that are more in tune with the needs of working parents and on the development of so-called "flexible" child care arrangements. Enhancing women's employment, in particular since the European Council of Lisbon and the creation of the European Employment Strategy, has moved so high on the policy agenda that the ministry in charge of family affairs introduced a measure in 2004 promoting the creation of *crèches* in private companies by providing them with tax deductions.[9]

The ministry also directed the CAFs to provide partial funding but in doing so created a potential conflict. According to the Education code[10] "*every child who*

---

[9] Established since 2004 (Borloo Law), the Family tax credit (Crédit d'impôt famille, CIF) is a financial incentive provided to companies to encourage them to develop family-friendly initiatives for their employees. The CIF stipulates that 25% of related expenses are deductible from taxes paid by the company up to a ceiling of 500,000 Euros per year and per company (Finance Law of 2004, art. 98). Within this regulatory framework, 4 categories of expenses are statutory:

– expenses linked to training programmes for employees on parental leave.
– supplements paid to employees on maternity or paternity leave or on child-sick leave.
– creation of their own crèches or contribution to the running of crèches with places reserved for the employees' children under three years of age.
– getting employees a refund on expenses related to exceptional childcare costs pertaining to unpredictable professional obligation outside the normal work schedules.
– CESU (a prepaid service voucher).

[10] Following the introduction of the law passed in July 10, 1989 on the regulation of children's attendance of nursery school.

reaches the age of three has the right to attend a nursery school as close as possible to his or her residence" in order to spare the child any fatigue related to long commuting time and potentially detrimental to his or her well-being. Therefore, when policy makers adopted this measure, they were drawing a veil over the fact that the average commuting time in France has increased dramatically over the last two decades (Crague, 2003). In his presentation in 2006 of the new "*Plan petite enfance*" (Childcare Program) (http://www.social.gouv.fr/htm/dossiers/dpm/index.htm) the minister in charge of family affairs acknowledged the development of non-standard work schedules and stated that the staff in public child care provision should work and be present "at various moments of the day, for instance very early in the morning and late in the evening". Disappointingly, he neglected to mention the effect this could have on a child's well being. In the same vein, the minister of Education, Xavier Darcos, after visiting a *crèche* in summer 2008, asked "Do we really need bac+5 (i.e. a 5-year university diploma) for changing nappies and settling children down for a nap?"

A final reason is that since the end of the nineteenth century, as we have already acknowledged, childcare policies have been at the forefront of social policy agenda. It would be no great stretch to assume that in French collective memory "quality of care" and concern about children's interests are somewhat taken for granted. It should also be pointed out that since its establishment in 2000, the office of the child ombudsman gives a report every year to the government. Among the issues which have been addressed are: child abuse; violence within the family; violence at school; prevention of delinquency; impact of poverty and parents' unemployment on children's welfare; influence of divorce and of the related custody arrangements made by the parents on their living conditions; and adoption of children by gay couples.

One report issued in 2003, critical of the fact that a growing number of children aged between two and three years old were already attending nursery school, placed the child ombudsman firmly in the middle of one of the enduring controversies among early childhood specialists. Its conclusion was that nursery schools were poorly adapted to the special needs of children in terms of biological rhythms, language learning, and cognitive development. Children of that age should therefore be taken care of in *crèches* or by registered childminders.[11] According to the Education Code children from underprivileged social backgrounds have priority access to nursery school as soon as they reach the age of two. However, the shortage of places in *crèches*, particularly in rural areas and small cities, and the fact that nursery school is free, has given parents living in socio-economically disadvantaged areas a strong incentive to ask for a place in nursery school.

---

[11] Staffing in "écoles maternelles" primarily consists of teachers (professeurs des écoles). In addition, classes usually include (at least for a half day) an assistant (agent spécialisé des écoles maternelles). In 2003, there was on average one teacher to every 27 children. In crèches, staffing standards are laid down nationally: 1 adult to 5 children who are not yet walking; and 1–8 for other children under 3 years.

Due to these reasons and others French family policy is straining under numerous tensions and is being forced to cope with a number of conflicting interests within the family. What is to be done to help promote the child's welfare and allow them spend adequate time with their parents? How can women be provided with the opportunities that allow them to stand on an equal footing with men in the labour market? Decision makers would therefore appear to be facing the following dilemmas.

On the one hand priority could be given to providing the services that will enable mothers to adapt to the realities of the world of work and to the demands of employers but this would be to draw a veil over the effects that organizational changes are having on family life and would very likely prove contrary to the principles on which French family policy is founded. There are numerous justifications for doing so (e.g., for the sake of gender equality on the labour market). On the other hand, and for the sake of protecting the interests of child well being (e.g., keeping in tune with biological rhythms), decision-makers could start refusing to rubber-stamp and support changes in working conditions, particularly the development of atypical and flexible working hours which are contributing to the growing disruption of the traditional rhythms of the family. The danger with this approach lies in the fact that there remains an enduring gender division of unpaid work in France. By taking this route they could in fact be helping to penalize certain categories of mothers in occupational terms, particularly the most poorly skilled, (or even helping to exclude them from the labour market altogether). Furthermore, all of these difficulties have been further exacerbated by the effects of the 35-hour laws on reducing working time.

3 Conclusion

Over the course of the eighties and nineties successive governments, whether right or left-wing, gave childcare policies a radical overhaul as a result of numerous societal pressures. The expansion of state-run childcare services went hand in hand with a rise in the rate of female participation in the labour force which in turn fuelled public demand for more public services. Currently, and despite a general tightening of purse strings in the social security administration, childcare policies have continued to see increases in funding and remain a growth area in the French welfare state (though geographical disparities regarding the supply of places in crèches and the number of registered childminders are persisting). This is an accurate reflection of the high priority the issue of a work/life balance occupies on the social and political agenda.

Unlike Germany, the UK or the Netherlands (Pfau-Effinger & Geissler, 2005), it is currently socially acceptable in France for a child under three years of age to be taken care of outside of the home in formal child care provision for the whole day while his or her parents are at work. The early socialization this provides is in fact considered to be of great value, particularly by the educated middle classes. The result is that amongst the member States of the European Union, France has one of the highest employment rates for mothers with young children and its fertility rates top the list for the EU along with Ireland.[12] Over the last few decades, the progressive introduction of measures and schemes to support "working mothers" and the modernization of child rearing norms have coalesced to justify in the eyes of couples, and more particularly women, both having children and being present on the labour market. At the same time, the right of fathers to make a commitment to family life has made its mark on the social and political debate, as we can see from the introduction of two weeks' statutory paternity leave, a measure which has had a strong symbolic impact. Nevertheless, as French family policy is still imbued by "maternalist" values, there has been little discussion whatsoever since the turn of the millennium about ways to increase father involvement in the family life.

The French parental leave scheme could also be viewed as a welfare measure which yields more leisure time and reduces pressure on families with young children, in particular low-income families. Through this scheme parents' social right to provide care to their young children has been validated and recognized (Kamerman & Kahn, 2002). Moreover, policies encouraging paid care outside the family have had benevolent effects when it comes to the inclusion of women in the work force, especially non-qualified or low-skilled immigrant women whose employment rate has been increasing rapidly and who receive, thanks to childcare allowances schemes, guarantees of social rights and a wage which does not fall under the minimum legal wage.

Nevertheless, the reforms periodically introduced since the mid-eighties in child care policies clearly illustrate the growing influence that employment policies have had over French family policy. Despite rhetoric promoting "freedom of choice", it is in fact the fight against unemployment and the development of "workfare" policies which have been given priority. That this has happened in a climate of unbalanced power relationships between employers and employees confirms that welfare state regimes are closely interrelated with different labour market institutions and policies (Esping-Andersen, 1999). The decision by policy makers to provide parents with more flexible childcare arrangements comes as a direct result of increasing demands from employers and in the process the rights of children have been somewhat swept by the wayside. When considering this scenario it is noteworthy that recent research has once again demonstrated that non-standard work schedules and long working hours may have detrimental effects on children's well-being and on the quality of interaction within the family (Strazdins, Clements, Korda, Broom, & D'Souza, 2006). Other research has shown that a more equal division of responsibility between parents in early childhood has numerous positive effects on the child's future well-being and success (Gregg & Washbrook, 2003).

In the context of rapid organizational changes in the workplace should not policy-makers be paying more attention to the well-being of children? Maximizing female participation in the labour market is not only desirable for ensuring women's financial independence, economic growth and to fight child poverty[13] but is in

---

[12] In 2006, 2.01 in France and 1.91 in Ireland (Eurostat, 2008).

[13] In nearly all European countries child poverty rates are significantly higher in single-earner families than in those with two earners. See Whiteford & Adema (2007).

fact required in order to comply with the EU gender equality policy. But could a new policy design simultaneously promote mothers' employment and enhance children's well-being (Ben-Arieh, 2008) by limiting the impact of current organizational changes in the workplace on their biological rhythms? Putting more emphasis on the quality of childcare provision and, in particular, on the enhancement of the professionalization of the childminders would also be an important issue to address (see Chapter 20 of this book). Better qualified childcare workers and ensuring that young children in nursery schools are in small groups with sufficient numbers of providers would therefore contribute to move from child welfare to children well-being.

* Estimations

References

Adema, W., & Thévenon, O. (2008). Les politiques de conciliation du travail et de la vie familiale en France au regard des pays de l'OCDE. *Recherches et Prévisions, 93*, 51–72.

Bailleau, G. (2007). *L'accueil collectif et en crèches familiales des enfants de moins de 6 ans en 2005*. Paris, DREES, Etudes et Résultats no. 548.

Ben-Arieh, A. (2008). Indicators and indices of children's well-being: Towards a more policy-oriented perspective. *European Journal of Education, 43*(1), 37–50.

Blanpain, N., & Momic, M. (2007). *Les assistantes maternelles en 2005*. Paris, DREES, Etudes et Résultats no. 581.

Bloemen, H. G., & Stancanelli, E. G. (2008). *How do parents allocate time? The effects of wages and income*. Discussion Paper Series No. 3679. Bonn, Germany: IZA (Institute for the Study of Labor).

Bressé, S., le Bihan, B., & Martin, C. (2007). *La garde des enfants en dehors des plages horaires standard*. Paris, DREES Etudes et Résultats, no. 551.

Bressé, S., & Galtier, B. (2006). La conciliation entre vie familiale et vie professionnelle selon le niveau de vie des familles. Paris, DREES, Etudes et Résultats, no. 465.

Caisse Nationale des Allocations Familiales (CNAF). (2008). *Les prestations familiales. Statistiques 2006*. Paris.

Crague, G. (2003). Des lieux de travail de plus en plus variables et temporaires. *Economie et Statistique, 369–370*, 25–37.

CREDOC. (2006). *Les allocataires de la Prestation d'Accueil du Jeune Enfant*. Paris: Report for the National Family Allowance Fund (CNAF).

Esping-Andersen, G. (1999). *Social foundations of postindustrial economies*. Oxford: Oxford University Press.

Eurostat (2008). *L'Europe en chiffres – L'annuaire d'Eurostat 2008*. Luxembourg.

Fagnani, J. (2006). Family policy in France. *International Encyclopedia of Social Policy, Routledge, 3*, 501–506.

Fagnani, J. (2007). Family policies in France and Germany: Sisters or distant cousins? *Community, Work and Family, 10* (1), 39–56.

Fagnani, J., & Letablier, M. T. (2004). Work and family life balance: The impact of the 35 hour laws in France. *Work, Employment and Society, 18* (3), 551–572.

Fagnani, J., & Letablier, M. T. (2005). Caring rights and responsibilities of families in the French welfare state. In B. Pfau-Effinger & B. Geissler (Eds.), *Care arrangements and social integration in European Societies* (pp. 153–172). Berlin: Policy Press.

Fagnani, J., & Math, O. (2008). Family packages in 11 European countries: Multiple approaches. In A. Leira & C. Saraceno (Eds.), *Childhood: Changing contexts. Comparative Social Research, 25*, 55–78.

Fagnani, J., & Math, A. (2009). France: Gender equality, a pipe dream? In S. Kamerman & P. Moss (Eds.), *The Politics of Parental leave Policies*. London, New York: Policy Press 103–117.

Gregg, P., & Washbrook, E. (2003). *The effects of early maternal employment on child development in the UK.* CMPO Working Paper Series 03/070.

Hall, P. (1993). Policy paradigms, social learning and the State: The case of economic Policy making in Britain. *Comparative Politics, 25*(3), 275–296.

Institut national de la statistique et des études économiques (INSEE). (2008). *Employment survey 2007.* Paris. http://www.insee.fr/fr/themes/detail.asp?reg_id=99&ref_id=fd-eec07

Kamerman, S., & Kahn, A. (Eds.). (2002). *Beyond child poverty: The social exclusion of children.* New York: Institute for Child and Family Policy, Columbia University.

Lesnard, L., & Chenu, A. (2003). *Disponibilité parentale et activités familiales. Les emplois du temps familiaux dans la France des années 1980 et 1990.* Paris, Report for the Haut Conseil de la Famille et de la Population.

Luc, J. N. (1999). *L'invention du jeune enfant au 19ème siècle. De la salle d'asile à l'école maternelle.* Paris: Belin.

Morgan, K. (2002). Forging the frontiers between state, church and family: Religious cleavages and the origins of early childhood education and care policies in France, Sweden and Germany. *Politics and Society, 30,* 113–148.

Pedersen, S. (1993). *Family, dependence, and the origins of the welfare state. Britain and France, 1914–1945.* Cambridge: University Press.

Perrons, D., Fagan, C., McDowell, L., Ray, K., & Ward, K. (Eds.). (2006). *Gender divisions and working time in the new economy: Changing patterns of work, care and public policy in Europe and North America.* Northampton, MA: Edward Elgar.

Pierson, P. (Ed.). (2001). *The new politics of the welfare state.* Oxford: Oxford University Press.

Pfau-Effinger, B., & Geissler, B. (Eds.). (2005). *Care arrangements and social integration in European Societies.* Berlin: Policy Press.

Renaudat, E. (2006). Les dernières réformes des modes de financement aux crèches. *Recherches et Prévisions, 85,* 76–82.

Ruault, M., & Audrey, D. (2003). *Les modes d'accueil des enfants de moins de six ans.* Paris, DREES, Etudes et Résultats, no. 235.

Strazdins, L., Clements, M. S., Korda, R., Broom, D. H., & D'Souza, R. (2006). Unsociable work? Non-standard work schedules, family relationships and children's well-being. *Journal of Marriage and the Family, 1,* 394–410.

Whiteford, P., & Adema, W. (2007). *What works best in reducing child poverty: A benefit or work strategy?* Working Paper No. 51. Paris: OECD.

Regional Case Studies—Child Well Being in Europe

Dominic Richardson

1 Introduction

Recent years have seen a growth in the literature comparing child well-being outcomes in advanced economies. UNICEF (2007), OECD (2009), the European Commission (2008), as well as efforts by academics (Bradshaw, Hoelscher, & Richardson, 2007; Bradshaw & Richardson, 2009) have contributed to the field. These comparisons are either entirely made up of European countries, or the major-ity of the countries compared are European. Because of these studies more is known about the regional relative standing of EU countries in terms of their child well-being, than children in any other region of the world.

Not only is more known about European child well-being in comparison to child well-being in other regions, but based upon the comparisons above, EU countries are more likely to have the highest levels of well-being amongst their children across a range of dimensions; a finding not easily explained by national wealth. In the UNICEF child well-being framework EU countries dominated the high-performing group and in the OECD child well-being publication EU countries dominate once again—specifically those in the north.

At the national-level a number of EU countries are now collecting wide-ranging data about the lives of their children. For example projects to monitor child well-being are underway in the UK, Ireland, France, and Italy. Regional comparisons for assessing the relative achievements of these projects are necessary. To assess whether the UK government's goal of making England "the best place in the world for our children and young people to grow up" (DCSF Children's Plan, 2007, p. 3) is achieved (or indeed achievable) comparative analysis of children's well-being is needed.

D. Richardson (✉)
OECD Social Policy Division, Paris, France
e-mail: Dominic.Richardson@OECD.org

The views expressed in this paper are those of the author alone, and not those of the OECD or any of its Member countries.

Child well-being is an increasingly important topic in research and policy circles at the EU level. European policymakers are looking beyond income poverty measures to assess children's well-being. With one eye on the role of parents in labour market and the work family-balance, and the other on human and social capital investment in the future generations, measurement of child well-being has an important role to play in informing policy design across member states. In recent years the European Commission has set up a task force to investigate the determinants of child poverty in the member states, with a view to understanding the disproportionate poverty outcomes experienced by children in Europe,[1] (European Commission, 2008). The Commission has also developed a project that will assess in greater detail the determinants of child poverty and social exclusion; the effectiveness of child policies in combating poverty and social exclusions; and, the possibility of using a reduced set of indicators that represent the multidimensional nature of child well-being.[2]

The first attempt at a multi-dimensional EU-wide comparison of child well-being was undertaken in 2005, in part to mark the UK presidency of the European Union, and in part as a response to the Luxembourg presidency efforts to mainstream child indicators to complement the so-called Laeken indicators (Bradshaw et al., 2007). An update of the EU child well-being index was published in 2009, with the purpose of accounting for new data; extending the comparison to the new members of the EU (Romania and Bulgaria), as well as Norway and Iceland; and to address criticisms of the earlier index though changes and improvements (Bradshaw & Richardson, 2009).[3]

The publication of the second European index of child well-being by Bradshaw & Richardson (2009) now provides a unique opportunity to test for changes in child well-being by indicators and dimensions in Europe. Comparing child well-being between two points in time can inform countries in regards to the early trends in terms of their relative standing in health, education and material outcomes amongst others. Furthermore analysis of the changes in well-being in Europe between 2003 and 2006 can inform attempts to assess policy effectiveness, and attempts to identify key indicators for a multi-dimensional representation of child well-being.

---

[1] In 2006 19% of European children lived in poverty, compared to only 16 percent of adults [Eurostat, November 2008] the poverty threshold is 60% of the median equivalised household income.

[2] Information on this project was provided in personal correspondences by István György Tóth and Andras Gabos from TARKI, Hungary (see http://www.tarki.hu/en/) who are managing the project on behalf of the European Commission.

[3] The work by Bradshaw and colleagues is undertaken in the form of a standard multi-dimensional comparison of equally weighted dimensions of commonly understood life outcomes such as health, education, housing, and so on (as defined by the organisation government ministries or academic fields). Methods to combine indicators into dimensions apply simple standardisation and normalisation techniques, equal weights, and are "cause" as oppose to "effect" models (the latter would require tests of internal reliability—see Bollen & Lennox, 1991). For more details see Bradshaw et al. (2007) and Bradshaw & Richardson (2009).

This chapter will look at the changes in the overall child well-being in EU countries between 2003 and 2006, as well as analyse changes in the relative positions of countries across the child well-being dimensions of health, education, subjective well-being, material well-being, risk and safety and housing. Convergences and divergences in child well-being outcomes by dimensions in Europe will also be discussed. Following sections will explore the absolute changes in both common and key indicators for measuring well-being in the period 2003–2006. The first task for this chapter, however, is to address the issues of comparability between the indices.

2 Comparing EU Child Well-Being Frameworks

In order to confidently show changes in child well-being by dimension in EU countries, issues of comparison between the frameworks need to be addressed first. Table 1 lists the indicators by dimension for the 2006 index and the changes made (by choice or necessity) from the 2003 index. Dates and sources for the indicators for both waves are also presented.

Between 2003 and 2006 three sources of data have changed. PISA 2000 data on family relationships, and PISA 2003 data on personal well-being and work aspirations, have been dropped from the 2006 index. Family relationships and personal well-being measures were not asked as part of the PISA survey background questionnaire for 2006. Although "work aspirations" questions were retained in PISA 2006, low response rates made it impossible to include the indicators in EU index for 2006. A second survey used in 2003, CivEd (the Civic Education study undertaken in 1999), has not been repeated. Until the results of the International Civic and Citizenship Education Study (ICCS) are made available it is not possible to assess the civic participation of children in the European Union and elsewhere (ICCS is in the field in 2009, see http://www.iea.nl/icces.html for more information). For this reason the 2006 EU child well-being index does not include a dimension on civic and political participation.

The first waves of the European Union Survey on Income and Living Conditions (EU SILC) have recently been made available to researchers. EU SILC collects household data on housing and environment conditions and income. Housing and environment indicators, which were originally sourced from the European Quality of Life Survey (EQLS) in 2003, were available in EU SILC 2006 with slight changes. In the 2006 index EU SILC data were used in favour of EQLS because direct access to EU SILC raw data was possible and housing data could be sourced from the same sample (using the same weighting system) that produces the child income poverty estimates. EU SILC also provided additional data to the material situation dimension in the 2006 index in the form of a subjective measure of families' material situation and a material deprivation measure. Together these replaced the Health Behaviour in School aged-Children survey (HBSC) Family Affluence data used in the 2003 index (Currie, 2004), which only referred to children aged 11–15.

Table 1 Changes in the child well-being frameworks 2003–2006

Dimension name	Component name	Indicator description	2007 date	2009 date	Source(s) and notes
Health	Child health from birth	Mortality rate, infant (per 1,000 live births)	2003	2006	World Development Indicators (2008)
		Low birth weight, as a percentage of total live births lower than 2.5 kg	c. 2003	c. 2006	OECD Health Database and European Health for All Database
	Immunisation	Immunization, measles (% of children ages 12–23 months)	2003	2006	World Development Indicators (2008)
		Child immunization rate, DPT3 (% of children ages 12–23 months)	2002	2006	World Development Indicators (2008)
		Child immunization rate, Pol3 (% of children ages 12–23 months)	2002	2006	HNP stats
	Children's health behaviour	Children who brush their teeth more than once a day	2001/02	2005/06	Health behaviour in school-aged children (Currie et al., 2008)
		Children who eat fruit daily	2001/02	2005/06	Health behaviour in school-aged children (Currie et al., 2008)
		Children who eat breakfast every school day	2001/02	2005/06	Health behaviour in school-aged children (Currie et al., 2008)
		Mean number of days children are physically active for one hour or more average of previous week and typical week	2001/02	2005/06	Health behaviour in school-aged children (Currie et al., 2008)
		Children who are overweight according to BMI	2001/02	2005/06	Health behaviour in school-aged children (Currie et al., 2008)
Subjective well-being	Personal well-being	Children who report high life satisfaction	2001/02	2005/06	Health behaviour in school-aged children (Currie et al., 2008)
		Percent of students who agree or strongly agree to "I feel like an outsider (or left out of things)"	2003	–	No new data available–indicator removed
		Percent of students who agree or strongly agree to "I feel awkward and out of place"	2003	–	No new data available—indicator removed
		Percent of students who agree or strongly agree to "I feel lonely"	2003	–	No new data available—indicator removed

Table 1 (continued)

Dimension name	Component name	Indicator description	2007 date	2009 date	Source(s) and notes
	Well-being at school	Children who feel pressured by schoolwork	2001/02	2005/06	Health behaviour in school-aged children (Currie et al., 2008)
		Young people liking school a lot 11, 13 and 15 years	2001/02	2005/06	Health behaviour in school-aged children (Currie et al., 2008)
	Self defined health	Children who rate their health as fair or poor	2001/02	2005/06	Health behaviour in school-aged children (Currie et al., 2008)
Children's relationships	*Quality of family relations*	*New indicator:* Child who find it easy to talk to their mothers	–	2005/06	Health behaviour in school-aged children (Currie et al., 2008). *Replaced indicators from PISA 2000 on talking to parents, and eating main meal with parents in 2007 framework.*
		New indicator: Child who find it easy to talk to their fathers	–	2005/06	Health behaviour in school-aged children (Currie et al., 2008). *Replaced indicators from PISA 2000 on talking to parents, and eating main meal with parents in 2007 framework.*
	Family structure	Young people living in "single parent" family structures 11, 13 and 15 years (%)—HBSC 2001/02	2001/02	–	Domain was dropped
		Young people living in "Stepfamily" family structures 11, 13 and 15 years (%)—HBSC 2001/02	2001/02	–	Domain was dropped
	Peer relationships	Children who agree that their classmates are kind and helpful	2001/02	2005/06	Health behaviour in school-aged children (Currie et al., 2008)
Material situation	*Deprivation*	*New indicator:* Percentage of household with children reporting an enforced lack of consumer durables	–	2006	European Union survey of income and living conditions—*Replaced Percentage of children reporting low affluence, according to FAS composite score 11, 13 and 15 years (%) from HBSC 2001/02*

Table 1 (continued)

Dimension name	Component name	Indicator description	2007 date	2009 date	Source(s) and notes
		New indicator: Percentage of household with children reporting economic strain	–	2006	European Union survey of income and living conditions—*Replaced Percentage of children reporting low affluence, according to FAS composite score 11, 13 and 15 years (%) from HBSC 2001/02*
		Percentage of pupils with less than 6 education possessions	2003	2006	OECD PISA Database 2006
		Percentage of pupils with less 10 books in the household	2003	2006	OECD PISA Database 2006
	Poverty	At risk of poverty rate (60% of median equivalised income after social transfers): 0–17 years	c. 2003	2006	European Union survey of income and living conditions
		Relative poverty gap (60% of median equivalised income): 0–17 years	c. 2003	2006	European Union Survey of Income and Living Conditions
	Worklessness	Children aged 0–17 living in jobless households: 0–17 years	2004	2006	European Union survey of income and living conditions
Risk and safety	*Violence and violent behaviour*	Young people who were involved in physical fighting at least once in the previous 12 months 11, 13 and 15 years	2001/02	2005/06	Health behaviour in school-aged children (Currie et al., 2008)
		Children who have bullied others at school at least twice in the past couple of months	2001/02	2005/06	Health behaviour in school-aged children (Currie et al., 2008)
	Child deaths	All child deaths: All under 19 deaths per 100,000 children: 3 year averages	c. 2002	c. 2005	WHO Mortality Database, July 2008 update
		Adolescent fertility rate (births per 1,000 women ages 15–19)	2003	2006	World Development Indicators, 2008
	Risk behaviours	15-year-olds who have had sexual intercourse	2001/02	2005/06	Health behaviour in school-aged children (Currie et al., 2008)

Table 1 (continued)

Dimension name	Component name	Indicator description	2007 date	2009 date	Source(s) and notes
		15-year-olds who used a condom at last sexual intercourse	2001/02	2005/06	Health behaviour in school-aged children (Currie et al., 2008)
		Children who smoke at least once a week	2001/02	2005/06	Health behaviour in school-aged children (Currie et al., 2008)—*Replaced ESPAD 2003 Cigarette smoking: Lifetime use 40 times or more (%)*
		13 and 15 year olds who have been drunk at least twice	2001/02	2005/06	Health behaviour in school-aged children (Currie et al., 2008)—*Replaced ESPAD 2003 Drunkenness: Lifetime 20 times or more (%)*
		15-year-olds who have ever used cannabis in their lifetime	2001/02	2005/06	Health behaviour in school-aged children (Currie et al., 2008)—*Replaced ESPAD 2003 Cannabis: Experience of use in Lifetime (%)*
		Inhalants: Experience of use in Lifetime (%)	2003	–	No new data available—indicator removed
Education	Attainment	Reading literacy achievement	2003	2006	OECD PISA Database 2006
		Mathematics literacy achievement	2003	2006	OECD PISA Database 2006
		Science literacy achievement	2003	2006	OECD PISA Database 2006
	Participation/enrolment	Full-time and part-time students in public and private institutions, by age: 15–19 as a % of 15 to 19-year-olds	2002	2005	OED Education at a Glance, 2007
		School enrollment, preprimary (% gross)	–	2006	World development indicators, 2008–*Replaced early years participation—children in registered childcare (% of children aged 0–2)—OECD*
	Aspirations	Percentage of the youth population not in education, not in the labour force or unemployed—age 15–19	2003	2005	OED Education at a Glance, 2007
		Proportion of pupils aspiring to low skill work—PISA (2000)	2000	–	No new data available—indicator removed

Table 1 (continued)

Dimension name	Component name	Indicator description	2007 date	2009 date	Source(s) and notes
Housing and environment	*Overcrowding*	Rooms per person in households with children	2003	2006	European Union survey of income and living conditions—*Replaced EQLS figures from 2003*
	Environment	*New indicator*: Households with children who report crime in the area is a problem	2003	2006	European Union survey of income and living conditions—*Replaced EQLS figures from 2003 on Households with children who think it is unsafe or very unsafe to walk around in their area at night*
		New indicator: Households with children reporting pollution or dirt are a problem in the area	2003	2006	European Union survey of income and living conditions—*Replaced EQLS figures from 2003 on Households with children reporting many physical environment problems*
	Housing problems	Households with children reporting more than one housing problems	2003	2006	European Union survey of income and living conditions—*Replaced EQLS figures from 2003*
Civic and political participation	*Civic participation*	Participation rates: young people reporting involvement in two of five social participations 14 years (%): CivEd. 1999	1999	–	No new data available—indicator removed
	Interest in politics	Political interest: young people reporting above the median involvement in political behaviours 14 years (%) CivEd. 1999	1999	–	No new data available—indicator removed

The health dimension in the 2006 index was updated using the same indicators and the same sources as those used for 2003. Unsurprisingly, data derived from international published series, such as the World Development Indicators, have proven to be more stable sources over the years than survey data, with the exception of HBSC surveys which has consistently asked the same questions across waves.

Thirty-one indicators are the same in both frameworks. In the health, material situation and education dimensions, fewer than two indicators have been dropped or replaced. In housing the indicators are the same, but sourced from a different survey. Risk and safety and subjective well-being have had four and three indicators dropped or replaced respectively. "Children who agree that classmates are kind and helpful" was the only child relationships indicator in the 2006 index that was also used in 2003. Family structure indicators were available but have been dropped from the analysis, and HBSC data on family relationships replaces data that had been previously sourced from PISA 2000.

Both of the European indices attempt to cover a range of outcomes for all children from birth to 18. This compromise is necessary because the availability of data for child well-being comparisons by age is limited. Surveys of children in the majority are taken towards the end of compulsory schooling, mainly because of assumptions regarding child capabilities, but also because of government interest in the transition of school to work (or childhood to adulthood). At the cross-national level this means that the only sources of data for children in early and middle childhood are series data, and then only when children are recorded via interaction with institutions such as hospitals or schools. This means that there is data for children's outcomes around the time of birth (mortality, birth weight and immunisations) and entry into and out of different levels of pre-schooling and schooling. One of the next big challenges for child well-being researchers is to identify and collect age-specific indicators for younger children across the range of child well-being dimensions.

The first EU child well-being framework included indicators of children's outcomes along 8 dimensions incorporating 51 indicators.[4] The results of this comparison are shown in Fig. 1. The second EU index was published in 2009, with fewer indicators (43) and dimensions (7), and is shown in Fig. 2. To compare the frameworks more readily the additional countries of Bulgaria, Romania, Iceland and Norway have been removed from calculations for Fig. 2. The reason being that scores are relative scores calculated on the basis of group mean and standard deviation; the inclusion of four extra countries will change these figures. Also the average ranks in Fig. 1 are produced after the civic and political participation ranks have been removed. At this stage remaining issues of comparability, for example where changes in sources and indicators have been unavoidable. However, how far these changes influence results (given two stages of aggregation and normalisation), and whether these differences represent true changes between the years or statistical anomalies is debateable.

---

[4] See Bradshaw et al. (2007) for methods involved in creating the child well-being index. Data for both frameworks can be requested directly from the author.

	Average rank	Health	Subjective Well-being	Children's Relationships	Material Situation	Risk & Safety	Education	Housing	Civic and political participation
Sweden	4.7	1	6	15	2	3	2	4	14
Netherlands	4.9	2	1	5	10	5	6	5	
Cyprus	5.5	5			1	2		14	1
Denmark	6.7	3	9	10	6	15	3	1	4
Finland	8.6	7	12	17	3	7	4	10	18
Spain	8.7	13	3	9	8	1	15	12	
Germany	9.9	10	7	12	12	11	9	7	10
Slovenia	10.3	15	8	4	4	18		13	13
Belgium	11.1	20	15	6	18	16	1	2	5
Ireland	12.1	18	5	8	19	20	7	8	
Italy	12.4	16	11	2	15	6	13	18	11
Luxembourg	12.4	11	20	19	5	9	20	3	
Austria	12.6	21	2	16	7	19	17	6	
France	13.0	14	13	14	11	10	14	15	
Malta	13.5	24	17	1	24	4		11	
Portugal	13.7	9	16	3	13	17	18	20	7
Czech Republic	13.7	4	14	22	9	21	10	16	17
Greece	14.0	25	4	11	17	8	16	17	2
Poland	14.0	6	19	13	23	11	5	21	6
Hungary	14.4	22	10	7	14	14	12	22	3
Slovak Republic	17.0	17	22		25	13	11	19	9
United Kingdom	18.3	23	18	23	20	22	13	9	8
Latvia	18.4	19	21	18	16	23	8	24	12
Estonia	20.7	12	23	26	21	24		23	15
Lithuania	20.7	8	24	20	21	25		25	16

Fig. 1 Child well-being index in Europe circa 2003
Note: The average rank in the table is calculated after the removal of the Civic and political participation dimension for reasons of comparability.
Source: Adapted from Bradshaw et al. (2007)

	Average rank	Health	Subjective Well-being	Children's Relationships	Material Situation	Risk & Safety	Education	Housing
Netherlands	3.3	2	1	1	5	3	4	7
Finland	4.4	6	6	6	1	7	3	2
Sweden	4.6	1	7	3	8	2	10	1
Denmark	7.3	3	5	7	7	14	12	3
Germany	9.4	14	10	5	10	5	8	14
Slovenia	9.4	9	13	2	3	11	11	17
Luxembourg	9.6	4	14	16	2	10	15	6
Ireland	10.0	11	8	11	18	13	5	4
Cyprus	10.4	5			12	1	25	9
Austria	10.9	23	2	4	6	20	16	5
Spain	11.3	10	4	14	16	4	19	12
Belgium	11.7	16	9	15	13	18	1	10
France	13.1	17	12	24	9	9	13	8
Estonia	13.1	8	17	8	11	23	2	23
Czech Republic	13.9	7	18	23	4	19	6	20
Italy	15.3	13	15	18	15	6	22	18
Slovakia	15.9	15	11	19	14	22	17	13
Greece	16.3	25	3	20	17	17	21	11
Portugal	16.3	18	19	10	19	8	24	16
Poland	16.7	12	22	13	24	16	9	21
Malta	16.8	24	24	17			12	7
Hungary	17.3	22	21	9	21	15	14	19
United Kingdom	18.0	20	16	12	22	21	20	15
Latvia	21.0	19	20	22	20	24	18	24
Lithuania	22.6	21	23	21	23	25	23	22

Fig. 2 Child well-being index in Europe circa 2006
Source: Adapted from Bradshaw & Richardson (2009)

Notwithstanding issues of comparability and data selection/restriction both indices have broadly the same leaders and the same laggards, and few overall changes to group standings are seen. The Northern EU countries of Sweden, the Netherlands, Denmark and Finland perform well in both frameworks. The Baltic

States and EU new members, Latvia, Lithuania, perform badly on both scales. Hungary and the UK are also poor performers, even though in the case of the latter the country is among the richest in the world, and both countries are relatively high investors in children.

Between 2003 and 2006 a number of countries have seen large changes in their average child well-being ranks; leading to a change in their high, middle or low order group standing. Estonia and Slovakia are now middle third countries, where previously they were bottom third. The southern EU countries of Malta and Portugal are now bottom third countries, having moved down from the middle third. Countries moving up from the middle third to top third include Luxembourg and Ireland. Movement in the other direction, from top to middle, includes Spain and Cyprus.

3 Comparing Dimensions of Well-Being in EU Countries

As noted above the content of the frameworks changed somewhat between the years 2003 and 2006. Some indicators were no longer available, and some indicators were removed or replaced, which begs the question: Which of the dimensions comparable in terms of broad relative trends?

Table 2 compares directly the dimension scores calculated by each framework. Both correlation coefficients and range of the dimension scores are shown. It is clear that with the exception of children's relationships (the dimension with the most substantial changes) that the results compare well between the 2 years, particularly in terms of health measures, risk and safety and housing.

In regards to the dimension ranges showed there is evidence of convergence in dimension-level outcomes for subjective well-being, material situation, and to a lesser extent education.[5] Outcomes are becoming more unequal for children in different EU countries across the dimensions of health, risk and safety, and housing.

Table 2 Comparisons of country associations and dimension-score ranges between 2003 and 2006 by child well-being dimension

	Correlation coefficient 2003–2006	Range 2003	Range 2006
Health	0.84**	39.0	41.2
Subjective well-being	0.73**	46.0	39.8
Children's relationships	0.32	39.2	39.1
Material situation	0.70**	35.7	31.0
Risk behaviours	0.87**	36.7	41.2
Education	0.77**	31.2	30.7
Housing and environment	0.82**	33.2	44.3

** denotes a significant association of $p < 0.05$.
Source: Authors calculations from data published in Bradshaw et al. (2007) and Bradshaw & Richardson (2009).

---

[5] Scales used to calculate ranges are normalised using z scores and the normalised to a mean of 100 and a standard deviation of 10. Ten points in a range is equivalent to a standard deviation from the EU average in each dimension.

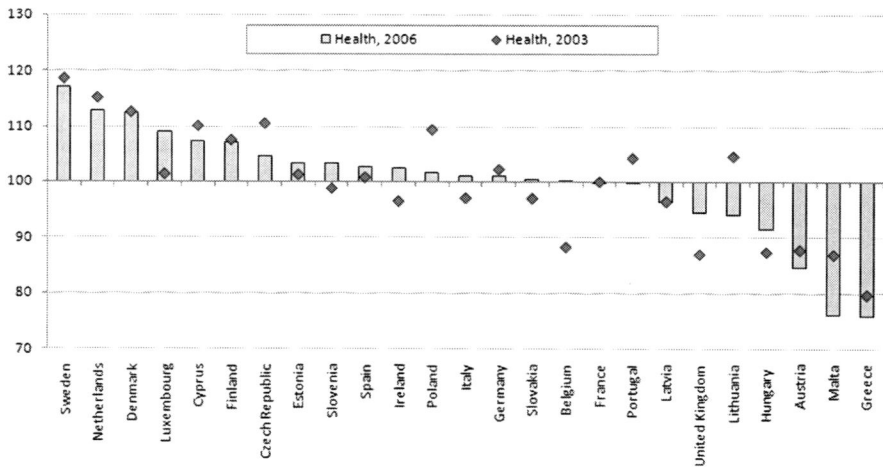

Fig. 3 Comparison of the health dimensions in Europe
Source: Adapted from Bradshaw et al. (2007) and Bradshaw & Richardson (2009)

The following section looks in more detail at the dimensions of well-being for children in Europe across the two frameworks.[6]

Figure 3 compares the results of the health dimensions from the 2003 and 2006 frameworks. Countries performing relatively well in 2003 remain in the top performing group in 2006. Broadly the same is true for poor performing countries, with the exception of Belgium whose below average child well-being in the health dimension is now slightly above the EU average.

Health outcomes for children in Europe are getting more unequal; the range of results widening slightly (see Table 2). Moreover, the inequality is driven by countries falling further below the EU standard rather than by gains being made by the high performing countries (it is important to remember that results refer to *relative inequality*—absolute measures will be dealt with in the following section). Indeed, the majority of high performing countries show a drop in relative advantage over the EU average in the 3 years following the 2003 index.

Countries getting better in terms of child health well-being include Hungary, the United Kingdom, and Ireland and Luxembourg. Countries showing relative declines in the health well-being of their children in the period 2003–2006 include Malta, Lithuania, Portugal, Poland and the Czech Republic.

Changes in the subjective well-being dimension are shown in Fig. 4. In terms of between-country inequality on this measure, Table 2 has shown a reduction by over half a standard deviation on the European average; or substantial evidence of convergence in regards to subjective well-being of children in Europe.

---

[6] Given the wholesale changes to the children's relationship dimension this measure is not included in the analysis.

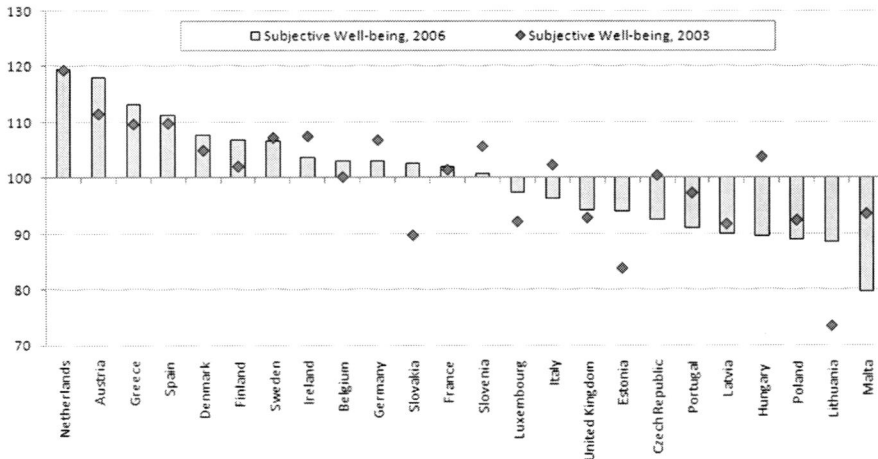

Fig. 4 Comparison of the subjective well-being dimensions in Europe
Source: Adapted from Bradshaw et al. (2007) and Bradshaw & Richardson (2009)

Partly this convergence can be explained by the three worst performing countries in 2003 (Lithuania, Estonia and Slovakia) making gains on other EU countries, at a time when only smaller improvements since 2003 are made for high performing countries.

Austria is one example of a country that was relative high performer in 2003 that has continued to make gains in this dimension.

Countries that show lower levels of subjective well-being since 2003 include Ireland, Germany, Slovenia and Hungary. Subjective well-being in Malta was low in 2003, and has dropped considerably in the 3 years since.

If one was able, and it was justified, to weight indicators on the pure basis of policy interest in the child well-being analyses, then material situation would be most important of all. Not only are the measures of child income poverty the most widely accepted indicator of children's outcomes amongst European policymakers, but recent efforts to go beyond poverty began with attempts to assess material deprivation.

The well-being of children in Europe in the material sense is getting more equal between countries (see Table 2), even though for the majority of low performing countries, things are not getting better, or in other words most are falling further below the average European standard. The convergence in outcomes on the material well-being dimension is driven by large relative gains in Slovakia, Estonia, and the Czech Republic; and similarly large losses in Sweden, Cyprus and Spain (Fig. 5).

Changes in the risk and safety amongst children in EU countries between 2003 and 2006 are outlined in Fig. 6. Table 2 shows that of all dimensions the pattern seen in 2006 is most similar to that seen in 2003 ($r = 0.87$, $p < 0.01$) for the risk and safety dimension. Comparison of the changes in the range of outcomes in

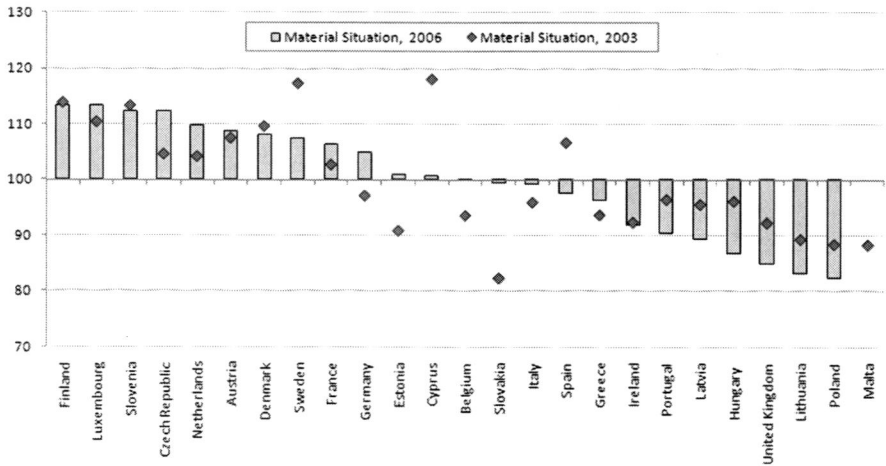

Fig. 5 Comparison of the material situation dimensions in Europe
Source: Adapted from Bradshaw et al. (2007) and Bradshaw & Richardson (2009)

terms of risk and safety shows that differences between the best performing and worst performing countries are increasing; a result driven in the main by the Baltic countries of Lithuania, Latvia and Estonia, that remain at the low end of the chart, and on average see their relative levels of risk and safety getting worse.

Although the association between the risk and safety dimensions in 2003 and 2006 is high, most countries are showing small changes up or down. Relative levels

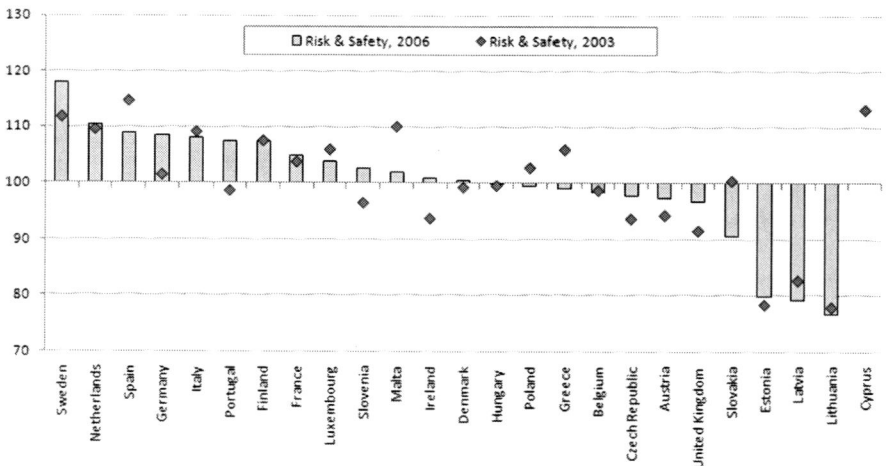

Fig. 6 Comparison of the risk and safety dimensions in Europe
Source: Adapted from Bradshaw et al. (2007) and Bradshaw & Richardson (2009)

of children's risk and safety are improving in Sweden Germany and Portugal. Spain, Malta, Greece and Slovakia have seen levels of risk and safety worsens in relative terms over the period 2003–2006.

Along with material situation, outcomes in child educational well-being are more equal in Europe than outcomes measured by the dimensions of health, housing, risk and safety or subjective well-being. Between 2003 and 2006 all countries can be found in a range of just over 3 standard deviations of the scale. Large improvements in educational well-being relative to the European average are seen in the Czech Republic, France, Luxembourg and Austria. Large declines are seen in Sweden, Denmark, Latvia the UK and Portugal (Fig. 7).

Figure 8 shows the changes in the housing dimension as measured using 2003 and 2006 data. Though the data are from different sources, the questions refer to the same well-being concepts, and the two dimensions correlate strongly ($r = 0.82$, $p < 0.01$). The main difference in changing sources has been the sensitivity of the EU SILC derived indicators to extreme cases, which results in 33% increase in the range of results (from 3.3 standard deviations to 4.4).

The majority of EU countries show an increase in the relative standing of their housing and environmental conditions for children in relation to the EU average standard. Improvements in Finland, Slovakia and Lithuania are most marked. Six countries show a marked decline in their relative EU performance on the housing and environment dimension. Five of which, Luxembourg, the Netherlands, Belgium, Germany and the UK were of a similar level above average in 2003. Latvia, the sixth country to show a fall in standing from 2003 to 2006, is now so far behind the rest of Europe to be considered a statistical outlier (more than 3 standard deviations below the mean).

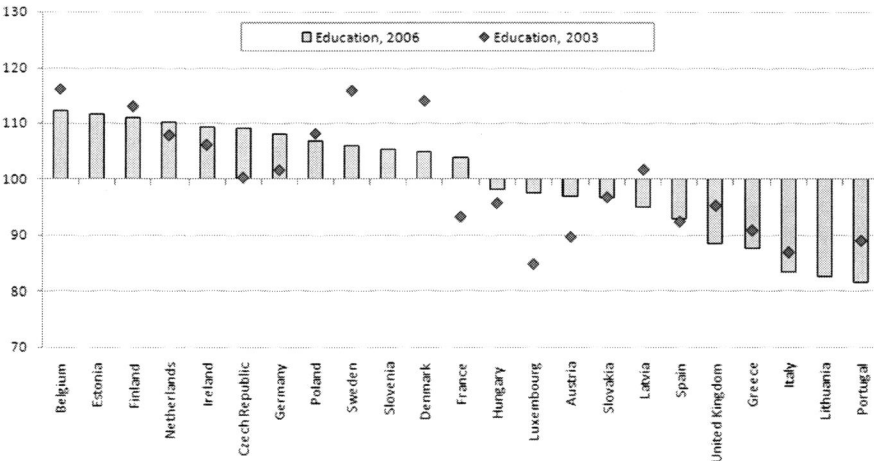

Fig. 7 Comparison of the education dimensions in Europe
Source: Adapted from Bradshaw et al. (2007) and Bradshaw & Richardson (2009)

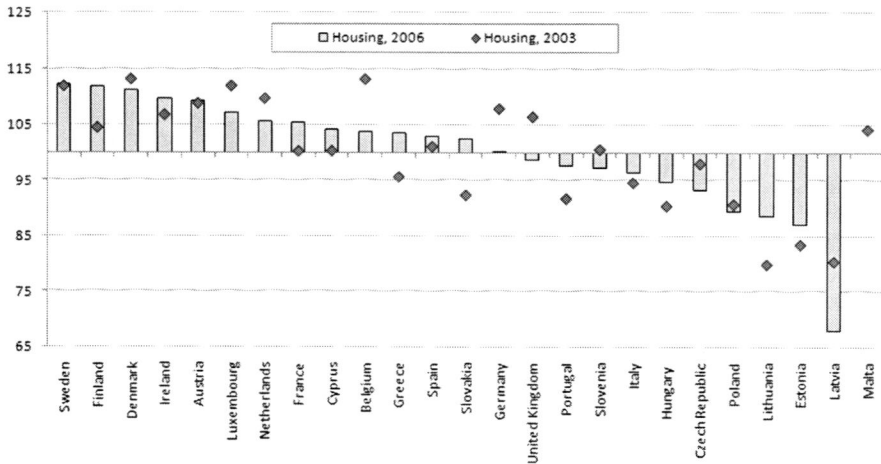

Fig. 8 Comparison of the housing and environment dimensions in Europe
Source: Adapted from Bradshaw et al. (2007) and Bradshaw & Richardson (2009)

4 Changes in Child Well-Being in Europe: Analysis of the Indicators

There are clearly some fluctuations in child well-being within and between EU countries when looking at broad representation of relative standings in health, subjective well-being, material situation, risk and safety, education and housing and environment. But two questions arise from this type of analysis: "How can comparisons of child well-being dimensions inform policy decisions?" and "Can these types of comparison be used to develop a reduced set of indicators?" These questions are important to address some the goals central to European plans for child research and policy.

4.1 How Can Comparisons of Child Well-Being Dimensions Inform Policy Decisions?

The short answer to this question is: they can't. Well, at least not on their own. To inform policy decisions one must refer to the underlying statistics that are used to build dimensions of well-being. Dimensions of well-being are used to bridge the conceptual understanding of child well-being as a comprehensive or holistic measure of child quality of life with the policy structures through which improvements to the lives of children can be made. Dimensions are useful for passing on a quick message of relative success or failure; they say *where* countries are in relation to comparators and competitors; but do not address *why* they are where they are, or indeed *what* or *how* to change. In order to answer the why, what and how questions, one must refer to the raw data.

This section of the chapter therefore moves to a more detailed inspection of the raw data at the European-level, and through this, provide some considerations for Europe in terms of which broad policy areas are succeeding in having positive outcomes for children, and which indicators might be considered in a reduced set designed for monitoring child well-being in Europe.

For policy purposes the monitoring of children's well-being outcomes is very important. Within our communities we can readily compare ourselves to neighbours and friends, and although our circumstances are not entirely the same, our goals often are similar and so we can learn from each other's choices and mistakes. Comparative child well-being indices allow governments to compare their achievements to other countries, and in doing so assess their overall approach, or prioritise areas for change. The reporting of trends at the same level is just as important. To start with it means that governments can assess the impact of their policy responses to problems earlier identified. Trends mean that government can reassess which countries they draw their policy lessons from, and predict (based on trends in other countries) future outcomes or the opportunity costs of prioritising their policy responses.

Table 3 shows the comparable indicators common to both frameworks, with the mean scores and standard deviations. All indicators that are incomparable between the years, because of changes in definition, description population coverage or source have been removed. The results give the best indicator-level assessment of European-wide changes in child well-being outcomes during the 2003–2006 period, and show both successes and failures in each of the dimensions of child well-being (the housing dimension has been removed because of the change in source affecting comparability).

Results for child health indicators show that the achievement in lowering infant mortality rates is offset to a degree by increases in the rates of children born with low birth weights. There will be a trade-off here to some degree as technological and skills developments mean low birth weight children are more like survive the birth process, and first year of life. The changes in the standard deviations show that the success in lower infant mortality rates is being achieved Europe-wide, whereas low birth weights are more unequally distributed than before. Vaccination rates change very little, with the exception of measles vaccinations which have increased on average in Europe countries, and across the board are more equal in member states in 2006 than in 2003. Child health behaviour results see increases in both positive and negative behaviour indicators. There has been an average increase in personal dental care and daily fruit consumption across Europe, with evidence that there is less inequality in these areas for children living in different EU countries. At the same time the average EU country shows that more children are overweight, and fewer children eat breakfast on a school day.

The biggest success in terms of child well-being in Europe is in the dimension of subjective well-being. The average EU country has more children reporting higher life and school satisfaction, and fewer children reporting ill health and school

Table 3 Changes in child well-being by indicators in Europe 2003–2006

		Mean		Standard deviation	
		c. 2003	c. 2006	c. 2003	c. 2006
Health	*Child health from birth*				
	Infant mortality rate (per 1,000 live births)	5.2	4.4	1.72	1.33
	Low birth weight, as a percentage of total live briths lower than 2.5 kg	6.2	6.3	1.29	1.38
	Immunisation				
	Immunization, measles (% of children ages 12–23 months)	91.4	93.0	7.45	5.32
	Child immunization rate, DPT3 (% of children ages 12–23 months)	94.9	94.9	4.62	4.54
	Child immunization rate, Pol3 (% of children ages 12–23 months)	95.2	95.1	4.55	4.71
	Childrens health behaviour				
	Children who brush their teeth more than once a day	59.3	62.8	14.64	12.87
	Children who eat fruit daily	33.6	34.8	8.52	6.12
	Children who eat breakfast every school day	65.3	62.5	11.31	11.26
	Children who are overweight according to BMI	11.9	13.3	4.54	4.86
	Personal well-being				
	Children who report high life satisfaction	84.9	85.7	4.88	4.14
Subjective well-being	*Well-being at school*				
	Children who feel pressured by schoolwork	37.0	36.3	13.12	11.40
	Young people liking school a lot 11, 13 and 15 years	23.4	24.7	8.12	8.50
	Self defined health				
	Children who rate their health as fair or poor	16.1	13.7	5.76	4.63

Table 3 (continued)

			Mean		Standard deviation	
			c. 2003	c. 2006	c. 2003	c. 2006
Children's relationships	*Peer relationships*	Children who agree that their classmates are kind and helpful	64.1	65.7	10.93	12.38
Material situation	*Deprivation*	Percentage of pupils with less 10 books in the household	7.6	9.2	3.22	3.59
	Poverty	Child poverty rate	17.6	16.6	6.01	5.84
		Child income poverty gap	21.4	25.9	7.05	5.15
	Worklessness	Children aged 0–17 living in jobless households: 0–17 years	8.0	8.5	3.75	3.77
Risk and safety	*Violence and violent behaviour*	Young people who were involved in physical fighting at least once in the previous 12 months 11, 13 and 15 years	40.0	40.2	6.03	6.27
	Child deaths	All child deaths: All under 19 deaths per 100,000 children: 3 year averages	16.8	14.3	9.52	6.81
	Risk behaviour	Adolescent fertility rate (births per 1,000 women ages 15–19)	17.3	11.9	8.73	5.59
		15-year-olds who have had sexual intercourse	22.9	24.9	5.45	5.56
		15-year-olds who used a condom at last sexual intercourse	75.7	77.9	6.75	6.58
Education	*Attainment*	Reading literacy achievement	494.2	489.8	18.12	20.26
		Mathematics literacy achievement	499.9	498.0	24.17	20.79
		Science literacy achievement	500.1	503.1	19.06	20.70
	Participation/enrolment	Full-time and part-time students, all institutions % of 15–19-year-olds	82.8	85.6	6.05	6.31
	Aspirations	NEET rate—age 15–19	7.3	6.0	3.02	2.41

Source: Adapted from Bradshaw et al. (2007) and Bradshaw & Richardson (2009).

pressures. Reduced levels of self-reported ill health are most marked both in terms of the European country average and standard deviation. The only indicator from children's relationships in both frameworks "finding their classmates kind and helpful" has also increased on average across the EU, but not for all EU children equally as shown by an increase in the standard deviation.

Indicators in the material situation dimension show that the average EU country has seen a reduction in child poverty, but an increase in educational deprivation (fewer books in the home of students), an increase in the number of children living in jobless households, and importantly an increase the child income poverty gap. Deviations for the average child poverty rate and child poverty gaps have also shrunk, meaning that as efforts to reduce the number of children in poverty in Europe have been successful across the board, equally there a has been a failure to address those in the most need is a Europe-wide issue.

Reported levels of risk and safety experiences are mixed. The average EU country has seen increasing numbers of 15 year olds having sex, but also higher rates of condom use and lower rates of teenage fertility. In the case of the former indicator the spread of country responses has increased around the average, though for teenage fertility and condom use, the average figures better represent an EU-wide trend. The remaining comparable indicators show that though there has been no true measurable increase or decrease in violent behaviour, child accidental deaths are down across the EU.

Education outcomes EU-wide have changed very little in the 3 years between 2003 and 2006. Average rates of reading and mathematics literacy have fallen slightly, and average rates of science literacy have increased slightly (though only 20 of the 25 EU countries took part on PISA in 2003 and 23 in 2006 following the inclusion of Estonia, Lithuania, and Slovenia). In terms of youth activity, namely NEET rates and education enrolment between 15 and 19 years of age, Europe has seen an improvement in the country average. In particular NEET rates have dropped from 7.3 to 6.0%.

4.2 Can These Types of Comparison be Used to Develop a Reduced Set of Indicators?

Table 4 below attempts to identify individual indicators that best represent well-being by the dimensions to which they contribute for each index. Simple correlation analysis is performed between indicators and their dimension aggregate score, and for each dimension the indicators with the highest correlation coefficient is shown. The purpose here is to identify indicators that could contribute to a reduced set of child well-being indicators.

The three strongest associates by dimension in both frameworks are the same: the proportion of children self reporting above high life satisfaction, under 19 accidental and non-accidental mortality rates, and children living in homes with more than one housing problem. There is some evidence therefore, that these indicators

Table 4 Indicators correlating most strongly to overall dimension scores for 2003 and 2006 child well-being frameworks

2006 framework		
Health	Child immunization rate for Polio (3rd dose)	0.73
Subjective well-being	Children who report high life satisfaction	0.87
Children's relationships	Children who find it easy to talk to their fathers	0.74
Material situation	Homes with children reporting an enforced lack of consumer durables	−0.75
Risk & safety	Rate of under 19 accidental and non-accidental deaths (3 year averages)	−0.84
Education	Mathematics literacy achievement	0.82
Housing and environment	Homes with children reporting more than one housing problems	−0.87
2003 framework		
Health	Low birth weight (less than 2.5 kg)	−0.58
Subjective well-being	Children who report high life satisfaction	0.88
Children's relationships	Young people living in single parent families	−0.75
Material situation	Child income poverty rate	−0.83
Risk & safety	Rate of under 19 accidental and non-accidental deaths (3 year averages)	−0.81
Education	Students in public and private educational institutions (15–19 year olds)	0.73
Housing and environment	Homes with children reporting more than one housing problems	−0.90

Source: Adapted from Bradshaw et al. (2007) and Bradshaw & Richardson (2009).

are relatively stable and robust proxies for child well-being dimensions that they contribute to.

Unfortunately due to the change in source for the housing indicators it does not make much sense to compare the raw data for this indicator. However data can be compared for the figures for child life satisfaction and under 19 accidental and non-accidental mortality rates.

The result of Tables 5 and 6 show that child well-being for these indicators in Europe is improving for the majority of countries. Only seven EU countries show a reduction in life satisfaction, and fewer still—four—show increases in unnecessary child deaths.

5 Summary

So what does this mean for child well-being in Europe, what is going on? First, the overall picture of child well-being in terms of European performance by high, low and middling groups has not changed a great deal. Only eight countries changed their group order. Of more concern is that those moving into lower groups are all Mediterranean countries (Cyprus, Spain, Portugal and Malta), typically countries

Table 5 Comparing changes in child life satisfaction reported in the EU indexes for 2003 and 2006

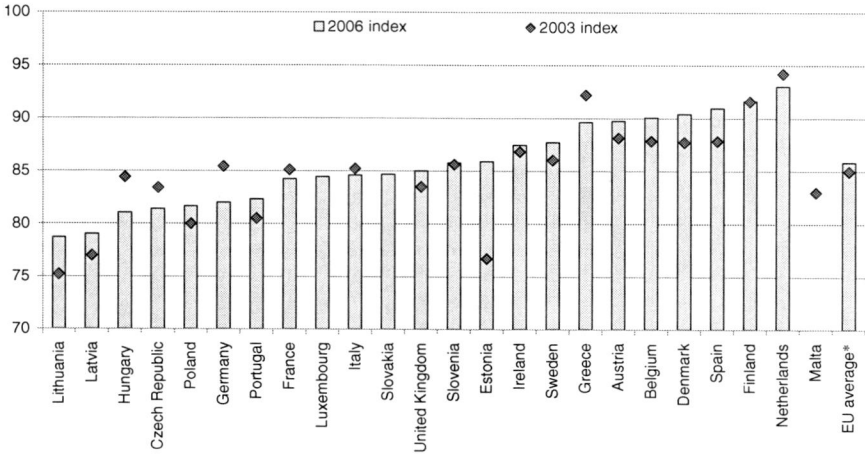

Note: 2006 updated the method of aggregated HBSC estimates by weighting the age and sex contributions to the aggregate. Significant difference between weight and unweighted estimates for life satisfaction were not found in 2006. No country estimate varied by more than $^1/_2$ a percentage point when using the weighted method: the average difference in the EU sample was 0.1 percentage points. EU estimates for 2003 and 2006 are averages for reporting countries in both waves.
Source: Bradshaw et al. (2007) and Bradshaw & Richardson (2009) calculations of HBSC 2001/02 data and 2004/05 data published in Currie et al. (2008) and Currie (2004).

Table 6 Comparing changes in child accidental and non-accidental deaths in the EU indexes for 2003 and 2006

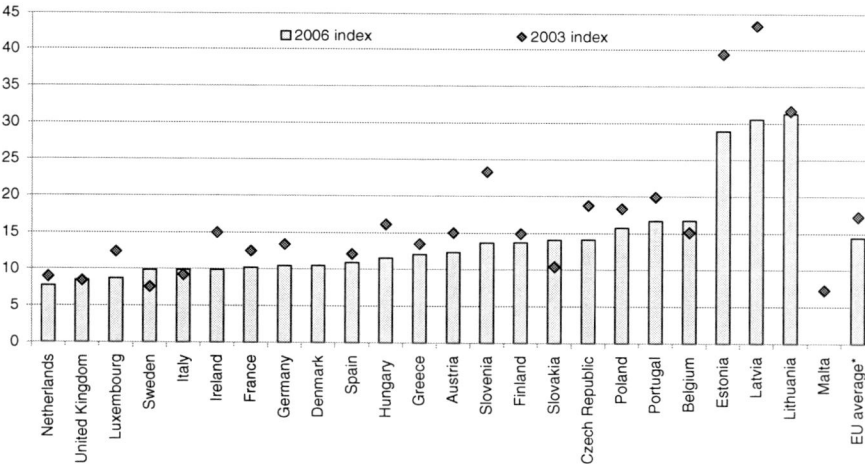

Note: Data are form the WHO mortality database for various years, and are 3 year average estimates of the most recent data available. EU estimates for 2003 and 2006 are averages for reporting countries in both waves.
Source: Bradshaw et al. (2007) and Bradshaw & Richardson (2009) calculations of World Health Organisation Mortality Database data published in 2005 and 2008 respectively.

with strong family cultures. Second, although there has been some European convergence in terms of equality of outcomes in material well-being and subjective well-being, European outcomes along the lines of health and risk behaviours are becoming more unequal. And finally where indicators that proxy dimensions of child well-being can be directly compared across the two indices (life satisfaction and child mortality) it is clear that child well-being is improving in the majority of European countries. And only one country, Italy, shows decreases in child well-being on both indicators.

Understanding child well-being changes over recent years can only take us so far if the goal is to improve the lives of children. The next step for child well-being analysts is to consider how this information about children's outcomes, and changes in the national standings, can be linked to policy choices and policy effort. One way of doing this could be to build panel datasets of children's outcomes and social contexts to complement data collected on social expenditure, and social security policies and services. With such data more can be learned through analysing longer term trends, as well as undertaking natural policy experiments. Whilst taking steps towards policy analysis, comparative child well-being analysts must however keep the focus on well-being outcomes, and ensure that policy effort is seen as a means to an end, rather than an end in itself. A comment made by Al Khan to the New York Post in 1965 is fitting here "I represent a concern for what is being accomplished, rather than what is being done... 'Services rendered' are not enough".[7] Comparative analysis of child well-being outcomes, some 40 years later, shows that the interest in "the accomplished" over "the rendered" for children continues to grow. And long may it continue!

References

Bollen, K., & Lennox, R. (1991). Conventional wisdom on measurement: A structural equation perspective. *Psychological Bulletin, 110*(2), 305–314.

Bradshaw, J., Hoelscher, P., & Richardson, D. (2007). An index of child well-being in the European Union. *Social Indicators Research, 80*(1), 133–177.

Bradshaw, J., & Richardson, D. (2009). An index of child well-being in Europe. *Child Indicators Research 2*(3), 319–351.

Department for Children Schools and Families. (2007). *The children's plan: Building brighter futures*. London, HMSO.

Currie, C., Roberts, C., Morgan. A., Smith, R., Settertobulte, W., Samdal, O., & Rasmussen, V.B. (2004). Young people's health in context. *Health behaviour in school-aged children study (HBSC): International report from the 2001/2002 study*. World Health Organization, Regional Office for Europe. http://www.euro.who.int/eprise/main/who/InformationSources/Publications/Catalogue/20040601_1

Currie, C., Roberts, C., Morgan, A., Smith, R., Settertobulte, W., Samdal, O., & Rasmussen, V. B. (2008). Inequalities in young people's health: Health behaviour in school-aged children (HBSC): International Report from the 2005/2006 Survey. *Health Policy for Children and Adolescents, No. 5*. Copenhagen: World Health Organization, Regional Office for Europe.

---

[7] http://www.nytimes.com/2009/02/22/nyregion/22kahn.html?_r=1

http://www.euro.who.int/eprise/main/WHO/InformationSources/Publications/Catalogue/20080617_1

European Commission (Social Protection Committee). (2008). *Child poverty and well-being in the EU: Current status and way forward.* Luxembourg: Office for Official Publications of the European Communities. http://www.libertysecurity.org/IMG/pdf_ke3008251_en.pdf

Eurostat. (2008). *Populations and social conditions: Living conditions and welfare statistics.* http://epp.eurostat.ec.europa.eu/pls/portal/url/page/SHARED/PER_POPSOC. Accessed August 2008.

OECD PISA. (2008). Programme for International Student Assessment (PISA) International Database 2006. http://pisa2006.acer.edu.au/. Accessed March 2008.

OECD. (2009). *Doing Better for children.* OECD: Paris.

UNICEF. (2007). *Child poverty in perspective: An overview of child well-being in rich countries.* Innocenti report card 7. UNICEF: Florence.

World Development Indicators. (2006). World Bank dataset. http://ddp-ext.worldbank.org/ext/DDPQQ/member.do?method=getMembers&userid=1&queryId=135

Part VI
Conclusion

Child, Family, and State: The Relationship Between Family Policy and Social Protection Policy

Sheila B. Kamerman

1 Introduction

Children are the largest age group in the world's population and the most vulnerable group economically, socially, and physically. Given the extensive demographic and social changes in recent years, there is a search for new policy strategies for protecting children and promoting child and family well-being. Even when there is economic growth and political commitment to children, and as essential as these are, more is needed. In particular, knowledge regarding which policy strategies are most effective is essential, if the goal is to do better by children.

Family policy, a holistic approach to evaluating social policies affecting children and their families usually regardless of income, is one such strategy (Kamerman, 2009; Kamerman & Kahn 1997, 1978).[1] Social protection, government actions that protect individuals, especially the most vulnerable and disadvantaged, against defined social risks, is a second such strategy.[2] Together they constitute two different yet related and complementary approaches to designing social policies. How they differ, what they constitute, and what values they maximize are the focus of this brief paper. The paper begins with a discussion of family policy, followed by a parallel discussion of social protection policy, which in turn highlights where the two interact. The paper concludes with a reminder of why both approaches are needed.

2 Family Policy

2.1 Definition

The term "family policy" was used first in European social policy discussions to describe what government does to and for children and their families. The term

S.B. Kamerman (✉)
School of Social Work, Columbia University, New York, USA
e-mail: sbk2@columbia.edu

---

[1] This discussion also draws on Kamerman (2009).

[2] This section draws on various papers prepared for UNICEF.

S.B. Kamerman et al. (eds.), *From Child Welfare to Child Well-Being*, Children's Well-Being: Indicators and Research 1, DOI 10.1007/978-90-481-3377-2,
© Springer Science+Business Media B.V. 2010

was used, in particular, to describe those public policies—such as laws, regulations, administrative policies—that are designed to affect the situation of families with children—or individuals in their family roles—and those that have clear, though possibly unintended, consequences for such families. Characteristic of family policy internationally is first, concern for all children and their families, not just poor families or families with problems, although these and other family types may receive special attention; and second, an acknowledgment that doing better by children requires help for parents and the family unit as well.

The increased attention to family policy during the last 30 years derives from the developments that either threaten this role of the family or are believed to do so. Demographic and social trends suggesting changes in the family as an institution and changes in the roles of family members have been the primary catalysts in generating support for family policies. Noteworthy among these are: increased longevity and proportion of aged in the population, deferred age of marriage, lower fertility, increased divorce, increased out-of-wedlock births and lone mother families, declining availability of extended families, and rising rates of female labor force participation.

As I have noted elsewhere (Kamerman & Kahn, 1978; Kamerman & Kahn, 1997; Kamerman, 2009), family policies may be explicit or implicit. Explicit family policy includes those policies and programs deliberately designed to achieve specific objectives regarding children, individuals in their family roles or the family unit as a whole. (This does not necessarily mean general agreement as to the objective, but only that the actions are directed toward the family; various actors may have different goals in mind.). Nor does it require agreement on the definition of "family". Indeed, greater progress can often be made by not getting caught up in issues of definition—and instead, acknowledging that there are many different definitions and they vary across countries and cultures. Explicit family policies may include population policies (pro-or anti-natalist), income security policies designed to assure families with children a certain standard of living, employment-related benefits for working parents, maternal and child health policies, child care policies, and so forth. Implicit family policy includes actions taken in other policy domains, for non-family related reasons, which have important consequences for children and their families as well. For example, policies regarding immigration—or HIV/AIDS—may have major consequences for children and their families, yet not directly target them.

Family policy is a sub-category of social policy and as such, can be viewed as a policy field or domain, a policy instrument, or as a criterion by which all social policies can be assessed as to their consequences for family and child well-being.

The *family policy field* includes those laws that are clearly directed at families, such as family law; child or family allowances; social assistance benefits contingent on the presence of children; maternity and parenting benefits; tax benefits for dependants; and child care or early childhood care and education services.

Family policy can also be an *instrument* to achieve other objectives in other social policy domains. For example, family policy may be used to achieve labor market objectives, encouraging more women to enter (or to leave) the workforce. Family policies may be designed to encourage parents to bear more ∼ or fewer ∼ children and thus achieve a country's population goals. Thus, in family policy, the family may be both object and vehicle of social policy—both agent and target of social policy.

Family policy as "perspective" assumes that sensitivity to effects and consequences for families informs the public debate about all social policies. Finally, family policy as perspective is concerned with monitoring a broad range of actions in terms of their potential or actual impact on children and their families. Viewing family policies from this vantage point is particularly important in those countries that do not have explicit family policies but rather a series of categorical policy initiatives directed toward different aspects of child and family functioning and designed to achieve different and sometimes contradictory objectives.

2.2 The Characteristics of Family Policy

Family policy therefore, in the sense discussed here, suggests:

- A view of the family as a central institution in the society;
- A definition of "family" that allows for drawing distinctions while encompassing a variety of types, structures, roles, and relationships, usually involving at least one adult and one child;
- A definition of "policy" that assumes a diversity and multiplicity of policies rather than a single, monolithic, comprehensive legislative act;
- A definition of "family policy" that, therefore, encompasses different types of families and policies and includes both the policy field and child and family well-being (or family impact) as a criterion for assessing the outcomes of relevant governmental and non-governmental policies.

Family policy instruments include cash and tax benefits; services; laws; and administrative directives. The major instruments are $\sim$ and here I highlight 8:

- Income transfers including child and family allowances, social insurance, social assistance, and tax policies, among others;
- Policies assuring time for parenting, including paid and job protected leaves from employment following childbirth or adoption, and during children's illnesses or school transitions;
- Early childhood education and care policies (ECEC), both services and various forms of cash and tax subsidies to extend access to ECEC services;
- The laws of inheritance, adoption, guardianship, child protection, foster care, marriage, separation, divorce, custody, and child support;
- Family planning and related contraceptive services;
- Personal social service programs;
- Housing allowances and policies;
- Maternal or family and child health services.

The roots of family policy (or *families* and *policies*) are found in Europe. The major developments occurred there first, and then the conceptual discussion moved to include other western countries as well. Among those countries with an explicit family policy today are the Nordic countries (Denmark, Finland, Norway, and Sweden), France and Germany. Implicit family policy can be derived from any country's social policies affecting children.

2.3 Family Policy as a Global Concept

Today the concept of family policy is a global one. It is used in both developed and developing countries, increasing over time, from a UN expert group in the 1980s, a European Union Observatory on Family Policies in the 1990s, to a conference in Hong Kong last year on "Strengthening Families". The key criterion is the presence of a child and the willingness (and capacity) for the society to invest in children. There is no country that does not recognize the centrality of the family in both short and long term societal developments—and as part of economic as well as social development. Families fulfill an essential societal role in reproduction, in socialization, in early education, in the promotion of good health, in preparing the next generation for adulthood. But families are changing—in composition and in structure—with women taking on new tasks in addition to their traditional caring roles. And the need for caring services is increasing as there are more elderly, and they are living longer in many countries. Family Policies have played a significant role in achieving countries' desired objectives, whether fertility-related, employment-related, facilitating poverty reduction, helping to reconcile work and family life, or linked to enhancing child well being. For families to carry out their traditional roles as well as new ones, they require help and support and sometimes supplementation ∼ and that is the role of government and of the various non-governmental organizations.

3 Social Protection

3.1 Definition

"Social protection" is a term used interchangeably in the literature with social policy, social welfare and/or social security, but seems increasingly to be used as a generic term that includes the other terms (Kamerman & Gatenio-Gabel, 2007). It is a term that includes those governmental actions or interventions (laws, regulations, funding) that provide individuals and/or families with a defined or minimum standard of living (cash or tax-benefit income and/or goods and services) regardless of the normal market pattern of distribution, often as a matter of legal right. It is designed to protect individuals against defined social risks including loss of income as a consequence of old age, death of a breadwinner, disability, sickness, unemployment, maternity, excessive costs of child rearing. It incorporates statutory as well as non-statutory measures and universal as well as selective or targeted measures. Social protection benefits and services are provided on the basis of non-market criteria such as need, contribution, employment status, age, or citizenship. The concept has emerged as a policy framework for dealing with poverty and vulnerability in developing as well as developed countries. A major issue has to do with the effectiveness of different social protection strategies.

In contrast to the emphasis on children, families with children, and universalism in family policies, social protection policies focus on a wider range of social risks and needs and on the vulnerable, the poor and disadvantaged. They are not limited to any particular age group or category and they emphasize means-testing as a primary strategy, and targeted policies.

The link between family policies and social protection lies with child-conditioned social protection or social protection policies affecting children. These latter policies include those interventions that are contingent on the presence of children, include attention to "new social risks", such as trafficking and HIV/AIDS *and* with, special attention to the poor and needy. UNICEF defines child-conditioned social protection as a basic human right, meaning that governments have an obligation to provide both economic and social support to the most vulnerable segments of their population, in particular children, Social protection strategies encompass cash and tax transfers (e.g., social insurance, social assistance, child-related demogrants) and economic support directed at the family or at the individual child and social services (e.g., family and community support, child protection, alternative care).

Child poverty is clearly at the forefront of concern in the developing countries despite variations across countries, and following this are the issues of access to health care, to education, and to adequate nutrition. (Minujin, Forthcoming; UNICEF, 2005) A UNICEF report stated that "human development and poverty reduction are pre-requisites" to achieving its key goals for child well-being: child survival, poverty and inequality reduction, social inclusion, elimination of hunger, increased access to education and health care, gender equality and empowerment, maternal health , safe water, and reduced incidence and impact of HIV/AIDS and other diseases. These concerns and problems are shared by the poorest countries, and largely affect the most vulnerable groups within the society. Children constitute the largest vulnerable group in most of these countries yet social protection for children remains far less developed than for certain other groups.

My objective here, would be to find evidence regarding what happened to children as a result of these social protection interventions? Did they avoid negative outcomes as a result? Increase positive outcomes? What aspects of the interventions made a difference? What factors strengthened countries' capacities for implementing interventions most effectively?

In recent years, the provision of cash benefits has become a key social protection strategy in developing countries, not just in the developed countries. One big difference has been the growing stress on linking cash benefits to particular behaviors, specifically, attendance at health clinics and enrollment and attendance at school. These "conditional" Cash Transfers (CCTs) were launched initially in Latin.

America but have been copied increasingly in Asia, Africa, and the CEE countries (Fiszbein & Schady, 2009; Gaenio-Gabel & Kamerman, Forthcoming). A debate has emerged regarding whether conditionality is essential or whether non-conditional benefits (as in South Africa, for example) at a decent level would not be as effective. In addition to an adequate benefit, reasonable conditions, and appropriate targeting, the major factors linked to a successful CCT program are an adequate supply of schools and health care centers; a social infrastructure adequate to cope with the administration and delivery of a categorical, cross-sector, means-tested benefit; and an identification of what the conditionality adds to the value of the cash benefit.

Other issues include: how vulnerability is defined apart from low income, the importance of, making the mother the beneficiary of the benefit, which promotes gender equity as well, making "carers" (grandparents, other relatives) eligible to receive the benefits when no parent is in the home, thus helping to support AIDS orphans and child-headed households, CCTs are not a magic bullet but may be an important component in a country's social protection package (World Bank, 2009).

CCTs have also been used to reduce child labor.

4 Conclusion

To conclude, I want to stress seven points:

1. The child problems/social risks are shared globally and there is beginning to be a global response but the major developments are regional. The primary intervention, the use of cash transfers, is not sufficient by itself to solve all the problems. Cash transfers are a component of a policy package but neither the full package, nor an alternative to other interventions, nor a panacea. There needs to be a more holistic approach to policies and programs that confront poverty and social exclusion including the reduction of income poverty along with ensuring access to health care, education, food aid, and social services.
2. The child conditioned social protection literature is dominated by the experiences and use of cash transfers, especially CCTs, and there is a significant gap with regard to the inclusion of social services interventions—protective services and supportive services including ECD/ECEC.
3. A large gap has to do with the lack of systematic data on child well-being including data on the policy responses and where possible, their effects, not just on the problems/risks.
4. Another gap has to do with the lack of comparable comparative data on social expenditures, especially child-conditioned social expenditures.
5. Still a third gap has to do with the lack of attention to the politics that facilitate or impede policy developments. What factors led to the rapid and widespread establishment of CCT policies and programs and what would be needed to broaden

that response to make for a holistic package? What factors led the European countries to enact parental leave policies, not just maternity policies?

6. And, finally, there is little discussion of children's rights and their entitlement to social protection.

As we approach the next anniversary of the International Year of the Family we will want to learn more about the changes that families are experiencing in different parts of the world, the problems they are confronting in their everyday lives, the ways that they are coping, and the innovative and creative responses of governments and other institutions in the society. Hopefully, in the intervening years between now and then we can agree on the major tasks for social protection and family policy attention and begin to address them, accumulating knowledge about the different experiences in different countries, Family policy, with its particular attention to a holistic policy approach to children and families with children, and social protection, with its emphasis on protecting against defined social risks for individuals, especially adults, are both needed.

There is no one model for either family policy or social protection although there are templates for each (as can be seen in the Appendix). The policy regimes vary across regions and countries. Nonetheless there are commonalities and there is lesson learning.

Maybe then, by the next anniversary, we will have learned more about what is happening to families—how governments are responding—what are the consequences for families ∼ as agents, targets and beneficiaries of family policies ∼ and which family policies may make a difference. That is a very full agenda, but we have to start someplace, so why not here, and now.

Acknowledgments This paper was presented at an Expert Meeting on "Family Policy in a Changing World: Promoting Social Protection and Intergenerational Solidarity" April 14–16, 2009, Doha, Qatar, under the Sponsorship of The United Nations Department of Economic and Social Affairs, Division for Social Policy and Development and the Doha International Institute for Family Studies and Development.

Appendix: The Most Extensive Child-Oriented Data Base is UNICEF's Annual State of the World's

Children Covering About 190 Countries

The most significant family data base is the OECD Family Data Base, first launched in 2006 and now updated to 2008, covering its current 30 member countries, and including 37 indicators. The structure of the Family Data Base does not include indicators that cover issues related to the position (and care needs) of elderly family members (e.g.) pensions or health care (a separate policy domain), or long term care of the aged. The indicators, which continue to be increased, are organized under four constructs:

1. The Structure of the Family

   - Families and children
   - Fertility indicators
   - Marital and partnership status

2. The Labor Market Position of Families

   - Families, children and employment status
   - Workplace hours and time for caring

3. Public Policies for Families and Children

   - Tax and cash benefits
   - Child related leaves
   - ECEC

4. Child Outcomes

   - Child health
   - Child poverty
   - Education

*The most significant social protection data base is the **ESSPROS** (European Social Statistics Social Protection) data base in the 27 country EU. It provides this classification of benefits in Europe: The benefits included are:*

    Sickness and health care including maternity
    Disability
    Old age
    Survivors
    Families and children
    Unemployment
    Housing
    Social exclusion

The Family-Children benefits include those that: provide financial support to households for bringing up children, financial assistance to people who support relatives, and provide social services specially designed to assist and protect the family, particularly children. They include cash benefits such as family or child allowances and tax benefits, maternity and parental leave benefits, and benefit s in kind such as ECEC, Home helps, and housing benefits.

References

Fiszbein, A., & Schady, N. (2009). *Conditional cash transfers*. Washington, DC: World Bank.
Kamerman, S. B., & Kahn, A. J. (Eds.). (1978). In *Family policy: Government and families in fourteen countries*. New York: Columbia University Press.

Kamerman, S. B., & Kahn, A. J. (Eds.). (1997). In *Family change and family policies in Great Britain, Canada, New Zealand and the United States*. New York: Oxford University Press.

Kamerman, S. B. (2009). Families and family policies: Developing a holistic family policy agenda. *Hong Kong Journal of Paediatrics, 14*(2), 115–121.

Minujin, A. & Delmonica, E. eds. Child Poverty: A Global Perspective Bristol, UK: Policy Press, Forthcoming.

UNICEF. (2005). *The state of the world's children 2006*.

Kamerman, S. B., and Gatenio-Gabel, S. (2007). Social protection for children and their families. In A. Minujin & E. Delamonica (Eds.), *Social protection initiatives for children, women and families*. New York: New School and UNICEF.

Breinigsville, PA USA
15 December 2010
251500BV00007B/43/P